REVIEW OF
NURSE
ANESTHESIA

REVIEW OF NURSE ANESTHESIA

John J. Nagelhout, CRNA, PhD
Director
School of Anesthesia
Kaiser Permanente
California State University Long Beach
Pasadena, California

W.B. SAUNDERS COMPANY
A Division of Harcourt Brace & Company
Philadelphia   London   Toronto   Sydney

W.B. SAUNDERS COMPANY
A Division of Harcourt Brace & Company

The Curtis Center
Independence Square West
Philadelphia, Pennsylvania 19106

Library of Congress Cataloging-in-Publication Data

Nagelhout, John J.
Review of nurse anesthesia/John J. Nagelhout.

p.   cm.

ISBN 0–7216–7531–X

1. Nurse anesthetists Examinations, questions, etc.   2. Anesthesia Examinations,
    questions, etc.   3. Operating room nursing Examinations, questions, etc.
    I. Title.   II. Title: Nurse anesthesia.
    [DNLM: 1. Anesthesia Nurses' Instruction. 2. Anesthesia Examination Questions.
    3. Anesthetics Nurses' Instruction. 4. Anesthetics Examination Questions.
    5. Nurse Anesthetists Examination Questions.   WO 218.2 N147r 1999]
RD82.N34 1999

617.9'6'076—dc21

DNLM/DLC   99–19474

REVIEW OF NURSE ANESTHESIA   ISBN 0–7216–7531–X

Printed in the United States of America.

Last digit is the print number: 9   8   7   6   5   4   3   2   1

PREFACE

Acquiring the knowledge necessary for a successful career in anesthesia is a continual process. Students build upon their nursing training and clinical practice in critical care when they enter graduate training in nurse anesthesia. Anesthesia training involves the acquisition of knowledge from both clinical and didactic venues. The purpose of this book is to provide a review and guide to a broad sampling of anesthesia-related knowledge. It is my intention that the material contained in this book will serve to reinforce already attained knowledge and to point to the areas where further study is necessary. Each question is referenced to the chapter in the text *Nurse Anesthesia*, where students may read further to gain a more thorough understanding of specific topic areas. The accompanying CD-ROM gives the user the opportunity to practice answering questions on the computer. Together, this book and its CD-ROM offer nurse anesthetists a comprehensive review tool for the CRNA examination.

JOHN J. NAGELHOUT, CRNA, PHD

ACKNOWLEDGMENTS

The production and success of this book required the collaborative efforts of many people. I wish to thank all of those who have contributed to the development and realization of this book. These include the staff of W.B. Saunders Company: Maura Connor-Murcar, Senior Editor; Victoria Legnini, Assistant Developmental Editor; and Frank Polizzano, Production Manager.

I would like to thank the following people for reviewing this book during its development: Naz Lalani, CRNA, MS; Denise Carrier, CRNA, MS; Ann Tulas, CRNA, MS; Fred Lazaga, CRNA, MS; Karen Pope, CRNA, MS; Michael Boytim, CRNA, MN; Donna Funke, CRNA, MS; and Mary Karlet, CRNA, PhD. Their efforts were invaluable in completing this book.

I would also like to thank Retta Smith for the many hours she worked in preparing the manuscript.

JOHN J. NAGELHOUT, CRNA, PhD

CONTENTS

◆　◆　◆

INTRODUCTION

Anesthesia is a discipline that borrows from many areas of basic science and medical and nursing practice. Successful completion of the National Certifying Exam for Nurse Anesthetists therefore requires a broad spectrum of knowledge encompassing a multidisciplinary set of skills in both the basic and clinical sciences. Students must draw on their previous nursing training and didactic and clinical experiences throughout the program and the long hours of concentrated studies in anesthesia. Certifying exams in general are meant to test a scope of knowledge necessary to acknowledge that a person has received adequate preparation to enter the specialty. Nurse anesthesia is no different in that the exam is meant to show the acquisition of a basic core of knowledge necessary to begin a successful career in clinical anesthesia.

This book was designed to help prepare for both the certifying exam and anesthesia practice. It is divided into subsections that mirror the Council on Certification content outline for the subject matter on the certifying exam. This allows for the proper amount of emphasis on each required area to ensure appropriate preparation for the exam. Each question in multiple-choice format has four answers, followed by a declarative statement that amplifies the answers. The questions are referenced to the appropriate chapter in the text *Nurse Anesthesia* to allow for further clarification in reading about the subject matter. I hope this provides an easy, systematic way to thoroughly prepare for the exam.

An exam consisting of 250 multiple-choice questions is included with the book, on disk, to help the reader to become familiar with taking an exam online and more comfortable with computerized testing.

The Council on Certification publishes basic information regarding computer adaptive testing and has graciously allowed me to reprint some commonly asked questions regarding the overall exam process. At the end of the chapter is the actual content outline that the Council uses to formulate the exam.

NATIONAL CERTIFICATION EXAMINATION FOR NURSE ANESTHETISTS

QUESTIONS AND ANSWERS*

INTRODUCTION

1. **What is Computerized Adaptive Testing (CAT)?**

   CAT is a method of administering tests that uses current technology and is based on the psychometric framework of Item Response Theory (IRT). With CAT, each candidate's test is individualized; it is assembled interactively as the candidate is tested. Test questions are stored in a large item bank and classified by content category and level of difficulty. After the candidate answers a question, the computer calculates an estimate of competence and chooses a next question of appropriate content and difficulty. This process is repeated for each question, thus creating an examination that is both tailored to each individual's knowledge and skills and fulfills the CCNA test plan requirements.

2. **What are the advantages of CAT compared to the paper and pencil test for NEC?**

   ✔ *Examination is individualized for each candidate*

   The adaptive algorithms target the difficulty of the test items to the ability of each candidate. When a candidate answers an item correctly, a more difficult item is presented and the estimate of ability is raised. When an item is answered incorrectly, an easier item is presented and the estimate of ability is lowered.

   The candidate has a less stressful testing environment and individualized testing conditions at the test administration site. Candidates sit at individual stations and take the test at their own pace.

   ✔ *More frequent and year round test administrations*

   The candidate is able to schedule a date, time, and location to take the NCE following completion of an accredited nurse anesthesia educational program and notice of eligibility by the CCNA. Candidates no longer need to wait for test dates and can test up to four times a year if necessary. Since certification is required in many states to practice, more immediate and repeated access to take the NCE is provided.

   ✔ *Prompt notification of certification status*

   The candidate's results and certification status are processed within four weeks after taking the NCE.

   ✔ *More efficient and accurate measurement of candidate's ability*

   CAT selects and administers only those items that provide the best measurement of each candidate's competence or ability level.

   ✔ *Enhanced security*

   Each candidate takes a different form of the examination, limiting exposure of the item bank and eliminating the need for hard copy of the NCE. Test administration site security measures include photo registration and videotaping of the session.

3. **If each candidate receives a different test, how can the NCE be fair to all candidates?**

---

*Council on Certification of Nurse Anesthetists. Questions and Answers, Content Outline for the National Certification Examination for Nurse Anesthetists. Park Ridge, IL. 1998. Reprinted with permission.

The CAT NCE is fair to all candidates. Each test conforms to the content outline, which assures inclusion of test questions in all of the major content areas. All questions are chosen from the same item bank. The passing score is identical for all candidates, indicating that the difficulty level to pass the NCE is consistent for all examinees. All candidates have the opportunity to demonstrate their ability or competence level, as the NCE will not end until a pass or fail decision is determined.

TAKING A TEST ON THE COMPUTER

4. **What if a candidate does not know how to use a computer?**

Prior knowledge of computers is **not** needed. Only three keys are needed to take the CAT NCE, the space bar and the ENTER and TAB keys. The space bar moves the cursor among the possible answers to a question. The enter key is used to select the answer. The tab key is used to select help or time information. Candidates may also choose to respond with number keys or a mouse. All other keys are turned off.

Previous research studies indicate that computer experience is not a factor in test performance. Only three keys are necessary during the entire test. The presentation of test questions on a computer screen and the use of a keyboard do not affect scores of candidates who have no prior computer experience.

5. **What happens if the candidate hits another key?**

While the candidate is taking the test, all unnecessary keys are turned off so nothing will happen if the candidate hits an extraneous key.

6. **Are there directions on the computer for taking the NCE?**

At the beginning of the examination, candidates must verify that their identification information and examination are correct as shown on the computer screen.

Pay careful attention to the identification number that appears on the screen. It is the AANA associate member number followed

by a series of zeroes in a social security number format. The CCNA uses the AANA associate member number only for ID purposes.

Next, the directions for entering responses will appear. Candidates should read these directions carefully before beginning the test. **There is no tutorial and there are no practice questions.** The examination begins with the appearance of the first exam question. There is a "help" screen which may be referred to at any time during the examination to refresh the candidate's memory as to how to enter responses.

7. **What happens if there is a computer problem or power failure?**

If a power failure occurs while a candidate is taking a test and the candidate has to restart his or her test on that same test day, it will be resumed at the point of interruption since the questions and answers are saved. However, if the test cannot be resumed on the same day and the candidate has to reschedule his or her test, a new test will be administered. There will be no charge to the candidate for rescheduling a test if the problem occurs at or is the result of a problem at the Sylvan Technology Center.

EXAMINATION INFORMATION

8. **What is the Sylvan Center like where the candidate will take the test?**

Test rooms at the Centers are similar to computer labs containing multiple cubicles with partitions between them. Because Sylvan Technology Centers provide a wide variety of testing services, it is likely that the certification candidate will not be the only person taking an examination in the test room. Other individuals taking other examinations may be present. Some examinations may require full use of the computer keyboard with accompanying keyboard noise. In addition, Sylvan personnel and other individuals may leave and enter the test room during the certification candidate's test period.

Sylvan Technology Centers will make every effort to keep movement of personnel and noise levels to a minimum during examination administrations. However, if a certification candidate believes that noise may be a distraction, he or she should consider bringing earplugs to use during the examination.

The Council will not grant a candidate's request for a private testing room at Sylvan Technology Centers, except where the candidate has a documented disability that requires such an accommodation.

9. **Who writes the examination questions?**

Three CRNAs and one anesthesiologist from the CCNA and an elected representative group of four CRNAs serve on the Examination Committee. This committee meets annually to write and review test questions for the approved item bank.

10. **What types of questions are included on the NCE?**

All of the questions will be multiple-choice questions. The current format of a question (stem) with four possible answers is used. Clinical situations, diagrams, graphs, monitor interpretation recordings are on the same screen as the question.

11. **How is the CAT NCE item bank reviewed and updated?**

The CRNA and physician members of the CCNA and examination committee review and update the item bank each year. The performance statistics for questions are continuously monitored by the CCNA and Computer Adaptive Technologies, Inc. (CAT, Inc.), the company that assists with the development and administration of the Certification and Self-Evaluation Examinations.

12. **How many questions are on the NCE?**

Each candidate takes a minimum of 90 test questions; 70 questions representing the NCE content outline and 10 pretest questions. The maximum number of questions is 160 questions (including 20 pretest questions).

13. **What is the purpose of the pretest questions?**

An important principle of test construction is that only questions that demonstrate ac-

ceptable performance should be used to compute examination scores. Questions that have never been used before have unknown performance characteristics, and it would be unfair to use such questions in computing examinees scores. Therefore, it is necessary to pretest new questions and evaluate their performance. There are 20 such questions on the certification examination. They appear throughout the examination and are not exclusively the first twenty or last twenty questions. Those questions that survive the complex evaluation process are retained for use on future examinations. The pretest questions are not used to score the examination.

14. **How much time is allowed to take the NCE?**

A maximum of three hours is allowed for the test period. Most candidates use less time to take a computerized adaptive test than a paper and pencil test.

15. **Can a candidate review or change his or her responses?**

Questions are presented one at a time on the computer screen. A question can be reviewed and responses can be changed until the candidate moves on to the next question. The candidate must answer each question as it is presented. Candidates can view each question as long as they like, and even change the answer of the item on the screen, but they cannot go back to previous questions. Psychometric research has shown that, in general, candidates do not significantly improve the estimate of their ability by reviewing and changing answers.

16. **How does the computer determine when a candidate's test is finished?**

The NCE will stop when:

- The maximum amount of questions (160) have been answered; or
- The time limit (3 hours) is reached; or
- The pass or fail status is clearly identified after the minimum number of questions (90) are answered.

17. **How is a pass/fail decision reached?**

A decision is made when one of the following conditions has been met:

- The candidate has clearly demonstrated competence. This decision may be reached at any point between 90 and 160 times.
- The candidate has clearly demonstrated incompetence. This decision may be reached at any point between 90 and 160 times.
- The maximum number of questions (160) have been administered. The pass/fail decision is based on whether the candidate's level of competence is above or below the pass/fail point.
- The maximum amount of time (3 hours) is reached. A fail decision is made if the candidate has not completed 90 questions. If the candidate has completed more than 90 questions, the pass/fail decision is based on whether the candidate's level of competence is above or below the pass/fail point.

18. How is the passing score determined?

The passing score is established by the CCNA. It is determined using the Angroff method. The passing point is the same for all candidates.

19. Can the candidate use a calculator or scratch paper during the test?

Calculators are not allowed during the test. NCE questions do not include calculations that require the use of a calculator. Scratch paper is provided by the Technology Center. No papers may be brought into the center by the candidate.

20. Why are candidates required to sign the Waiver of Liability and Agreement of Nondisclosure?

The NCE is the property of the Council on Certification and has been copyrighted by it.

Under the "Waiver of Liability and Agreement of Authorization, Confidentiality, and Nondisclosure," if any examinee, either directly or indirectly, discloses any question or any part of a question from the examination to any person or entity, the examinee may be subject to legal action that could result in monetary damages and/or disciplinary action, including denial or revocation of certification.

21. What does a candidate do if there are problems with the administration of the examination at the test center?

All test administrations are videotaped. Candidates have access to a proctor at the Sylvan Technology Centers. As a rule, if a problem occurs with the computer and the candidate has to restart his or her test on the scheduled test day, it will be resumed at the point of interruption since the questions and answers are saved. However, if the test cannot be resumed on the same day and the candidate has to reschedule his or her test, a new test will be administered. There will be no charge to the candidate for rescheduling a test if the problem occurs at or is the result of a problem at the Sylvan Technology Center.

Problems related to admission and/or administration of the examination should be reported as soon as possible, by fax, to the CCNA office. Any other problems relating to conditions at a test center must be reported in writing to the CCNA no later than three days after the examination date. Reports should include the candidate's full name, address, and signature, as well as a description of the conditions that caused a problem at the test center. After reviewing a report of a problem at a test center, the CCNA may, at its discretion, determine whether a new Certification Examination should be administered or other actions should be taken. Reports submitted from a program director will be considered only if these are accompanied by the candidate's report. Notice of test administration problems that are received after test results have been mailed are not considered by the Council.

REGISTRATION

22. How do candidates register to take the NCE?

Registration with the CCNA office can take place after the candidate has officially completed the anesthesia program. The program director sends all the necessary materials, including the official transcript, to the CCNA office. The candidate is responsible for completing the official application to take the Certification Examination. Upon receipt of the materials, the CCNA processes the applications and, where appropriate, grants certification eligibility status and sends a letter and certification eligibility card to the applicant. Eligibility materials, including the candidate's eligibility number, are sent in writing only by first class mail. Eligibility information is not given over the telephone or sent by Fax under any circumstances.

Upon receipt of written notification from the CCNA, the candidate can call Sylvan's National Registration Center to schedule an appointment to the NCE. The CCNA does not schedule appointments to the NCE.

Candidates should be aware that it may take up to 4 weeks for Sylvan to schedule an appointment depending on availability at the local Sylvan Technology Center. Remember that the GRE, GMAT, and N-CLEX examinations are also scheduled through Sylvan so immediate access for a particular time and site is not always possible.

Candidates should be aware that the months of June and July are very busy for Sylvan due to the administration of the N-CLEX for registered nurses, and October and November are busy due to the GRE and GMAT. Therefore, scheduling during these dates could be problematic. In addition, keep in mind that during the Christmas holidays, scheduling of examinations may present problems due to the holiday season, office closures, and decrease in personnel.

Because of the large volume of mail the CCNA receives, confirmation of receipt of transcripts, eligibility status, and letters to state boards of nursing and potential employers regarding eligibility status cannot be acknowledged immediately. Applicants are asked not to call the CCNA concerning the receipt or mailing of these materials.

23. **What kind of eligibility materials does the candidate receive from the CCNA?**

The eligibility candidate receives by first class mail a letter that contains information about registration, a certification eligibility card, and the 1998 CCNA Candidate Handbook. The information on the eligibility card is to schedule an appointment to take the examination with Sylvan's National Registration Center. The eligibility letter contains

the 800 number to call Sylvan's National Registration Center.

24. **How long after a student completes the program does it take to register to take the NCE?**

The registration process with the CCNA should be completed within 4 weeks after the Council receives official notification of the student's program completion and all the required materials. **It may take up to 4 weeks for Sylvan to schedule an appointment depending on the availability at the local Sylvan Technology Center.**

25. **How does a candidate request confirmation of eligibility to be sent to a state board or prospective employer?**

All requests for verification eligibility letters to state boards of nursing and potential employers are addressed *at the time the application is processed.* Candidates should not make any commitments to prospective employers that depend on immediate verification from the Council since requests are handled at the time the application is processed and will not be handled at any other time. Any other requests for verification of eligibility that were not received with the application are handled as time permits, not on an immediate basis.

Candidates can expect all requests for letters of eligibility and forms for state boards and employees to be processed **within 4 weeks** from the time the official application and all required materials to take the examination are received in the CCNA office.

However, if the official transcript has to be returned to the program director for corrections, this time may be longer and candidates should check with their program directors for information concerning their transcript.

26. **Are there any time limits for students to take the test?**

The certification eligibility card expires **three** months from the date of issue. During this time, the candidate must schedule and take the NCE.

If a candidate does not schedule an appointment with Sylvan's National Registration

Center and take the NCE by the expiration date on the certification eligible card, he or she must restart the registration process and pay the full fee.

27. What is the NCE fee?

The 1999 NCE fee is $500. Only certified checks or money orders are acceptable. **Personal checks are not accepted.**

28. How is the candidate identified at the testing center?

When a candidate arrives at the Sylvan Technology Center, he or she must present to the proctor the certification eligible card from the CCNA and two separate forms of valid I.D., one of which must be a photo and signature-bearing identification card (e.g., driver's license). Candidates who appear without photo identification are not permitted to take the NCE and are required to reapply and pay the full registration fee for another examination. The certification eligibility card must be an original, not a photocopy.

29. How do candidates notify the Council of a name or address change before the examination date?

Candidates will not be able to request a name change once the Council has sent the eligibility file to Sylvan. The name that the candidate used on the official CCNA application form is the name that is submitted to Sylvan on the eligibility file. Therefore, when the candidate appears at the test center, *the name on the original CCNA eligibility card and two pieces of identification* (one of which must be a photo and signature-bearing identification) *must all match.* Candidates will not be allowed to test if their eligibility card does not bear the same first and last name as their eligibility file at the Sylvan Center.

Candidates will not be able to record a name or address change at Sylvan Technology Centers. Because the CCNA needs to keep their files updated, if a candidate changes his or her name and/or address after eligibility materials have been mailed, the CCNA should be notified by fax or mail of the change.

30. Will there be a problem being admitted to the examination if a candidate's name has changed?

As long as the candidate's photo identification matches the name that was submitted on the official CCNA application form and sent to Sylvan, there will not be a problem being admitted to the examination.

31. How often can a candidate repeat the NCE?

Each candidate is allowed to repeat the NCE, if necessary, up to four times a calendar year. Candidates can schedule the NCE throughout the year.

32. How long must a candidate who failed the NCE wait before retesting?

Candidates should allow for a minimum time period of thirty days between examinations for the CCNA to review and process the necessary information.

TEST PREPARATION

33. How should a candidate prepare for the NCE?

The best way to prepare is through serious and consistent attention to the clinical and didactic aspects of the candidate's nurse anesthesia educational program. It is important to exercise problem-solving skills and develop appropriate anesthesia care plans throughout the anesthesia educational program.

In addition, candidates can organize comprehensive review or study programs for themselves based on the areas contained in the content outline. Unquestionably, it is difficult to remember everything learned during the anesthesia program. But candidates should not assume that they can pass the examination without adequate review and preparation. Candidates should take part in a study review group with classmates and ask their program directors and other instructors for additional suggestions. For instance, some candidates might benefit from attending a test-taking and/or stress management workshop at a local college or university.

The CCNA has a demonstration disk available for faculty and students that shows how the test will look on the computer.

Another good way to prepare for the NCE is to take the Self-Evaluation Examination (SEE) at some time while enrolled in the nurse anesthesia program.

The CCNA does not recommend, sponsor, or endorse any particular review course or review materials.

34. **What is the SEE and why is it important?**

The SEE is administered on the computer at the Sylvan Technology Centers.

Taking the SEE will give candidates the opportunity to experience an on-line computerized adaptive test, including understanding test directions and help screens, and responding to test questions with the keyboard or a mouse.

The SEE helps prepare candidates for the test-taking conditions that will be encountered during the NCE, and many of the questions on the SEE related to clinical practice. For example, the SEE provides information about a case or type of patient, and candidates are asked to make a judgment about the correct management.

In one national study, a positive correlation was found between the scores on the SEE and those on the NCE. Students who attained higher scores on the SEE also scored higher on the NCE. Further study of this correlation is planned.

35. **How can candidates be certain they have reviewed everything that might be asked on the NCE?**

Program directors have a copy of the examination content outline that can be a great help to candidates. A copy of the content outline also appears in the *Candidate Handbook* and in the *1998 NCE Questions and Answers*. Candidates should review the content outline with the director and ask for assistance on areas that are new or that were not included in the classroom instruction they received. For example, continuous quality improvement (CQI) in anesthesia is now a part of practice, and questions regarding it should be expected on an examination that certifies nurse anesthetists.

36. **Are the majority of questions taken from any particular textbook?**

There is no single book that serves as a resource. Just as anesthesia practice is vast and varied, so are the resources for learning. The principal anesthesia textbooks used in anesthesia educational programs should provide information related to all the major content areas on the NCE. Research articles and review books are not used as references.

37. **Is there any other material candidates should review prior to taking the NCE?**

Candidates should review the *1998 CCNA Candidate Handbook* and the materials sent with their eligibility card very carefully. These materials contain everything candidates need to know about administration of the NCE. It is the candidate's responsibility to be familiar with the contents of the *1998 CCNA Candidate Handbook* as well as the information sent with the eligibility notice.

EXAMINATION RESULTS

38. **How is the NCE scored?**

The CAT NCE is scored based on the candidates performance relative to the difficulty of items administered.

39. **When do candidates receive their NCE results?**

The CCNA will notify candidates of their certification status within four weeks to assure that all other certification criteria have been met. Candidates do not receive on-screen results at the test administration site.

You are strongly advised not to make commitments to prospective employers that depend on your receiving test results any sooner than **4 weeks from the day after you test.** The Council on Certification of Nurse Anesthetists sends results to candidates within 24 hours after the results are processed in the CCNA office and this can be up to 4 weeks. It is important to remember that not everyone who tests on the same day at the same center will receive the results from the CCNA at the same time because the information is not transmitted to us in that manner. Therefore, calls to the CCNA requesting information on when an applicant will receive test results will not be returned until the end of the 4-week reporting period.

If you request results to be sent by overnight mail, it means that your results will be sent by Fed Ex within 24 hours after the results are processed in the office. It does not guarantee a quicker processing of results.

40. What information does the candidate receive after taking the NCE?

Candidates receive a test result report. If the candidate passes the NCE, he or she receives notification of passing, a certification card, and a certificate attesting to the new status of Certified Registered Nurse Anesthetist (CRNA). If the candidate fails the NCE he or she receives notification of not passing and, in addition, his or her total scaled score and diagnostic score information for the five content areas.

41. Where is the test result sent?

The test results are sent to the name and address on the candidate's eligibility letter unless the candidate has notified the CCNA in writing of a different name or address.

42. How are hand scoring requests handled for the NCE?

With CAT, all information is recorded directly into the computer, thus eliminating the need for hand scoring. However, an individual record is maintained for each candidate, and failing candidates can request *in writing* that their examination results be individually reviewed by contacting the Council on Certification of Nurse Anesthetists, 222 S. Prospect Avenue, Park Ridge, IL 60068, within 6 months of the candidate's test date. The *1998 CCNA Candidate Handbook* provides additional detailed information.

43. Who receives a report of test results?

Test results are released to the candidate and his or her program director. Written authorization must be provided for the release of the results to anyone else. The only information that is available regarding the examination and a candidate's performance on it is the test results received by the candidate. Because of the need to maintain test security, test questions and answers are not available for review. Neither the CCNA nor the testing agency provides a list of the test questions.

44. What if a candidate fails the NCE?

The NCE may be repeated up to four times a year. To reapply, candidates must submit an application to retake the examination, proof of current licensure, and the application fee. Questions concerning employment in a particular state prior to certification should be addressed to the Board of Nursing of that state.

45. What percentage of first-time takers fail the NCE?

The percentage of first time takers failing the NCE over the past ten years is as follows.

Year	June	December
87		17.4%
88	15.9%	20.0
89	10.7	18.1
90	14.8	15.8
91	16.5	14.4
92	15.0	9.3
93	9.9	14.3
94	11.3	10.0
95	9.3	5.2
April–December 1996		10.2%
January–June 1997		10.3%
July–December 1997		7.2%
January–June 1998		8.5%
July–December 1998		8.8%

46. Is there any recourse for challenging a question if a candidate believes that his or her answer is supported by current references?

Questions for which two or more answers may be acceptable, or which are ambiguous in any clinical situation have been deleted from the item bank. Only one answer will be clearly correct. A candidate can write to the CCNA about any question he or she believes was ambiguous.

47. Will I receive results faster if I pay the Fed Ex fee?

Fed Ex service means that the candidate's test results will be sent by Federal Express within 24 hours after the results have been processed in the CCNA office. It does not guarantee quicker processing of results.

COUNCIL ON CERTIFICATION OF NURSE ANESTHETISTS EXAMINATION CONTENT OUTLINE

The following topical outline is provided to assist candidates in preparing for the Certification Examination. It is a guide only that suggests topics and topical areas to generate and categorize examination questions. It is not all-inclusive, with some elements applying to more than one area. The Council reserves the right to determine examination content, to classify examination questions, and to determine the percentage of test questions from each topical area. The approximate percentages of questions in each major content area are provided below.

CONTENT OUTLINE

30% of Questions

I. Basic science
  A. Anatomy, physiology, and pathophysiology
    1. Cardiovascular
       a. Arrhythmias
       b. Ischemic heart disease/angina
       c. Myocardial infarction
       d. Hypertension
       e. Congestive heart failure
       f. Shock
       g. Valvular heart disease
       h. Cardiomyopathy
       i. Peripheral vascular disease
       j. Pacemaker
       k. Pericardial processes/tamponade
    2. Respiratory
       a. COPD/emphysema/obstructive
       b. Reactive airway conditions/ asthma
       c. Pneumonia
       d. Tuberculosis
       e. Pulmonary embolism
       f. Cor pulmonale
       g. Pulmonary hypertension
       h. Upper respiratory infection
       i. Sarcoidosis/restrictive
       j. Adult respiratory distress syndrome
       k. Intrapleural (hemo/pneumo-thorax)
    3. Central nervous system
       a. Seizures
       b. CVA/vascular lesions
       c. Hydrocephalus
       d. Parkinson's
       e. Multiple sclerosis
       f. Myasthenia gravis
       g. Alzheimer's/dementia
       h. Demyelinating disease
       i. Intracranial hypertension
       j. Autonomic hyperreflexia/ dysautonomia
       k. Neuropathy/myopathy
       l. Coma
       m. Mental disorders
       n. Spinal cord injury
    4. Musculoskeletal
       a. Fractures
       b. Arthritis
       c. Muscular dystrophy
       d. Scoliosis
    5. Endocrine
       a. Diabetes mellitus
       b. Diabetes insipidus
       c. Hypo/hyperthyroid
       d. Cushing's disease
       f. Pituitary dysfunction
       g. Pheochromocytoma
       h. Acromegaly
       i. Hypo/hyperaldosteronism

6. Hepatic
    a. Hepatitis
    b. Cirrhosis/portal hypertension
    c. Hepatic failure
7. Renal
    a. Urolithiasis/kidney stones
    b. Acute renal failure
    c. Chronic renal failure
8. Hematologic
    a. Anemia
    b. Sickle cell/hemoglobinopathies
    c. Polycythemia/leukemia
    d. AIDS/HIV
    e. Coagulopathies
9. Gastrointestinal
    a. Ulcer disease
    b. Ulcerative colitis
    c. Diaphragmatic hernia
    d. Hiatal hernia/gastric reflux
    e. Gallstones/gallbladder disease
    f. Pancreatitis
    g. Splenic disorders
    h. Carcinoid syndrome
10. Other conditions
    a. Cancer
    b. Obesity
    c. Glaucoma/open globe
    d. Hypothermia
    e. Hyperthermia
    f. Major trauma
    g. Critical care
    h. Smoking
    i. Substance abuse (alcohol and drugs)
    j. Airway difficulties
    k. Collagen/lupus erythematosus
    l. Immunosuppression/malnutrition
B. **Pharmacology**
    1. General principles
        a. Pharmacodynamics
        b. Pharmacokinetics
        c. Anaphylaxis
        d. Drug interactions
    2. Inhalation anesthetics
    3. Intravenous anesthetics
        a. Barbiturates
        b. Opioids (agonist/antagonist)
        c. Benzodiazepines
        d. Other
    4. Local anesthetics
        a. Esters
        b. Amides
    5. Muscle relaxants/antagonists

6. Autonomic and cardiovascular drugs
7. Others
    a. CNS drugs
    b. Diuretics
    c. Autocoids
C. **Chemistry, biochemistry, physics**

5% of Questions

II. **Equipment, instrumentation, and technology**
    A. **Anesthetic delivery systems**
        1. High/low pressure gas sources
        2. Regulators/manifolds
        3. Flowmeters, valves, floats
        4. Vaporizers
        5. Proportioning systems
        6. Pressure failure safety devices
        7. "Fail-safe" devices
        8. Ventilator
        9. Carbon dioxide absorbent
        10. Anesthetic circuits
        11. Pneumatic and electronic alarm devices
        12. Flow-over systems
        13. Jet ventilation
        14. Infusion devices
    B. **Airway equipment**
    C. **Monitoring devices**
        1. Central nervous system
            a. Electroencephalogram
            b. Evoked potential
            c. Intracranial pressure
        2. Cardiovascular
            a. Electrocardiogram
            b. Arterial pressure monitoring
            c. Noninvasive blood pressure monitoring
            d. Transesophageal echocardiography
            e. Central venous pressure monitoring
            f. Pulmonary artery pressure monitoring/SVO$_2$
            g. Cardiac output
        3. Precordial/esophageal stethoscope/Doppler
        4. Respiratory monitoring
            a. Apnea monitor
            b. Capnography
            c. Mass spectrometry
            d. Pulse oximetry

  e. Airway pressure
  f. Respirometer
  g. Blood gas analysis
 5. Peripheral nerve stimulator
 6. Renal monitoring
 7. Temperature monitoring
 8. Maternal/fetal monitoring devices
 9. Others
  a. Blood warmers
  b. Warming blanket
  c. Heat moisture exchanger
  d. Heated humidifier

III. Basic principles of anesthesia
 A. **Preoperative assessment**
 B. **Preparation of patient**
 C. **Fluid/blood replacement**
 D. **Positioning**
 E. **Interpretation of data**
  1. Lab tests
  2. Diagnostic data
  3. Intraoperative monitoring data
 F. **Airway management**
  1. Mask
  2. Intubation
  3. Cricothyrotomy
  4. Fiberoptics
 G. **Local/regional anesthesia**
  1. Infiltration
  2. Regional blocks
   a. Subarachnoid
   b. Epidural
   c. Brachial plexus
   d. Transtracheal
   e. IV regional (Bier)
   f. Retrobulbar/peribulbar
   g. Ankle
   h. Digital
   i. Femoral/sciatic
 H. **Monitored anesthesia care/conscious sedation**
 I. **Pain management**
  1. Epidural analgesia
  2. Infiltration nerve blocks
  3. Intrathecal narcotics
 J. **Others**
  1. Hypotensive
  2. Hypothermia
  3. Intraoperative wake up
 K. **Postanesthesia care/respiratory therapy**

IV. Advanced principles of anesthesia
 A. **Surgical procedures and procedures related to organ systems**
  1. Intra-abdominal
   a. Gallbladder
   b. Liver
   c. Pancreas
   d. Spleen
   e. Stomach
   f. Renal/adrenal
   g. Diaphragm
   h. Laparoscopy
   i. Intestine
   j. Herniorrhaphy
   k. Bladder
   l. Abdominal/gyn
   m. Prostate
  2. Extrathoracic
   a. Breast biopsy
   b. Mastectomy
   c. Plastic and/or reconstructive
   d. mediastinoscopy/open lung biopsy
  3. Extremities
   a. Lower
   b. Upper
   c. Total joint replacements
  4. Genital and urologic
   a. Penis/testes
   b. Transurethral resection
   c. Cystoscopy
   d. D and C
   e. Vaginal hysterectomy
  5. Head
   a. Extracranial
    (1) Cranioplasty
    (2) Rhizotomy
    (3) Ear
    (4) Eye
    (5) Face
    (6) Nose
   b. Intracranial
    (1) Decompression (burr holes)
    (2) Space-occupying lesion
    (3) Vascular
    (4) Transsphenoidal
    (5) CSF shunts
   c. Oropharyngeal
    (1) Endoscopy
    (2) Fractures
    (3) Tonsils and adenoids/ peritonsillar abscess
    (4) Orthodontic/dental
    (5) Pharynx
    (6) Reconstructive and/or plastic

CHAPTER 1

Basic Science

◆ ◆ ◆

1. Symptoms of anemia are unlikely to manifest in a healthy patient until the hemoglobin value falls below:

   A. 6 g/dL
   B. 8 g/dL
   C. 7 g/dL
   D. 9 g/dL

2. Sickling may occur with the sickle cell disease when the PO_2 falls below how many mm Hg?

   A. below 70 mm Hg
   B. below 60 mm Hg
   C. below 80 mm Hg
   D. below 50 mm Hg

3. In the patient with sickle cell disease, what percentage of the total hemoglobin pool is hemoglobin S?

   A. greater than 70%
   B. greater than 50%
   C. greater than 60%
   D. greater than 80%

4. The major vascular flow of blood to the liver is through the:

   A. portal artery
   B. portal vein
   C. hepatic vein
   D. hepatic artery

5. From what vessel does the hepatic artery rise?

   A. renal artery
   B. splenic artery
   C. celiac artery
   D. gastric artery

6. Approximately what percentage of cardiac output goes through the liver?

   A. 15%
   B. 25%
   C. 20%
   D. 10%

7. Which process is used the least by the liver in biotransformation?

   A. oxidation
   B. reduction
   C. synthesis
   D. hydrolysis

8. The blood/gas partition coefficient is an indication of an inhalation anesthetic's:

   A. lipid solubility
   B. protein binding
   C. potency
   D. speed of induction and emergence

9. What agents should be used with caution when administering halothane anesthesia?

   A. alpha$_1$ agonists
   B. catecholamines
   C. beta$_2$ agonists
   D. angiotensin-converting enzyme inhibitors

10. The addition of halogen to an inhalation anesthetic structure:

    A. increases blood solubility
    B. increases lipid solubility
    C. decreases potency
    D. decreases flammability

11. The ventilatory pattern known as "rocking boat ventilation" is caused by:

    A. loss of intercostal muscle function
    B. loss of diaphragm muscle function
    C. loss of abdominal muscle function
    D. loss of accessory muscle function

12. Which inhalation anesthetic inhibits methionine synthetase by oxidizing the cobalt atom of vitamin B_{12}?

    A. sevoflurane
    B. nitrous oxide
    C. halothane
    D. isoflurane

13. What results from damage to the posterior pituitary?

A. acromegaly, which reflects excess secretion of growth hormone in an adult

B. syndrome of inappropriate secretion of antidiuretic hormone, which reflects the absence of ADH

C. diabetes insipidus, which reflects the absence of ADH

D. Addison's disease, which reflects the absence of cortisol and aldosterone

14. In a patient with oliguric renal failure the urine output:

A. decreases to < 30 mL/h

B. decreases to < 0.5 mL/kg/h

C. decreases to < 15 mL/kg/h

D. decreases to < 500 mL/d

15. What is the principal mechanism of anterior pituitary hormonal control?

A. negative feedback

B. positive feedback

C. the stimulation of mitosis and cell division in various tissues

D. via somatostatins

16. The two hormones secreted by the posterior pituitary gland are:

A. antidiuretic hormone (ADH) and cortisol

B. ADH and follicle-stimulating hormone (FSH)

C. ADH and oxytoxcin

D. ADH and luteinizing hormone (LH)

17. What are the initial and maintenance doses of dantrolene for malignant hyperthermia, and what is the therapeutic blood level?

A. Initial dose is 5 mg, maintenance dose is 2-mg/kg boluses up to a maximum total dose of 10 mg/kg, and therapeutic blood level is 2.5 mg/mL.

B. Initial dose is 5 mg/kg, maintenance dose is 2.5-mg/kg boluses up to a maximum of 20 mg/kg and therapeutic blood level is 5 μg/mL.

C. Initial dose is 2.5 mg/kg, maintenance dose is 0.5 mg/kg, and therapeutic blood level is 25 mg/kg.

D. Initial dose is 2.5 mg/kg, maintenance dose is 1- to 2-mg/kg boluses up to a maximum total dose of 10 mg/kg, and therapeutic blood level is 2.5 μg/mL.

18. What is the earliest sign of malignant hyperthermia?

A. increase in end-tidal CO_2

B. tachycardia

C. increased temperature

D. tachypnea

19. What is the most sensitive sign of malignant hyperthermia?

A. increased temperature

B. tachycardia

C. increase in end-tidal CO_2 during constant ventilation

D. overheated CO_2 absorber

20. What is the mortality rate for malignant hyperthermia?

A. 100%

B. 10%

C. 50%

D. 25%

21. What syndrome can mimic malignant hyperthermia?

A. Eaton-Lambert syndrome

B. sudden death syndrome

C. neuroleptic malignant syndrome

D. Kearns-Sayre syndrome

22. What is the ASA physical status classification of a patient with an incapacitating disease that is a constant threat to life, such as heart failure or renal failure?

A. ASA 5

B. ASA 3

C. ASA 4

D. ASA 2

23. What is the ASA physical status classification of a patient with a mild systemic disease such as mild diabetes mellitus, controlled hypertension, anemia, chronic bronchitis, or morbid obesity?

A. ASA 2

B. ASA 3

C. ASA 4

D. ASA 5

24. Cyclosporine for immunosuppressant therapy exerts its effect by:

A. suppressing T cells
B. blocking histamines
C. activating beta cells
D. enhancing steroids

25. What is the best position for a postoperative tonsillectomy patient?

A. lateral position with head lower than hips
B. supine position with head of bed elevated 30°
C. lateral position with head elevated 30°
D. prone with head turned to side and lower than hips

26. Why should the legs be lowered slowly from the lithotomy position?

A. to prevent hip dislocations
B. The speed at which the legs are lowered is not important, only that they are lowered together.
C. to avoid hypotension
D. to prevent nerve injuries

27. Ephedrine stimulates:

A. alpha receptors only
B. beta receptors only
C. alpha and beta receptors
D. dopamine receptors

28. Acids tend to be most highly ionized at:

A. low pH
B. high pH
C. pH 7.0
D. equal at all pH levels

29. Which enzyme catalyzes the final step in acetylcholine synthesis?

A. carbonic anhydrase
B. adenylcyclase
C. choline acetyltransferase
D. glutamic transferase

30. Acetylcholine is the neurotransmitter in all of the following sites except:

A. neuromuscular junction
B. preganglionic sympathetic neurons
C. postganglionic sympathetic receptors
D. preganglionic parasympathetic neurons

31. How many grams of reduced hemoglobin are necessary for cyanosis to occur?

A. 5 mg/100 mL
B. 5 g/1000 mL
C. 5 mg/1000 mL
D. 5 mg/100 mL

32. What is the most common cause of pancreatitis?

A. hepatitis
B. malnutrition
C. alcoholism
D. diabetes

33. How much oxygen is carried by each gram of hemoglobin when saturated?

A. 3%
B. 1.34 mL
C. 5%
D. 2 mL

34. What coagulation factor is deficient in hemophilia A?

A. Factor X
B. Factor VII
C. Factor VIII
D. Factor IV

35. What is the most important plasma protein binding of drugs?

A. globulin
B. albumin
C. fibrinogen
D. glycine

36. What percentage of CO_2 is carried in simple solution?

A. 10%
B. 5%
C. 2%
D. 4%

37. What is the abnormality associated with megaloblastic anemia?

    A. vitamin B_{12} deficiency
    B. presence of Hgb S
    C. short red blood cell span
    D. bone marrow depression

38. The stimulation of what sensory nerve triggers laryngospasm?

    A. hypoglossal
    B. recurrent laryngeal nerve
    C. superior laryngeal nerve
    D. vagus

39. What muscle tenses the vocal cords?

    A. thyroarytenoid
    B. cricothyroid
    C. lateral cricoarytenoids
    D. oblique arytenoids

40. What is the afferent nerve pathway for the carotid sinus body?

    A. glossopharyngeal
    B. vagus
    C. accessory
    D. hypoglossal

41. What hormone plays a primary role in regulating vascular volume?

    A. cortisol
    B. aldosterone
    C. thyrotropin
    D. parathyroid hormone

42. Explain why anephric or renal failure patients exhibit anemia.

    A. These renal patients have altered calcium levels, which alters the bone marrow's ability to produce large quantities of red blood cells.
    B. The lack of either vitamin B_{12} or folic acid necessary for red blood cell maturation is common in renal patients.
    C. The kidneys normally reabsorb ferritin (which is necessary for the formation of hemoglobin) as the glomerular filtrate passes through the renal tubular system. The inability of these renal patients to reabsorb ferritin is the contributory factor to anemia.
    D. The kidneys normally manufacture and secrete erythropoietin, a hormone that stimulates red blood cell production. These renal patients are lacking erythropoietin and therefore have fewer red blood cells.

43. The addition of a fluorine atom to a hydrocarbon results in:

    A. decreased stability
    B. increased flammability
    C. more potency
    D. increased stability

44. Acetylcholine is what type of ammonium compound?

    A. quaternary
    B. primary
    C. tertiary
    D. secondary

45. Muscle relaxants commonly contain what type of chemical group in their structure?

    A. tertiary base
    B. quaternary base
    C. secondary acid
    D. primary base

46. Which of the following beta blockers produces vasodilation?

    A. propranolol
    B. labetolol
    C. esmolol
    D. metoprolol

47. Sodium dantrolene's mechanism of action involves which of the following structures?

    A. myosin filaments
    B. sarcoplasmic reticulum
    C. neuromuscular junction
    D. actin filaments

48. What is an anesthetic consideration in the patient receiving $MgSO_4$?

    A. increased requirements of inhalational agent
    B. up-regulation of acetylcholine receptors
    C. reduced muscle relaxant doses
    D. severe hypertension

49. Which drug commonly inhibits the hepatic metabolism of many other substances?

    A. neostigmine
    B. glycopyrrolate
    C. atropine
    D. cimetidine

50. Basic compounds tend to be the most highly ionized:

A. in a high pH
B. they do not ionize
C. at a low pH
D. at physiologic pH

51. Sudden withdrawal from the antihypertensive drug clonidine may produce:

A. bradycardia
B. tachyphylaxis
C. severe rebound hypertension
D. severe hypotension

52. The well-established drug interaction between monoamine oxidase inhibitors and meperidine may produce:

A. hypothermia
B. tachycardia
C. hyperpyrexia
D. bradycardia

53. In the patient with diabetes insipidus, which of the following is a commonly found problem?

A. lethargy
B. hypernatremia
C. hyponatremia
D. anuria

54. Cocaine would be expected to produce which of the following?

A. vasodilation
B. dysphoria
C. blockade of norepinephrine reuptake
D. spinal anesthesia

55. Addition of epinephrine to local anesthetics is contraindicated in which of the following situations?

A. congestive heart failure
B. intravenous regional anesthesia
C. hypotension
D. axillary block

56. Cyclic adenosine monophosphate, a second messenger in many cells, causes what to occur in motor nerves?

A. releases neurotransmitters
B. opens calcium channels
C. stimulates intercellular enzymes
D. increases action potentials

57. The average blood volume in premature neonates is:

A. 110 mL/kg
B. 95 mL/kg
C. 65 mL/kg
D. 40 mL/kg

58. The average blood volume in a full-term neonate is:

A. 105 mL/kg
B. 95 mL/kg
C. 85 mL/kg
D. 40 mL/kg

59. What is the average blood volume in healthy infants?

A. 100 mL/kg
B. 85 mL/kg
C. 90 mL/kg
D. 80 mL/kg

60. What is the average blood volume for an adult male?

A. 95 mL/kg
B. 65 mL/kg
C. 75 mL/kg
D. 55 mL/kg

61. Which of the following vasoactive substances is not commonly released from carcinoid tumors?

A. serotonin
B. kalikrein
C. calcitonin
D. histamine

62. Which of the following exerts the longest duration of action when given epidurally?

A. fentanyl
B. meperidine
C. sufentanil
D. morphine

63. The definition of multiple endocrine neoplasia (MEN) is:

    A. a disorder involving pituitary tumor formation
    B. a group of syndromes characterized by tumor formation in various endocrine organs
    C. a muscular dystrophy involving multiple proximal muscle groups
    D. another name for pheochromocytoma

64. A patient with carpal tunnel syndrome has sustained injury to which of the following nerves?

    A. ulnar nerve
    B. radial nerve
    C. median nerve
    D. brachial nerve

65. How does the P_{50} differ between sickle cell hemoglobin (HbS) and normal hemoglobin (HbA)?

    A. The P_{50} is the same for both.
    B. HbS has less affinity for oxygen.
    C. HbS has greater affinity for oxygen.
    D. Clinically the difference is insignificant.

66. The normal red blood cell survival is 120 days; what is the sickle cell survival?

    A. 90 days
    B. 1 week
    C. the same as normal red blood cells
    D. 1015 days

67. An excess secretion of glucocorticosteroids from the adrenal cortex produces:

    A. Addison's disease
    B. diabetes
    C. pheochromocytoma
    D. Cushing's disease

68. Hypersecretion of aldosterone by the adrenal cortex is referred to as:

    A. Cushing's syndrome
    B. Conn's syndrome
    C. Addison's disease
    D. diabetes

69. Destruction of the adrenal gland resulting in a combination of mineralocorticoid and glucocorticoid deficiency is known as:

    A. Cushing's syndrome
    B. carcinoid syndrome
    C. diabetes
    D. Addison's disease

70. What is the most common cause of secondary adrenal insufficiency?

    A. increased ACTH secretion from the pituitary
    B. iatrogenic administration of exogenous glucocorticoids
    C. missed dose of exogenous corticosteroids
    D. general anesthesia with etomidate administration

71. Acute adrenal insufficiency or addisonian crisis is a medical emergency characterized by all of the following, except:

    A. circulatory collapse
    B. decreased mentation
    C. fever
    D. hyperglycemia

72. What happens when a drug that is a weak base is administered to an acidotic patient?

    A. More drug is nonionized.
    B. Less drug is nonionized.
    C. The pK_a increases.
    D. The pK_a decreases.

73. What is the total CO_2 content of arterial blood?

    A. 100 mL CO_2/dL blood
    B. 48 mL CO_2/dL blood
    C. 25 mL CO_2/dL blood
    D. 12 mL CO_2/dL blood

74. How much CO_2 is produced by cellular metabolism in a resting 70-kg person?

    A. 100,150 mL CO_2/min
    B. 5075 mL CO_2/min
    C. 200,250 mL CO_2/min
    D. over 500 ml CO_2/min

75. All of the following respiratory abnormalities are associated with scoliosis except:

    A. increased chest wall compliance
    B. decreased PaO_2 and increased $PaCO_2$
    C. pulmonary hypertension
    D. decreased lung volumes

76. The central chemoreceptors are primarily sensitive to:

    A. increased PCO_2
    B. hypotension
    C. H^+ ions or pH
    D. increased PaO_2

77. The peripheral chemoreceptors are primarily sensitive to:

    A. increased PCO_2
    B. decreased PCO_2
    C. decreased PaO_2
    D. H^+ ions

78. What is the significance of brown fat?

    A. Large amounts of iron are stored here.
    B. It is a source of nonshivering thermogenesis in infants.
    C. Obese patients have increased amounts of brown fat.
    D. It is the origin of sweating in infants before 1 year of age.

79. Which of the following is not considered a triggering agent of malignant hyperthermia?

    A. desflurane
    B. halothane
    C. succinylcholine
    D. propofol

80. Which electrolyte augments nondepolarizing muscle relaxants?

    A. sodium
    B. magnesium
    C. phosphorus
    D. potassium

81. Oxygen consumption of a neonate is how many times greater than in an adult?

    A. 2
    B. 1
    C. 3
    D. 4

82. Which of the following is not true regarding the neonate's kidney function?

    A. Glomerular filtration rate is increased.
    B. Urine output is high.
    C. Renal blood flow is decreased.
    D. Excretion of renal-eliminated drugs is delayed.

83. What is the average glomerular filtration rate for a term neonate?

    A. 120 mL/min $\times$ 1.7/m
    B. 20 mL/min $\times$ 1.7/m
    C. 100 mL/min $\times$ 1.7/m
    D. 50 mL/min $\times$ 1.7/m

84. In equipotent doses, which of the following produces the most cardiac depression?

    A. thiopental
    B. etomidate
    C. propofol
    D. midazolam

85. At what percentage should the neonate's hematocrit be maintained to optimize tissue oxygenation?

    A. 50%
    B. 45%
    C. 25%
    D. 40%

86. The primary function of surfactant is to:

    A. maintain alveolar stability
    B. dilate bronchi
    C. promote mucociliary transport
    D. allow diffusion of gases

87. Surfactant is produced in specialized cells called:

    A. alveolar cells
    B. type II pneumocytes
    C. hyaline membrane cells
    D. alveolar cells

88. Which of the following is not a risk in preterm neonates?

    A. respiratory distress syndrome
    B. retrolental fibroplasia
    C. hypercalcemia
    D. intracranial hemorrhage

89. To reduce the risk of retinopathy (retrolental fibroplasia) in susceptible neonates, at what should the PaO_2 be maintained?

    A. as close to 100 mm Hg as possible
    B. between 80 and 90 mm Hg
    C. between 60 and 80 mm Hg
    D. less than 60 mm Hg

90. Total renal blood flow decreases what percent each decade of adult life?

    A. 15%
    B. 10%
    C. 5%
    D. 1%

91. All of the following statements are true regarding the pulmonary system of the geriatric patient except:

    A. Closing volume decreases.
    B. Functional residual capacity increases.
    C. Residual volume increases.
    D. Vital capacity decreases.

92. All of the following statements are true regarding the renal function of the geriatric patient except:

    A. Renal blood flow decreases.
    B. Glomerular filtration rate decreases.
    C. Ability to concentrate the urine is impaired.
    D. Serum creatinine level increases.

93. All are physiologic changes that put the geriatric patient at risk for developing hypothermia except:

    A. deficient thermostat control
    B. ineffective shivering mechanisms
    C. decreased heat production
    D. increased heat loss

94. All the following are signs and symptoms of thyroid storm except:

    A. bradycardia
    B. hyperpyrexia
    C. hypertension followed by hypotension
    D. alteration in consciousness

95. Marked deficiency in circulating levels of thyroid hormone during fetal development can lead to:

    A. Addison's disease
    B. cretinism
    C. thyroid storm
    D. thyroid goiter

96. The patient with myxedema would likely exhibit which of the following signs or symptoms:

    A. heat intolerance
    B. sunken facial structures
    C. hypertension
    D. slowed mentation

97. Fibrinogen is synonymous with what clotting factor?

    A. Factor II
    B. Factor VIII
    C. Factor I
    D. Factor IX

98. The extrinsic pathway integrity can be measured by what test?

    A. prothrombin time
    B. partial thromboplastin time
    C. bleeding time
    D. activated clotting time

99. The intrinsic pathway is normally tested by which laboratory test?

    A. activated clotting time
    B. bleeding time
    C. prothrombin time
    D. partial thromboplastin time

100. The most common reaction to occur after nonautologuous blood transfusion is:

A. allergic reaction
B. hemolytic reaction
C. febrile reaction
D. activation of the clotting cascade

101. Intracellular fluid volume represents what percent of total body weight?

A. 40%
B. 20%
C. 60%
D. 80%

102. Extracellular fluid volume represents what percent of total body weight?

A. 20%
B. 40%
C. 60%
D. 5%

103. The predominant intracellular cation is:

A. PO_4^-
B. Na^+
C. K^+
D. Cl^-

104. Water represents what percent of total body weight?

A. 60%
B. 80%
C. 50%
D. 90%

105. The predominant extracellular cation is:

A. Cl^-
B. K^+
C. PO_4^-
D. Na^+

106. Clinical manifestations of hypernatremia include all except:

A. seizures
B. hyporeflexia
C. hyperreflexia
D. thirst

107. The most common cause of hyperkalemia is:

A. drugs
B. excess potassium intake
C. insulin deficiency
D. catecholamine insufficiency

108. Hyperkalemia may result from all of the following except:

A. mineralocorticoid deficiency
B. insulin excess
C. renal tubular dysfunction
D. catecholamine insufficiency

109. Hemophilia A is characterized by deficiency of which blood factor:

A. VII
B. X
C. XI
D. VIII

110. Bleeding time is a measurement of the:

A. thrombin time
B. platelet function only
C. platelet number and function
D. time to clot lysis

111. A normal bleeding time is:

A. 1 to 2 minutes
B. 3 to 8 minutes
C. 10 minutes
D. 12 to 15 minutes

112. The atrial contraction component generally accounts for what percentage of ventricular filling?

A. 20% but may increase to 40% with pathology
B. 40% in all individuals
C. varies from 30% to 60%
D. accounts for 100%

113. In regard to the pathophysiology of aortic insufficiency, all of the following are true except:

A. It is usually rheumatoid in origin.
B. Concentric hypertrophy develops.
C. Compliance is increased.
D. Bradycardia increases regurgitant flow.

114. In regard to the pathophysiology behind mitral stenosis:

    A. Pulmonary hypertension is common.
    B. Right-sided heart failure is an uncommon finding.
    C. Atrial fibrillation is an uncommon concurrent finding.
    D. Pulmonary vascular resistance is decreased.

115. In chronic mitral regurgitation all of the following are true except:

    A. Left ventricular systolic pressure decreases.
    B. Left ventricle shows signs of overload.
    C. Pulmonary hypertension is common.
    D. Concentric hypertrophy occurs.

116. All of the following are hormonal changes commonly found with stress or trauma except:

    A. increased cortisol
    B. decreased glucagon
    C. hyperglycemia
    D. increased catecholamines

117. The most common metabolic complication of total parenteral nutrition is:

    A. alkalosis
    B. hyperkalemia
    C. acidosis
    D. hyperglycemia

118. What causes the first (S_1) heart sound?

    A. aortic valves
    B. closure of the mitral and tricuspid valves
    C. closure of the aortic and pulmonic valves
    D. closure of the semilunar valves

119. What causes the second (S_2) heart sound?

    A. closure of the aortic and pulmonic valves
    B. closure of the mitral and tricuspid valves
    C. closure of the mitral valve only
    D. closure of the atrioventricular valves

120. In myocardial infarction, which area of the heart is usually damaged first?

    A. transmural myocardium
    B. epicardium
    C. subendocardium
    D. endocardium

121. The coronary arteries are perfused during what phase of the cardiac cycle:

    A. presystolic
    B. systole
    C. diastole
    D. postdiastolic phase

122. The main determinants of cardiac output are all of the following except:

    A. compliance
    B. preload
    C. afterload
    D. body surface area

123. Normal cardiac index is:

    A. 2.5–4.0
    B. 2.0–5.0
    C. 1.5–2.5
    D. 2.5–6.0

124. Normal ejection fraction is:

    A. 0.4–0.6
    B. 0.4–1.0
    C. 0.6–0.7
    D. 0.7–0.9

125. Normal systemic vascular resistance (SVR) is:

    A. 900–1200 dynes/cm/sec
    B. 1200–1500 dynes/cm/sec
    C. 1000–1200 dynes/cm/sec
    D. 1500–2000 dynes/cm/sec

126. Normal pulmonary vascular resistance (PVR) is:

    A. 100–500 dynes/cm/sec
    B. 100–300 dynes/cm/sec
    C. 50–150 dynes/cm/sec
    D. 200–600 dynes/cm/sec

127. The reflex that causes an increase in arterial pressure secondary to cerebral ischemia is:

    A. chemoreceptor reflex
    B. Bezold-Jarisch reflex
    C. Cushing's reflex
    D. Bainbridge reflex

128. The reflex in which noxious stimuli to the ventricular wall causes hypotension and bradycardia is:

    A. Bezold-Jarisch reflex
    B. Cushing's reflex
    C. Bainbridge reflex
    D. Müller maneuver

129. Peripheral chemoreceptors sensitive to decreasing oxygenation are located in the:

    A. peripheral chemoreceptors
    B. carotid body
    C. aortic arch
    D. carotid and aortic bodies

130. During a Valsalva maneuver:

    A. venous return to the right ventricle decreases
    B. venous pressure in the extremities decreases
    C. cardiac output increases
    D. intrathoracic pressure decreases

131. The heart receives approximately what percentage of cardiac output?

    A. 10%
    B. 4%
    C. 20%
    D. 25%

132. The primary effect of atrial natriuretic factor is:

    A. increased heart rate
    B. direct peripheral vasoconstriction
    C. suppression of antidiuretic hormone
    D. increased cardiac output

133. All of the following are true of the oculocardiac reflex except:

    A. Traction on the lateral rectus muscle may stimulate it.
    B. Traction on the medial rectus muscle will stimulate it.
    C. Afferent fibers travel the trigeminal nerve.
    D. Efferent fibers travel the vagus nerve.

134. What is the normal stroke volume in milliliters of a 70-kg man?

    A. 75–110 mL
    B. 50–75 mL
    C. 100–120 mL
    D. 60–90 mL

135. An increase in atrial pressure causes a reflex increase in heart rate known as:

    A. Cushing's reflex
    B. vasomotor reflex
    C. Bainbridge reflex
    D. Stanley reflex

136. Aortic and carotid chemoreceptors are sensitive to all except:

    A. increased H^+
    B. modest hypotension with systolic BP > 90 mm Hg
    C. increased CO_2
    D. decreased P_{AO_2}

137. Angiotensin I is converted to angiotensin II:

    A. in the kidney tubules
    B. in the juxtamedullary cells
    C. in the adrenal glands
    D. in the lung

138. Angiotensin II causes all of the following except:

    A. vasoconstriction
    B. retention of potassium
    C. retention of salt
    D. aldosterone secretion

139. Hypertension of unknown origin is:

    A. essential hypertension
    B. neurogenic hypertension
    C. malignant hypertension
    D. spontaneous hypertension

140. All the following are true of heart rate except:

   A. It is not strongly influenced by humoral stimulation.
   B. It is primarily determined by the sinus node.
   C. Parasympathetic stimulation causes bradycardia.
   D. Sympathetic stimulation causes tachycardia.

141. All of the following are characteristics of fetal hemoglobin (HbF) except:

   A. Newborns have 70% to 90% HgF.
   B. Its affinity for oxygen is greater than that of adult hemoglobin.
   C. It is released more readily to the tissues.
   D. The P_{50} of HgF is 20 mm Hg.

142. Normal newborn hemoglobin is:

   A. 18–19 g/dL
   B. 14–15 g/dL
   C. 10–12 g/dL
   D. 8–10 g/dL

143. All the following congenital heart lesions result in an increased pulmonary blood flow except:

   A. atrial septal defect
   B. tetralogy of Fallot
   C. ventricular septal defect
   D. patent ductus arteriosus

144. The safe dose of epinephrine for local infiltration in a child anesthetized with halothane is:

   A. 0.1 mg/kg
   B. 0.1 µg/kg
   C. 10 µg/kg
   D. 0.001 mg/kg

145. All the following are true of infants' physiology of temperature homeostasis except:

   A. They rely on shivering thermogenesis.
   B. They lack insulating subcutaneous fat.
   C. They lose heat rapidly.
   D. They have a large surface area relative to body weight.

146. Flow through the ductus arteriosus is insignificant by:

   A. 2 to 3 days
   B. 2 hours
   C. 15 hours
   D. 5 to 7 days

147. All of the following are true of the neonate except:

   A. Peripheral vascular resistance is dramatically increased.
   B. Systemic vascular resistance is dramatically increased.
   C. Blood flow to the lungs increases as the cord is cut.
   D. Flow through the ductus reverses.

148. Neonates exposed to hypoxemia suffer all of the following except:

   A. systemic vasoconstriction
   B. pulmonary vasodilation
   C. bradycardia
   D. reduced cardiac output

149. Newborns fatigue more easily during periods of increased respiration due to:

   A. decreased levels of type I muscle fibers
   B. increased levels of type I muscle fibers
   C. decreased levels of type II muscle fibers
   D. increased levels of type II muscle fibers

150. Slow-twitch, highly oxidative, fatigue-resistant muscle fibers are type:

   A. III
   B. IV
   C. II
   D. I

151. The principal surfactant in the lung is:

   A. lysine
   B. sphingomyelin
   C. lecithin
   D. glycine

152. All the following are true of the infant airway except:

A. The larynx is at level C6.
B. The epiglottis is stiff and "U"-shaped.
C. The tongue is large.
D. The larynx is relatively anterior.

153. Retinopathy of prematurity is more common in all of the following except:

A. infants who have had major surgery
B. infants exposed to high levels of oxygen
C. gestational age < 44 weeks
D. weight < 1000 g

154. Surfactant production occurs at:

A. 32 weeks
B. 24 weeks
C. 22 weeks
D. 34 to 36 weeks

155. Surfactant is produced by:

A. type II pneumocytes
B. type I and II pneumocytes
C. type I pneumocytes
D. All pneumocytes are capable of producing surfactant.

156. Decreased levels of surfactant in the preterm infant lead to all of the following except:

A. decreased compliance
B. decreased work of breathing
C. collapse of alveoli
D. impaired gas exchange

157. All of the following are true of caudal block except:

A. The injection is made in the epidural space.
B. The catheter is advanced cephalad at a 45° angle to the skin.
C. A triangle is drawn using the sacral hiatus and the posterior superior iliac spine.
D. The bevel of the needle faces posteriorly.

158. The preferred anticholinergic in pediatrics is:

A. glycopyrrolate
B. atropine
C. scopolamine
D. hydroxyzine

159. All of the following are components of tetrology of Fallot except:

A. atrial septal defect
B. right ventricular hypertrophy
C. overriding aorta
D. pulmonary stenosis

160. Concurrent use of what eye drops can result in prolongation of succinylcholine or mivacurium?

A. pilocarpine
B. timolol
C. cyclopentolate
D. echothiophate iodide

161. Anesthetic management for the infant who presents for pyloric stenosis repair includes all of the following except:

A. rehydration
B. rapid sequence induction with cricoid pressure
C. avoid nitrous oxide
D. insertion of a nasogastric tube before induction

162. The most common reason a child needs to be admitted after a planned same-day surgery procedure is:

A. sore throat
B. vomiting
C. sleep apnea
D. excessive lethargy

163. All of the following are known triggers of malignant hyperthermia except:

A. sevoflurane
B. succinylcholine
C. halothane
D. vecuronium

164. The majority of blood flow to the liver is derived from the:

A. portal vein
B. hepatic artery
C. vena cava
D. mesenteric artery

165. All of the following are true of the oculo-cardiac reflex except:

    A. The afferent pathway is CN III.
    B. The efferent pathway is CN X.
    C. It fatigues easily.
    D. It can be prevented by prophylactic use of atropine.

166. Maintaining normal body temperature is more difficult in infants than in adults because of all of the following except:

    A. larger surface-to-volume ratio
    B. increased total body water
    C. increased metabolic rate
    D. lack of sufficient body fat

167. All of the following are true of the kidneys at birth except:

    A. decreased concentrating ability
    B. decreased glomerular filtration rate
    C. decreased sodium excretion
    D. increased renal blood flow

168. The primary reason increased doses of muscle relaxants are necessary in infants is:

    A. immature hepatic system
    B. decreased extracellular fluid volume
    C. increased volume of distribution
    D. increased glomerular filtration rate

169. All of the following are characteristic symptoms of laryngotracheobronchitis except:

    A. high fever
    B. airway obstruction
    C. slow onset
    D. barking cough

170. Laryngotracheobronchitis most often affects:

A. toddlers
B. children younger than 6 years
C. There is no age significance.
D. children younger than 2 years

171. All of the following are true of epiglottitis except:

    A. It is accompanied by drooling.
    B. Its cause is viral.
    C. It is less common than croup.
    D. Affected children insist on sitting up.

172. The maximum dosage of IV dantrolene is:

    A. 5 mg/kg
    B. 2.5 mg/kg
    C. 10 mg/kg
    D. 1 mg/kg

173. An infant born with a scaphoid abdomen, profound arterial hypoxemia, and a shift of the mediastinum most likely has:

    A. congenital diaphragmatic hernia
    B. tracheoesophageal fistula
    C. pyloric stenosis
    D. patent ductus arteriosus

174. The infant with pyloric stenosis manifests all of the following except:

    A. hypochloremia
    B. hypokalemia
    C. dehydration
    D. acidosis

175. Infants are at increased risk for retinopathy of prematurity up to:

    A. 36 weeks
    B. 44 weeks
    C. 48 weeks
    D. 50 weeks

176. A half-empty "E" N20 cylinder has a psi of:

    A. 750
    B. 500
    C. 1100
    D. 325

177. Cardiac output is altered in infants by:

  A. systemic vasoconstriction
  B. increasing stroke volume
  C. increasing heart rate
  D. right-to-left shunt

178. All of the following are true of the pediatric pulmonary system except:

  A. smaller airways
  B. increased airway resistance
  C. higher closing volumes
  D. larger alveoli

179. All of the following are secreted by the adrenal medulla except:

  A. cortisol
  B. dopamine
  C. epinephrine
  D. norepinephrine

180. Catecholamines are found in:

  A. organs of Zuckerkandl
  B. chromaffin cells
  C. preganglionic fibers of the sympathetic nervous system
  D. adrenal cortex

181. The most common symptom associated with pheochromocytoma is:

  A. palpitations
  B. excessive sweating
  C. elevated basal metabolic rate
  D. hypertension

182. Select the true statement regarding muscle relaxation in patients with myasthenia gravis:

  A. Resistance to succinylcholine is common.
  B. Patients have an increased number of acetylcholine receptors postjunctionally.
  C. Nondepolarizing muscle relaxants should not be used.
  D. Recovery from succinylcholine is shortened.

183. A diastolic murmur is characteristic of:

  A. floppy valve syndrome
  B. aortic stenosis
  C. aortic insufficiency
  D. mitral stenosis

184. All of the following produce systolic murmurs except:

  A. aortic insufficiency
  B. mitral insufficiency
  C. aortic stenosis
  D. mitral stenosis

185. The main blood supply to the lumbar area of the spinal cord is by means of the:

  A. posterior radicular artery
  B. artery of Adamkiewicz
  C. epidural veins
  D. neuromedullary arteries

186. Normal cerebral blood flow is:

  A. 30 mL/100 g/min
  B. 40 mL/100 g/min
  C. 70 mL/100 g/min
  D. 50 mL/100 g/min

187. Blood flow that is in excess of metabolic need is:

  A. luxury perfusion
  B. intracerebral steal
  C. inverse steal
  D. reverse perfusion

188. What kind of electrocautery practice or use is safest for patients who have pacemakers?

  A. electrocautery be used in short bursts no more frequent than every 10 seconds
  B. electrocautery current be as low as possible
  C. electrocautery ground plate be placed as far as possible from the pulse generator
  D. all of the above

189. The vapor pressure of a liquid is most dependent on the:

A. atmospheric pressure
B. specific heat of the container
C. temperature
D. conductivity of the container

190. Identify four characteristics of the circle system:

    A. conservation of gases, heat, and moisture and minimal operating room pollution, and control of anesthetic depth
    B. conservation of gases, heat, and moisture and minimal exhaustion of CO_2 absorber
    C. maximum humidification efficiency of gas usage, minimal operating room pollution, and economy
    D. all of the above

191. Where does the fresh gas flow enter the breathing circuit in the circle system?

    A. between the absorber and inspiratory valve
    B. between the absorber and expiratory valve
    C. between the reservoir bag and absorber
    D. between the reservoir bag and inspiratory valve

192. What two blood products increase factor VIII?

    A. Fresh frozen plasma and platelets
    B. cryoprecipitate and fresh frozen plasma
    C. packed red blood cells and platelets
    D. packed red blood cells and fresh frozen plasma

193. What cellular structure is responsible for metabolizing anesthetic gases?

    A. reductive metabolism
    B. hepatic microsomes
    C. oxidative metabolism
    D. alveolar diffusion

194. Anesthetic partial pressure in the brain depends on:

    A. solubility of the agent
    B. minimal alveolar concentration of the agent
    C. second gas effect
    D. anesthetic partial pressure in the alveoli

195. What nerve is a part of the afferent pathway in the oculocardiac reflex?

    A. trigeminal
    B. vagus
    C. gasserian
    D. trochlear

196. The apneustic center is located in the

    A. hypothalamus
    B. pons
    C. medulla
    D. spinal cord

197. Dorsal root nerves are:

    A. cholinergic
    B. adrenergic
    C. motor
    D. sensory

198. Approximately 90% of the blood supply to the brain is supplied by the:

    A. external carotid artery
    B. internal carotid artery
    C. vertebral artery
    D. middle cerebral artery

199. The adrenal medulla secretes approximately _____ % epinephrine and _____ % norepinephrine.

    A. 40; 60
    B. 80; 20
    C. 60; 40
    D. 20; 80

200. The relationship between ventricular contraction strength and myocardial muscle fiber length is known as:

    A. Henry's law
    B. law of Laplace
    C. law of synergistic function
    D. Frank-Starling law

201. Phrenic nerve innervation to the diaphragm comes from:

    A. lumbar spinal cord
    B. medulla
    C. cervical spinal cord
    D. pons

202. Aortic stenosis is recognized by its characteristic:

A. diastolic murmur at the second right intercostal interspace
B. systolic murmur at the second right intercostal interspace
C. diastolic murmur at the left fourth intercostal interspace
D. diastolic murmur at the left fourth intercostal interspace

203. Addison's disease and aldosterone deficiency results in:

A. renal Na^+ loss and acidosis
B. renal Cl^- loss and alkalosis
C. renal H^+ loss and acidosis
D. renal K^+ loss and alkalosis

204. Acetylcholine is a neurotransmitter for all the following except:

A. preganglionic sympathetic neurons
B. preganglionic parasympathetic neurons
C. postganglionic sympathetic receptors on the heart
D. postganglionic parasympathetic receptors on the heart

205. The rate-limiting step in the biosynthesis of endogenous catecholamines is:

A. metabolism of tyrosine to dopa
B. metabolism of dopa to dopamine
C. metabolism of phenylalanine to tyrosine
D. metabolism of norepinephrine to epinephrine

206. The adrenal cortex secretes hormones of which chemical class?

A. peptide
B. glycoprotein
C. amine
D. steroid

207. The patient with myxedema would likely exhibit which of the following signs or symptoms?

A. heat intolerance
B. hypocholesterolemia
C. hyperactivity
D. slowed mentation and puffy face

208. The structural unit of the thyroid gland is the:

A. chief cell
B. follicle
C. colloid
D. parafollicular cell

209. The structural layer of the arteries that allows dilation and constriction is:

A. tunica intima
B. tunica media
C. tunica adventitia
D. vasa vasorum

210. Which two veins form the portal vein?

A. hepatic and splenic
B. pancreatic and superior mesenteric
C. superior and inferior mesenteric
D. superior mesenteric and splenic

211. The first branches of the ascending aorta are:

A. innominate arteries
B. carotid arteries
C. vertebral arteries
D. coronary arteries

212. What is responsible for the majority of venous drainage of the myocardium?

A. anterior cardiac veins
B. thebesian veins
C. coronary sinus
D. posterior cardiac vein

213. When does maximal left coronary artery filling occur?

A. early systole
B. early diastole
C. late systole
D. late diastole

214. Which area of the myocardium is most susceptible to ischemic injury during episodes of reduced oxygen supply?

A. subendocardium
B. inferior endocardium
C. anterior wall tissue
D. posterior endocardium

215. Cyanosis is a regular feature of:

A. coarctation of the aorta
B. patent ductus arteriosus
C. tetralogy of Fallot
D. simple interventricular septal defect

216. The relative humidity in the operating room providing enough conductivity in open surfaces to carry away static changes is:

A. 50–60%
B. 60–70%
C. 70–80%
D. 80–90%

217. A line isolation monitor (LIM) is a device that continuously monitors:

A. macro shock potentials
B. circuit breaker in the operating room
C. integrity of isolated power systems
D. contact and grounding of patients

218. Increased need for intraoperative narcotics to maintain anesthesia depth in patients taking phenobarbital may be an example of:

A. zero order kinetics
B. enzyme inhibition
C. enzyme induction
D. mercapturic acid synthesis

219. The maximum amount of air that can be inhaled from the resting end-expiratory level is:

A. tidal volume
B. vital capacity
C. inspiratory capacity
D. inspiratory reserve volume

220. Stimulation of _____ receptors inhibits further norepinephrine release from presynaptic storage sites.

A. alpha$_1$
B. beta$_1$
C. alpha$_2$
D. beta$_2$

221. An anesthetic agent with low blood/gas partition coefficient would result in:

A. slow induction, rapid emergence
B. slow induction, slow emergence
C. rapid induction, slow emergence
D. rapid induction, rapid emergence

222. Which is not a sign or symptom of atropine poisoning?

A. cutaneous flush
B. mydriasis
C. hyperpyrexia
D. sedation

223. The boiling point of a liquid is defined as the temperature at which the vapor pressure of the liquid equals:

A. atmospheric pressure
B. its critical temperature
C. its critical pressure
D. its specific heat

224. Under normal conditions, 70% to 85% of the circulating blood volume lies within the:

A. arteries
B. arterioles
C. capillaries
D. veins

225. Blood is supplied to the anterior portion of the left ventricle by the:

A. circumflex artery
B. right coronary artery
C. left coronary artery
D. anterior descending artery

226. The ratio between blood concentration and concentration in the gaseous phase of an agent is:

A. diffusion ratio
B. partition coefficient
C. Avogadro's constant
D. exchange ratio

1. ANSWER: **C**

   Rationale: Compensatory mechanisms will prevent symptoms from occurring as long as the anemia is slowly developing and chronic until the hemoglobin value falls to approximately 7 g/dL or below.
   Reference: Gerbasi, F.R. (1997). Chapter 41: Hematology and Anesthesia. In J. Nagelhout & K. Zaglaniczny (Eds.), *Nurse Anesthesia.* Philadelphia: W.B. Saunders.

2. ANSWER: **D**

   Rationale: Low concentrations of oxygen precipitate hemoglobin into elongated crystals, which results in the sickle cell crisis.
   Reference: Gerbasi, F.R. (1997). Chapter 41: Hematology and Anesthesia. In J. Nagelhout & K. Zaglaniczny (Eds.), *Nurse Anesthesia.* Philadelphia: W.B. Saunders.

3. ANSWER: **A**

   Rationale: Hemoglobin S is caused by an abnormal composition of the beta chains, which in a person with sickle cell disease frequently exceeds 70%.
   Reference: Gerbasi, F.R. (1997). Chapter 41: Hematology and Anesthesia. In J. Nagelhout & K. Zaglaniczny (Eds.), *Nurse Anesthesia.* Philadelphia: W.B. Saunders.

4. ANSWER: **B**

   Rationale: About 1100 mL of blood flows from the portal vein into the liver sinusoids each minute in addition to 350 mL that flows into the sinusoids from the hepatic artery. This is approximately 29% of the cardiac output.
   Reference: Palmer, T.J. (1997). Chapter 10: Hepatobiliary and Gastrointestinal Disturbances. In J. Nagelhout & K. Zaglaniczny (Eds.), *Nurse Anesthesia.* Philadelphia: W.B. Saunders.

5. ANSWER: **C**

   Rationale: The hepatic artery brings blood to the liver from the celiac artery and accounts for approximately 25% of total hepatic blood flow but 45% to 50% of the oxygen supply. The other main vessel supplying blood to the liver is the hepatic vein.
   Reference: Palmer T.J. (1997). Chapter 10: Hepatobiliary and Gastrointestinal Disturbances. In J. Nagelhout & K. Zaglaniczny (Eds.), *Nurse Anesthesia.* Philadelphia: W.B. Saunders.

6. ANSWER: **B**

   Rationale: Twenty-five to 29 percent of the cardiac output flows to the liver per minute through the portal vein and sinusoids of the hepatic artery.
   Reference: Palmer T.J. (1997). Chapter 10: Hepatobiliary and Gastrointestinal Disturbances. In J. Nagelhout & K. Zaglaniczny (Eds.), *Nurse Anesthesia.* Philadelphia: W.B. Saunders.

7. ANSWER: **D**

   Rationale: Hydrolysis generally occurs outside the liver in plasma, tissues, and red blood cells.
   Reference: Troop, M. (1997). Chapter 16: Pharmacokinetics. In J. Nagelhout & K. Zaglaniczny (Eds.), *Nurse Anesthesia.* Philadelphia: W.B. Saunders.

8. ANSWER: **D**

   Rationale: Blood/gas partition coefficient is an indication of the uptake of anesthetic into the lungs and thus into the brain; therefore, it is a measure of the speed of onset of an anesthetic.
   Reference: Nagelhout, J.J. (1997). Chapter 17: Uptake and Distribution of Inhalation Anesthetics. In J. Nagelhout & K. Zaglaniczny (Eds.), *Nurse Anesthesia.* Philadelphia: W.B. Saunders.

9. ANSWER: **B**

   Rationale: Halothane synthesizes the myocardium to sympathomimetic medications; therefore, catecholamines and catecholamine-like drugs should be used with extreme caution.

Reference: Kossick, M.A. (1997). Chapter 18: Inhalation Anesthetics. In J. Nagelhout & K. Zaglaniczny (Eds.), *Nurse Anesthesia.* Philadelphia: W.B. Saunders.

10. ANSWER: **D**

Rationale: The addition of halogens chlorine, fluorine, bromine, or iodine drug molecules results in a decrease in flammability owing to an increased stability of the molecule.

Reference: Hall, S.M. (1997). Chapter 4: Chemistry and Physics for Anesthesia. In J. Nagelhout & K. Zaglaniczny (Eds.), *Nurse Anesthesia.* Philadelphia: W.B. Saunders.

11. ANSWER: **A**

Rationale: With improper intercostal muscle strength the chest is unable to expand during inspiration, resulting in chest retraction in abdominal breathing. This combination of strained abdominal expansion and intercostal paralysis mimics a boat rocking in water.

Reference: Rojo, J. & Iacopelli, M. (1997). Chapter 39A: Respiratory Pathophysiology. In J. Nagelhout & K. Zaglaniczny (Eds.), *Nurse Anesthesia.* Philadelphia: W.B. Saunders.

12. ANSWER: **B**

Rationale: Prolonged or chronic exposure to high concentrations of nitrous oxide may result in an inhibition of methionine synthetase sometimes referred to as "bone marrow suppression." This phenomenon usually occurs with prolonged exposure in debilitated patients and is not a consideration with routine use in healthy patients.

Reference: Kossick, M.A. (1997). Chapter 18: Inhalation Anesthetics. In J. Nagelhout & K. Zaglaniczny (Eds.), *Nurse Anesthesia.* Philadelphia: W.B. Saunders.

13. ANSWER: **C**

Rationale: The posterior pituitary gland secretes antidiuretic hormone and oxytocin. Lack of ADH results in diabetes insipidus.

Reference: Karlet, M.C. & Sebastian, L.A. (1997). Chapter 12: The Endocrine System. In J.

Nagelhout & K. Zaglaniczny (Eds.), *Nurse Anesthesia.* Philadelphia: W.B. Saunders.

14. ANSWER: **B**

Rationale: Oliguria is usually defined in the acutely stressed patient as a urine output of less than 0.5 mL/h, which averages to about 35 mL/h. This is higher in stressed patients than in nonstressed patients. Nonstressed patients are usually defined as having a urine output of less than 17 mL/kg per hour.

Reference: Ouelette S.M. (1997). Chapter 11: Renal Anatomy, Physiology, and Pathophysiology, and Anesthesia. In J. Nagelhout & K. Zaglaniczny (Eds.), *Nurse Anesthesia.* Philadelphia: W.B. Saunders.

15. ANSWER: **A**

Rationale: The anterior pituitary hormones are influenced by releasing factors and the amount of each hormone at the target organ. This is referred to as a negative feedback control system.

Reference: Karlet, M.C. & Sebastian, L.A. (1997). Chapter 12: The Endocrine System. In J. Nagelhout & K. Zaglaniczny (Eds.), *Nurse Anesthesia.* Philadelphia: W.B. Saunders.

16. ANSWER: **C**

Rationale: The posterior pituitary gland secretes antidiuretic hormone, also referred to as vasopressin. The other hormone is oxytocin, which is involved in uterine contraction during childbirth.

Reference: Karlet, M.C. & Sebastian, L.A. (1997). Chapter 12: The Endocrine System. In J. Nagelhout & K. Zaglaniczny (Eds.), *Nurse Anesthesia.* Philadelphia: W.B. Saunders.

17. ANSWER: **D**

Rationale: Dantrolene should be mixed with distilled water based on heart rate, body temperature, and $PaCO_2$. Therapeutic levels of dantrolene usually persist for 4 to 6 hours after this IV dose.

Reference: Karlet, M.C. (1997). Chapter 40: Musculoskeletal Pathophysiology and Anesthesia. In J. Nagelhout & K. Zaglaniczny (Eds.), *Nurse Anesthesia.* Philadelphia: W.B. Saunders.

18. ANSWER: **B**

Rationale: An increase in end-tidal carbon dioxide may be masked by hyperventilation; therefore, tachycardia is frequently the earliest sign exhibited by a patient developing this disorder. Tachypnea is also frequently masked by controlled ventilation and anesthetic drugs.

Reference: Karlet, M.C. (1997). Chapter 40: Musculoskeletal Pathophysiology and Anesthesia. In J. Nagelhout & K. Zaglaniczny (Eds.), *Nurse Anesthesia.* Philadelphia: W.B. Saunders.

19. ANSWER: **C**

Rationale: An increase in carbon dioxide resulting from hypermetabolism is often the most sensitive sign; however, it may be masked by controlled ventilation, leaving the cardiovascular symptoms the first to be noted.

Reference: Karlet, M.C. (1997). Chapter 40: Musculoskeletal Pathophysiology and Anesthesia. In J. Nagelhout & K. Zaglaniczny (Eds.), *Nurse Anesthesia.* Philadelphia: W.B. Saunders.

20. ANSWER: **B**

Rationale: Although the number of reported cases have increased, the mortality rate has decreased, reflecting a greater awareness, early diagnoses, and better treatment.

Reference: Karlet, M.C. (1997). Chapter 40: Musculoskeletal Pathophysiology and Anesthesia. In J. Nagelhout & K. Zaglaniczny (Eds.), *Nurse Anesthesia.* Philadelphia: W.B. Saunders.

21. ANSWER: **C**

Rationale: Neuroleptic malignant syndrome is caused by the use of psychoactive drugs. Dopamine antagonist and serotonin agonist and antagonist can produce this syndrome. It usually does not result in rigidity; however, the other signs may be similar to those of malignant hyperthermia.

Reference: Karlet, M.C. (1997). Chapter 40: Musculoskeletal Pathophysiology and Anesthesia. In J. Nagelhout & K. Zaglaniczny (Eds.), *Nurse Anesthesia.* Philadelphia: W.B. Saunders.

22. ANSWER: **C**

Rationale: A patient with a major systemic disorder such as heart failure or renal failure represents a high risk for general anesthesia.

Reference: Kachnij, J.M. (1997). Chapter 28: Preoperative Evaluation and Preparation of the Patient. In J. Nagelhout & K. Zaglaniczny (Eds.), *Nurse Anesthesia.* Philadelphia: W.B. Saunders.

23. ANSWER: **A**

Rationale: A patient with a chronic systemic mild disease, generally well controlled, represents only a slightly increased risk for general anesthesia.

Reference: Kachnij, J.M. (1997). Chapter 28: Preoperative Evaluation and Preparation of the Patient. In J. Nagelhout & K. Zaglaniczny (Eds.), *Nurse Anesthesia.* Philadelphia: W.B. Saunders.

24. ANSWER: **A**

Rationale: Cyclosporine selectively depresses the activity of helper T cells and CD4 lymphocytes by inhibiting production of interleukin-2, and other cytokines.

Reference: Scarsell, J. (1997). Chapter 54A: Anesthesia for Heart Transplantation. In J. Nagelhout & K. Zaglaniczny (Eds.), *Nurse Anesthesia.* Philadelphia: W.B. Saunders.

25. ANSWER: **A**

Rationale: The lateral head-down position is commonly referred to as the "tonsil position"; this helps prevents aspiration of blood and secretions on the vocal cord that result in laryngospasm.

Reference: Hill, F.C., Jr. & Kopecky, J.F. (1997). Chapter 47: Anesthesia for Ear, Nose, Throat, and Maxillofacial Surgery. In J. Nagelhout & K. Zaglaniczny (Eds.), *Nurse Anesthesia.* Philadelphia: W.B. Saunders.

26. ANSWER: **C**

Rationale: Gradually lowering the legs from the lithotomy position prevents stress on the lumbar spine as well as allowing gradual accommodation to the change in venous return, thereby avoiding hypotension.

Reference: Monti, E.J. (1997). Chapter 32: Positioning for Anesthesia and Surgery. In J. Nagelhout & K. Zaglaniczny (Eds.), *Nurse Anesthesia.* Philadelphia: W.B. Saunders.

27. ANSWER: **C**

Rationale: Ephedrine has multiple mechanisms of action, including alpha and beta receptor stimulation, indirect catechol-amine release, as well as central stimulant activity.

Reference: Alisoglu, R. (1997). Chapter 23: Cardiac Pharmacology. In J. Nagelhout & K. Zaglaniczny (Eds.), *Nurse Anesthesia.* Philadelphia: W.B. Saunders.

28. ANSWER: **B**

Rationale: Acids tend to be ionized or to become charged in a very basic pH. An acid plus a base will yield a salt plus water.

Reference: Troop, M. (1997). Chapter 16: Pharmacokinetics. In J. Nagelhout & K. Zaglaniczny (Eds.), *Nurse Anesthesia.* Philadelphia: W.B. Saunders.

29. ANSWER: **C**

Rationale: Acetylcholine is synthesized from choline and acetic acid. The enzyme responsible for synthesis is choline acetyltransferase.

Reference: Haas, R.E. & Erway, R.L. (1997). Chapter 22: Neuromuscular Blocking Agents, Reversal Agents, and Their Monitoring. In J. Nagelhout & K. Zaglaniczny (Eds.), *Nurse Anesthesia.* Philadelphia: W.B. Saunders.

30. ANSWER: **C**

Rationale: The cholinergic sites in the sympathetic and parasympathetic systems include both ganglia of the sympathetic and parasympathetic nervous system. The postganglionic effector sites of the parasympathetic nervous system include muscarinic receptors and the neuromuscular junction. The sympathetic end organs secrete norepinephrine.

Reference: Alisoglu, R. (1997). Chapter 23: Cardiac Pharmacology. In J. Nagelhout & K. Zaglaniczny (Eds.), *Nurse Anesthesia.* Philadelphia: W.B. Saunders.

31. ANSWER: **D**

Rationale: Cyanosis will occur when oxygen saturation falls below 80%, which results from a PO_2 of less than 53. At this point more than 5 g of hemoglobin will be reduced.

Reference: Gerbasi, F.R. (1997). Chapter 41: Hematology and Anesthesia. In J. Nagelhout & K. Zaglaniczny (Eds.), *Nurse Anesthesia.* Philadelphia: W.B. Saunders.

32. ANSWER: **C**

Rationale: Alcoholism is the most frequent cause of pancreatitis; therefore, patients should be evaluated for malnutrition, abnormal liver function, and signs of alcohol withdrawal.

Reference: Palmer, T.J. (1997). Chapter 10: Hepatobiliary and Gastrointestinal Disturbances. In J. Nagelhout & K. Zaglaniczny (Eds.), *Nurse Anesthesia.* Philadelphia: W.B. Saunders.

33. ANSWER: **B**

Rationale: The blood of a normal person contains approximately 15 g of hemoglobin in each 100 mL of blood, and each gram is combined with a maximum of 1.34 mL of oxygen.

Reference: Gerbasi, F.R. (1997). Chapter 41: Hematology and Anesthesia. In J. Nagelhout & K. Zaglaniczny (Eds.), *Nurse Anesthesia.* Philadelphia: W.B. Saunders.

34. ANSWER: **C**

Rationale: Factor VIII is missing in a person who has classic hemophilia, for which reason it is called the antihemophilic factor or antihemophilic factor A.

Reference: Gerbasi, F.R. (1997). Chapter 41: Hematology and Anesthesia. In J. Nagelhout & K. Zaglaniczny (Eds.), *Nurse Anesthesia.* Philadelphia: W.B. Saunders.

35. ANSWER: **B**

Rationale: The three major plasma proteins are albumin, globulin, and fibrinogen. Albumin provides the colloid osmotic pressure in the plasma. It binds drugs because of its ability to accept both positive and negative charges of a variety of chemical types.

Reference: Troop, M. (1997). Chapter 16: Pharmacokinetics. In J. Nagelhout & K. Zaglaniczny (Eds.), *Nurse Anesthesia.* Philadelphia: W.B. Saunders.

36. ANSWER: **B**

Rationale: PCO_2 of 40 mm Hg is approximately 5% of the 760 mm Hg total at 1 atmosphere.

Reference: Hall, S.M. (1997). Chapter 9: Respiratory Anatomy and Physiology. In J. Nagelhout & K. Zaglaniczny (Eds.), *Nurse Anesthesia.* Philadelphia: W.B. Saunders.

37. ANSWER: **A**

Rationale: Vitamin B_{12} deficiency leads to abnormal formation of red blood cells. They grow large, are odd shaped, and are called megaloblastic.
Reference: Gerbasi, F.R. (1997). Chapter 41: Hematology and Anesthesia. In J. Nagelhout & K. Zaglaniczny (Eds.), *Nurse Anesthesia*. Philadelphia: W.B. Saunders.

38. ANSWER: **C**

Rationale: The superior laryngeal nerve provides sensory supply to the larynx between the epiglottis and vocal cord. The cricothyroid muscle is supplied by the external laryngeal nerve and adducts the vocal cords.
Reference: Chipas, A. (1997). Chapter 33: Airway Management. In J. Nagelhout & K. Zaglaniczny (Eds.), *Nurse Anesthesia*. Philadelphia: W.B. Saunders.

39. ANSWER: **B**

Rationale: The cricothyroid muscle is responsible for closing the vocal cords in response to sensory stimulation from the superior laryngeal nerve.
Reference: Chipas, A. (1997). Chapter 33: Airway Management. In J. Nagelhout & K. Zaglaniczny (Eds.), *Nurse Anesthesia*. Philadelphia: W.B. Saunders.

40. ANSWER: **A**

Rationale: The neural output from the carotid body reaches the respiratory center by way of the afferent glossopharyngeal nerve. Output from the aortic bodies travels to the medulla via the vagus nerve.
Reference: Morgan, R.O., Jr. (1997). Chapter 8: The Cardiovascular System. In J. Nagelhout & K. Zaglaniczny (Eds.), *Nurse Anesthesia*. Philadelphia: W.B. Saunders.

41. ANSWER: **B**

Rationale: Aldosterone is the major regulator of extracellular volume and potassium hemostasis through the rate of absorption of sodium and secretion of potassium in the tissues.
Reference: Karlet, M.C. & Sebastian, L.A. (1997). Chapter 12: The Endocrine System. In J.

Nagelhout & K. Zaglaniczny (Eds.), *Nurse Anesthesia*. Philadelphia: W.B. Saunders.

42. ANSWER: **D**

Rationale: Eighty to 90 percent of all erythropoietin is produced in the kidneys; the remainder is produced in the liver. An anephric or renal failure patient lacks sufficient quantity to stimulate red blood cells, which results in anemia.
Reference: Ouelette S.M. (1997). Chapter 11: Renal Anatomy, Physiology, and Pathophysiology, and Anesthesia. In J. Nagelhout & K. Zaglaniczny (Eds.), *Nurse Anesthesia*. Philadelphia: W.B. Saunders.

43. ANSWER: **D**

Rationale: Fluorine is one of the most reactive halogens. It produces exceptionally stable bonds that resist separation by chemical or thermal means.
Reference: Hall, S.M. (1997). Chapter 4: Chemistry and Physics for Anesthesia. In J. Nagelhout & K. Zaglaniczny (Eds.), *Nurse Anesthesia*. Philadelphia: W.B. Saunders.

44. ANSWER: **A**

Rationale: Acetylcholine has four carbons attached to the nitrogen molecule, making it a quaternary compound.
Reference: Haas, R.E. & Erway, R.L. (1997). Chapter 22: Neuromuscular Blocking Agents, Reversal Agents, and Their Monitoring. In J. Nagelhout & K. Zaglaniczny (Eds.), *Nurse Anesthesia*. Philadelphia: W.B. Saunders.

45. ANSWER: **B**

Rationale: Like acetylcholine, muscle relaxants contain at least one and most commonly two quaternary ammonium molecules within their structure. This promotes binding to the cholinergic receptor.
Reference: Haas, R.E. & Erway, R.L. (1997). Chapter 22: Neuromuscular Blocking Agents, Reversal Agents, and Their Monitoring. In J. Nagelhout & K. Zaglaniczny (Eds.), *Nurse Anesthesia*. Philadelphia: W.B. Saunders.

46. ANSWER: **B**

Rationale: All beta-blocking drugs produce vasoconstriction except for labetalol, which also possesses alpha-receptor blocking properties, producing vasodilation.

Reference: Alisoglu, R. (1997). Chapter 23: Cardiac Pharmacology. In J. Nagelhout & K. Zaglaniczny (Eds.), *Nurse Anesthesia*. Philadelphia: W.B. Saunders.

47. ANSWER: **B**

Rationale: Dantrolene produces skeletal muscle relaxation by a direct action on excitation-contraction coupling by decreasing the release of calcium from the sarcoplasmic reticulum.

Reference: Karlet, M.C. (1997). Chapter 40: Musculoskeletal Pathophysiology and Anesthesia. In J. Nagelhout & K. Zaglaniczny (Eds.), *Nurse Anesthesia*. Philadelphia: W.B. Saunders.

48. ANSWER: **C**

Rationale: An increase in magnesium in skeletal muscle leads to relaxation. Addition of a nondepolarizing muscle relaxant may yield prolonged paralysis; reduced doses of muscle relaxants are indicated.

Reference: Fiedler, M.A. & Shaw, B. (1997). Chapter 13: Obstetric Anesthesia. In J. Nagelhout & K. Zaglaniczny (Eds.), *Nurse Anesthesia*. Philadelphia: W.B. Saunders.

49. ANSWER: **D**

Rationale: Cimetadine inhibits oxidative drug metabolism by forming a tight complex with heme iron of cytochrome P450.

Reference: Troop, M. (1997). Chapter 16: Pharmacokinetics. In J. Nagelhout & K. Zaglaniczny (Eds.), *Nurse Anesthesia*. Philadelphia: W.B. Saunders.

50. ANSWER: **C**

Rationale: Basic compounds will tend to donate charges in an acid environment and visa versa. Therefore, they will be most ionized at a low pH.

Reference: Troop, M. (1997). Chapter 16: Pharmacokinetics. In J. Nagelhout & K. Zaglaniczny (Eds.), *Nurse Anesthesia*. Philadelphia: W.B. Saunders.

51. ANSWER: **C**

Rationale: Clonidine, an antihypertensive, has severe withdrawal reactions when stopped abruptly. Patients should continue to take clonidine throughout the perioperative period.

Reference: Alisoglu, R. (1997). Chapter 23: Cardiac Pharmacology. In J. Nagelhout & K. Zaglaniczny (Eds.), *Nurse Anesthesia*. Philadelphia: W.B. Saunders.

52. ANSWER: **C**

Rationale: A severe drug interaction may occur from a metabolite of meperidine when meperidine is given to a patient receiving monoamine oxidase inhibitors. The reaction may also involve serotonin and commonly results in hyperthermia, hypertension, respiratory depression, skeletal muscle rigidity, seizures, and coma.

Reference: Chick, M. (1997). Chapter 21: Opioid Agonists and Antagonists. In J. Nagelhout & K. Zaglaniczny (Eds.), *Nurse Anesthesia*. Philadelphia: W.B. Saunders.

53. ANSWER: **B**

Rationale: Hypernatremia is one of the most common symptoms of diabetes insipidus. It results from excretion of high amounts of dilute urine, allowing sodium levels to rise as the patient's osmolarity increases.

Reference: Karlet, M.C. & Sebastian, L.A. (1997). Chapter 12: The Endocrine System. In J. Nagelhout & K. Zaglaniczny (Eds.), *Nurse Anesthesia*. Philadelphia: W.B. Saunders.

54. ANSWER: **C**

Rationale: Cocaine has the unique ability of local anesthetics to block the reuptake of norepinephrine. This leads to vasoconstriction along with the topical anesthetic effect.

Reference: Williams, J.R. (1997). Chapter 20: Local Anesthetics. In J. Nagelhout & K. Zaglaniczny (Eds.), *Nurse Anesthesia*. Philadelphia: W.B. Saunders.

55. ANSWER: **B**

Rationale: Epinephrine should not be given during intravenous regional anesthesia because of the vascular systemic effects that may be produced both locally in the arm by vasoconstriction and systemically when the cuff is released.

Reference: Williams, J.R. (1997). Chapter 20: Local Anesthetics. In J. Nagelhout & K. Zaglaniczny (Eds.), *Nurse Anesthesia*. Philadelphia: W.B. Saunders.

56. ANSWER: **B**

Rationale: Cyclic adenosine monophosphate opens calcium channels, causing synaptic vesicles to fuse with the nerve membrane and release acetylcholine.

Reference: Karlet, M.C. (1997). Chapter 40: Musculoskeletal Pathophysiology and Anesthesia. In J. Nagelhout & K. Zaglaniczny (Eds.), *Nurse Anesthesia*. Philadelphia: W.B. Saunders.

57. ANSWER: **B**

Rationale: The average blood volume is the highest in premature neonates and decreases through infancy and adulthood.

Reference: Dobbins, P. & Hall, S.M. (1997). Chapter 14: Pediatric Anesthesia. In J. Nagelhout & K. Zaglaniczny (Eds.), *Nurse Anesthesia*. Philadelphia: W.B. Saunders.

58. ANSWER: **C**

Rationale: See question 57.

Reference: Dobbins, P. & Hall, S.M. (1997). Chapter 14: Pediatric Anesthesia. In J. Nagelhout & K. Zaglaniczny (Eds.), *Nurse Anesthesia*. Philadelphia: W.B. Saunders.

59. ANSWER: **D**

Rationale: See question 57.

Reference: Dobbins, P. & Hall, S.M. (1997). Chapter 14: Pediatric Anesthesia. In J. Nagelhout & K. Zaglaniczny (Eds.), *Nurse Anesthesia*. Philadelphia: W.B. Saunders.

60. ANSWER: **C**

Rationale: See question 57.

Reference: Dobbins, P. & Hall, S.M. (1997). Chapter 14: Pediatric Anesthesia. In J. Nagelhout & K. Zaglaniczny (Eds.), *Nurse Anesthesia*. Philadelphia: W.B. Saunders.

61. ANSWER: **C**

Rationale: Carcinoid syndrome is a complex of signs and symptoms caused by the secretion of vasoactive substances serotonin, kallikrein, and histamine from enterochromaffin tumors. Most of these tumors are located in the gastrointestinal tract, but they may be present elsewhere and cause a variety of clinical manifestations.

Reference: Palmer, T.J. (1997). Chapter 10: Hepatobiliary and Gastrointestinal Disturbances. In J. Nagelhout & K. Zaglaniczny (Eds.), *Nurse Anesthesia*. Philadelphia: W.B. Saunders.

62. ANSWER: **D**

Rationale: Depending on dose, the effects of morphine can last up to 24 hours when given by this route. The effects of the other three drugs generally last a maximum of 6 to 8 hours.

Reference: Chick, M. (1997). Chapter 21: Opioid Agonists and Antagonists. In J. Nagelhout & K. Zaglaniczny (Eds.), *Nurse Anesthesia*. Philadelphia: W.B. Saunders.

63. ANSWER: **B**

Rationale: Multiple endocrine neoplasia is a group of syndromes characterized by tumor formation throughout the endocrine system. Hypertension can result that is similar to that found in pheochromocytoma. The patients are typically young adults with a family history of this disorder.

Reference: Karlet, M.C. & Sebastian, L.A. (1997). Chapter 12: The Endocrine System. In J. Nagelhout & K. Zaglaniczny (Eds.), *Nurse Anesthesia*. Philadelphia: W.B. Saunders.

64. ANSWER: **C**

Rationale: Carpal tunnel syndrome results from strain on the median nerve affecting the palmar surface of the first three digits.

Reference: Monti, E.J. (1997). Chapter 32: Positioning for Anesthesia and Surgery. In J. Nagelhout & K. Zaglaniczny (Eds.), *Nurse Anesthesia*. Philadelphia: W.B. Saunders.

65. ANSWER: **B**

Rationale: Functionally, sickle cell hemoglobin has a lower affinity for oxygen than normal hemoglobin ($P_{50} = 31$ mm Hg) as well as a decreased solubility; on deoxygenation the sickle cell polymerizes and precipitates inside the red blood cell, causing sickling.

Reference: Gerbasi, F.R. (1997). Chapter 41:
Hematology and Anesthesia. In J. Nagelhout &
K. Zaglaniczny (Eds.), *Nurse Anesthesia.*
Philadelphia: W.B. Saunders.

66. ANSWER: D

Rationale: Red cell survival is reduced to 10 to 15 days, compared with normal red blood cells, owing to the more fragile state of sickle hemoglobin.
Reference: Gerbasi, F.R. (1997). Chapter 41:
Hematology and Anesthesia. In J. Nagelhout &
K. Zaglaniczny (Eds.), *Nurse Anesthesia.*
Philadelphia: W.B. Saunders.

67. ANSWER: D

Rationale: An excess of corticosteroids produces Cushing's syndrome, which is characterized by muscle wasting and weakness, osteoporosis, obesity, glucose intolerance, hypertension, and mental status changes.
Reference: Karlet, M.C. & Sebastian, L.A. (1997).
Chapter 12: The Endocrine System. In J.
Nagelhout & K. Zaglaniczny (Eds.), *Nurse
Anesthesia.* Philadelphia: W.B. Saunders.

68. ANSWER: B

Rationale: Primary aldosteronism is also referred to as Conn's syndrome. Clinical manifestations include hypertension, hypervolemia, hyperkalemia, muscle weakness, and metabolic acidosis.
Reference: Karlet, M.C. & Sebastian, L.A. (1997).
Chapter 12: The Endocrine System. In J.
Nagelhout & K. Zaglaniczny (Eds.), *Nurse
Anesthesia.* Philadelphia: W.B. Saunders.

69. ANSWER: D

Rationale: Primary adrenal insufficiency is also referred to as Addison's disease. Clinical manifestations include hypotension, hypovolemia, hyperkalemia, and metabolic acidosis.
Reference: Karlet, M.C. & Sebastian, L.A. (1997).
Chapter 12: The Endocrine System. In J.
Nagelhout & K. Zaglaniczny (Eds.), *Nurse
Anesthesia.* Philadelphia: W.B. Saunders.

70. ANSWER: B

Rationale: Adrenal insufficiency is generally iatrogenic. It is a result of inade-quate ACTH secretion by the pituitary. Acute adrenal insufficiency can be precipitated by infection, trauma, and surgery.
Reference: Karlet, M.C. & Sebastian, L.A. (1997).
Chapter 12: The Endocrine System. In J.
Nagelhout & K. Zaglaniczny (Eds.), *Nurse
Anesthesia.* Philadelphia: W.B. Saunders.

71. ANSWER: D

Rationale: The clinical features of this medical emergency include all of those listed except hyperglycemia. Hypoglycemia is a common manifestation in steroid-dependent patients.
Reference: Karlet, M.C. & Sebastian, L.A. (1997).
Chapter 12: The Endocrine System. In J.
Nagelhout & K. Zaglaniczny (Eds.), *Nurse
Anesthesia.* Philadelphia: W.B. Saunders.

72. ANSWER: B

Rationale: When a base is in an acidotic environment it tends to ionize; therefore, less drug is nonionized or in a lipid-soluble form.
Reference: Troop, M. (1997). Chapter 12:
Pharmacokinetics. In J. Nagelhout & K.
Zaglaniczny (Eds.), *Nurse Anesthesia.* Philadelphia:
W.B. Saunders.

73. ANSWER: B

Rationale: The total CO_2 contents of arterial blood is made up of the sum of dissolved carbon dioxide and bicarbonate.
Reference: Hall, S.M. (1997). Chapter 9:
Respiratory Anatomy and Physiology. In J.
Nagelhout & K. Zaglaniczny (Eds.), *Nurse
Anesthesia.* Philadelphia: W.B. Saunders.

74. ANSWER: C

Rationale: At rest, certain tissues generate less CO_2 than others; for example, the heart results in high CO_2 production versus other areas. However, total production resulting from aerobic metabolism in the body approximates 200 to 250 mL of CO_2 per minute.
Reference: Hall, S.M. (1997). Chapter 9:
Respiratory Anatomy and Physiology. In J.
Nagelhout & K. Zaglaniczny (Eds.), *Nurse
Anesthesia.* Philadelphia: W.B. Saunders.

75. ANSWER: **A**

Rationale: Scoliosis is a lateral rotation and curvature of the spine and a deformity of the rib cage. It affects both cardiac and respiratory functions. Reduced lung volumes, pulmonary hypertension, decreased PO_2, and increased PCO_2 are commonly prevalent. Chest wall compliance is decreased.

Reference: Rojo, J. & Iacopelli, M. (1997). Chapter 39A: Respiratory Pathophysiology. In J. Nagelhout & K. Zaglaniczny (Eds.), *Nurse Anesthesia*. Philadelphia: W.B. Saunders.

76. ANSWER: **C**

Rationale: Central chemoreceptors are thought to lie on the anterolateral surface of the medulla and respond to changes in hydrogen ion concentrations in cerebrospinal fluid.

Reference: Hall, S.M. (1997). Chapter 9: Respiratory Anatomy and Physiology. In J. Nagelhout & K. Zaglaniczny (Eds.), *Nurse Anesthesia*. Philadelphia: W.B. Saunders.

77. ANSWER: **C**

Rationale: The carotid bodies are the principal peripheral chemoreceptors in humans and are sensitive to changes in PO_2, PCO_2, pH, and arterial perfusion. Reductions in PO_2 produce the most sensitive changes in chemoreceptors.

Reference: Hall, S.M. (1997). Chapter 9: Respiratory Anatomy and Physiology. In J. Nagelhout & K. Zaglaniczny (Eds.), *Nurse Anesthesia*. Philadelphia: W.B. Saunders.

78. ANSWER: **B**

Rationale: Nonshivering thermogenesis is an increase in metabolic heat production without an increase in mechanical muscular work. It occurs principally through metabolism of brown fat, which comprises 2% to 6% of an infant's total body weight.

Reference: Dobbins, P. & Hall, S.M. (1997). Chapter 14: Pediatric Anesthesia. In J. Nagelhout & K. Zaglaniczny (Eds.), *Nurse Anesthesia*. Philadelphia: W.B. Saunders.

79. ANSWER: **D**

Rationale: Inhalation anesthetics (except for nitrous oxide) and succinylcholine are potent triggers of malignant hyperthermia. The induction agents are not considered triggers; therefore, propofol is safely administered.

Reference: Karlet, M.C. (1997). Chapter 40: Musculoskeletal Pathophysiology and Anesthesia. In J. Nagelhout & K. Zaglaniczny (Eds.), *Nurse Anesthesia*. Philadelphia: W.B. Saunders.

80. ANSWER: **D**

Rationale: Magnesium augments nondepolarizing muscle relaxants and, to a lesser extent, succinylcholine. The mechanism for this effect is not known, but it may be related to a decrease in calcium level resulting from an increased magnesium concentration.

Reference: Haas, R.E. & Erway, R.L. (1997). Chapter 22: Neuromuscular Blocking Agents, Reversal Agents, and Their Monitoring. In J. Nagelhout & K. Zaglaniczny (Eds.), *Nurse Anesthesia*. Philadelphia: W.B. Saunders.

81. ANSWER: **A**

Rationale: The most important difference physiologically between the pediatric patient and the adult patient is oxygen consumption. Oxygen consumption of the neonate is greater than 6 mL/kg, which is twice that of a 70-kg adult.

Reference: Dobbins, P. & Hall, S.M. (1997). Chapter 14: Pediatric Anesthesia. In J. Nagelhout & K. Zaglaniczny (Eds.), *Nurse Anesthesia*. Philadelphia: W.B. Saunders.

82. ANSWER: **D**

Rationale: The decrease in renal function that is common among neonates can also delay the excretion of drugs that are dependent on the kidney for elimination. This effect usually normalizes within 6 months.

Reference: Dobbins, P. & Hall, S.M. (1997). Chapter 14: Pediatric Anesthesia. In J. Nagelhout & K. Zaglaniczny (Eds.), *Nurse Anesthesia*. Philadelphia: W.B. Saunders.

83. ANSWER: **B**

Rationale: The glomerular filtration rate is greatly decreased in term neonates but is increased nearly four-fold within 3 to 5 weeks. At term it is approximately 20 mL/min whereas within 3 to 5 weeks it has risen to approximately 60 mL/min.

Reference: Dobbins, P. & Hall, S.M. (1997). Chapter 14: Pediatric Anesthesia. In J. Nagelhout & K. Zaglaniczny (Eds.), *Nurse Anesthesia.* Philadelphia: W.B. Saunders.

84. ANSWER: **D**

Rationale: Propofol causes the most cardiac and respiratory depression of all induction drugs and should be used in reduced doses, if at all, in patients with cardiac disease and the elderly.

Reference: Fallacaro, N.A. & Fallacaro, M.D. (1997). Chapter 19: Intravenous Induction Agents. In J. Nagelhout & K. Zaglaniczny (Eds.), *Nurse Anesthesia.* Philadelphia: W.B. Saunders.

85. ANSWER: **D**

Rationale: Because of the decreased cardiac reserve of the neonate and the leftward shift in the oxygen-hemoglobin dissociation curve, it is useful to maintain the hematocrit at approximately 40% to ensure proper oxygenation.

Reference: Dobbins, P. & Hall, S.M. (1997). Chapter 14: Pediatric Anesthesia. In J. Nagelhout & K. Zaglaniczny (Eds.), *Nurse Anesthesia.* Philadelphia: W.B. Saunders.

86. ANSWER: **A**

Rationale: The function of surfactant is to stabilize alveolar membranes. Without surfactant, alveoli would collapse, leading to a right-to-left intrapulmonary shunt, hypoxia, and metabolic acidosis.

Reference: Hall, S.M. (1997). Chapter 9: Respiratory Anatomy and Physiology. In J. Nagelhout & K. Zaglaniczny (Eds.), *Nurse Anesthesia.* Philadelphia: W.B. Saunders.

87. ANSWER: **B**

Rationale: Surfactant is produced by type II pneumocytes. Before 26 weeks' gestation there are not enough type II cells to produce adequate surfactant but this is corrected by 35 weeks' gestation.

Reference: Hall, S.M. (1997). Chapter 9: Respiratory Anatomy and Physiology. In J. Nagelhout & K. Zaglaniczny (Eds.), *Nurse Anesthesia.* Philadelphia: W.B. Saunders.

88. ANSWER: **C**

Rationale: Fetal calcium stores are largely achieved through the last trimester. The preterm neonate commonly presents with hypocalcemia, which is defined as a plasma calcium concentration of less than 3.5 mEq/L.

Reference: Dobbins, P. & Hall, S.M. (1997). Chapter 14: Pediatric Anesthesia. In J. Nagelhout & K. Zaglaniczny (Eds.), *Nurse Anesthesia.* Philadelphia: W.B. Saunders.

89. ANSWER: **C**

Rationale: These guidelines have been established by the American Academy of Pediatrics and state that the administration of oxygen in premature infants should achieve 50 to 80 mm Hg. These levels are most likely to be safe with regards to retinopathy. To reduce the risk of retinopathy it is recommended that the PO_2 be maintained between 60 and 80 mm Hg. This can present a dilemma because these neonates are also prone to hypoxia. These low PO_2 levels must be tempered with the realization that hypoxia can lead to brain injury.

Reference: Dobbins, P. & Hall, S.M. (1997). Chapter 14: Pediatric Anesthesia. In J. Nagelhout & K. Zaglaniczny (Eds.), *Nurse Anesthesia.* Philadelphia: W.B. Saunders.

90. ANSWER: **B**

Rationale: Total renal blood flow decreases approximately 10% per decade in the adult years. The effect is primarily in the renal cortex with relative sparing of the renal medulla. As a result, glomerular filtration rate also decreases.

Reference: Martin-Sheridan, D. (1997). Chapter 42: Geriatrics and Anesthesia Practice. In J. Nagelhout & K. Zaglaniczny (Eds.), *Nurse Anesthesia.* Philadelphia: W.B. Saunders.

91. ANSWER: **A**

Rationale: Closing volumes and closing capacity increase with aging and approach the functional residual capacity. This and other changes associated with geriatrics account for their widening alveolar arterial gradient.

Reference: Martin-Sheridan, D. (1997). Chapter 42: Geriatrics and Anesthesia Practice. In J.

Nagelhout & K. Zaglaniczny (Eds.), *Nurse Anesthesia*. Philadelphia: W.B. Saunders.

92. ANSWER: D

Rationale: Serum creatinine concentration in the elderly remains within normal guidelines in spite of impaired glomerular filtration rate. The marked reduction in the proportion of muscle to total body mass progressively reduces creatinine load.

Reference: Martin-Sheridan, D. (1997). Chapter 42: Geriatrics and Anesthesia Practice. In J. Nagelhout & K. Zaglaniczny (Eds.), *Nurse Anesthesia*. Philadelphia: W.B. Saunders.

93. ANSWER: B

Rationale: The elderly patient is at a higher risk for hypothermia than the average adult. This is due to a decrease in the ability to retain heat. The shivering mechanism is still intact; however, temperature regulation is affected by the lack of heat production, and an increased heat loss.

Reference: Martin-Sheridan, D. (1997). Chapter 42: Geriatrics and Anesthesia Practice. In J. Nagelhout & K. Zaglaniczny (Eds.), *Nurse Anesthesia*. Philadelphia: W.B. Saunders.

94. ANSWER: A

Rationale: Thyroid storm is a medical emergency that carries a 10% to 50% mortality rate. Signs and symptoms include mental changes, arrhythmias, congestive heart failure, heat intolerance, fever, profuse swelling, nausea and vomiting, and diarrhea. Hypokalemia may be present. Treatment includes beta blockers, propylthiouracil, and sodium iodide.

Reference: Karlet, M.C. & Sebastian, L.A. (1997). Chapter 12: The Endocrine System. In J. Nagelhout & K. Zaglaniczny (Eds.), *Nurse Anesthesia*. Philadelphia: W.B. Saunders.

95. ANSWER: B

Rationale: Cretinism is a condition caused by extreme hypothyroidism during fetal life, infancy, and childhood. It is characterized especially by growth failure and mental retardation. Skeletal growth is more inhibited than soft tissue growth, giving the appearance of an obese, stocky, and short child.

Reference: Karlet, M.C. & Sebastian, L.A. (1997). Chapter 12: The Endocrine System. In J. Nagelhout & K. Zaglaniczny (Eds.), *Nurse Anesthesia*. Philadelphia: W.B. Saunders.

96. ANSWER: D

Rationale: Myxedema is caused by severe hypofunction of the thyroid gland. It is characterized by a generalized slowing of the metabolic function, swelling of the facial structures, cold intolerance, and drowsiness. Therapy includes thyroid hormone replacement.

Reference: Dobbins, P. & Hall, S.M. (1997). Chapter 14: Pediatric Anesthesia. In J. Nagelhout & K. Zaglaniczny (Eds.), *Nurse Anesthesia*. Philadelphia: W.B. Saunders.

97. ANSWER: C

Rationale: Fibrinogen is also known as clotting factor I. During blood coagulation fibrinogen is converted to fibrin by factor IIA.

Reference: Gerbasi, F.R. (1997). Chapter 41: Hematology and Anesthesia. In J. Nagelhout & K. Zaglaniczny (Eds.), *Nurse Anesthesia*. Philadelphia: W.B. Saunders.

98. ANSWER: A

Rationale: Formation of prothrombin activator by the extrinsic pathway is rapid, often within 15 seconds. The prothrombin time reflects the integrity of the extrinsic pathway.

Reference: Gerbasi, F.R. (1997). Chapter 41: Hematology and Anesthesia. In J. Nagelhout & K. Zaglaniczny (Eds.), *Nurse Anesthesia*. Philadelphia: W.B. Saunders.

99. ANSWER: D

Rationale: The intrinsic pathway proceeds slowly, usually requiring 2 to 6 minutes to cause clotting. A variety of inhibitors act at different sites in the intrinsic pathway. The partial thromboplastin time reflects the integrity of the intrinsic pathway.

Reference: Gerbasi, F.R. (1997). Chapter 41: Hematology and Anesthesia. In J. Nagelhout & K. Zaglaniczny (Eds.), *Nurse Anesthesia*. Philadelphia: W.B. Saunders.

100. ANSWER: **C**

Rationale: White blood cell or platelet sensitization is typically manifested as a febrile reaction. Such reactions are relatively common and occur in 1% to 3% of transfusions. They are characterized by an increase in temperature without evidence of hemolysis. Use of a 20- to 40-µm filter helps to reduce this reaction.

Reference: Gerbasi, F.R. (1997). Chapter 41: Hematology and Anesthesia. In J. Nagelhout & K. Zaglaniczny (Eds.), *Nurse Anesthesia*. Philadelphia: W.B. Saunders.

101. ANSWER: **A**

Rationale: Total body water is approximately 60% of total body weight or 42 L in a 70-kg person. The intercellular fluid volume constitutes 40% of total body weight, and the extracellular fluid volume constitutes 20% of body weight.

Reference: Litwack, K. & Keithley, J.K. (1997). Chapter 31: Fluids, Electrolytes, and Therapy. In J. Nagelhout & K. Zaglaniczny (Eds.), *Nurse Anesthesia*. Philadelphia: W.B. Saunders.

102. ANSWER: **A**

Rationale: See question 101.

Reference: Litwack, K. & Keithley, J.K. (1997). Chapter 31: Fluids, Electrolytes, and Therapy. In J. Nagelhout & K. Zaglaniczny (Eds.), *Nurse Anesthesia*. Philadelphia: W.B. Saunders.

103. ANSWER: **C**

Rationale: The predominant intracellular cation is potassium, with the intercellular concentration approximating 150 mEq/L. This contrasts to the amount of potassium in the extracellular concentration, which is approximately 4 mEq/L.

Reference: Litwack, K. & Keithley, J.K. (1997). Chapter 31: Fluids, Electrolytes, and Therapy. In J. Nagelhout & K. Zaglaniczny (Eds.), *Nurse Anesthesia*. Philadelphia: W.B. Saunders.

104. ANSWER: **A**

Rationale: Total body water, the distribution volume of sodium free water, approximates 60% of total body weight or 42 L in a 70-kg person.

Reference: Litwack, K. & Keithley, J.K. (1997). Chapter 31: Fluids, Electrolytes, and Therapy. In J. Nagelhout & K. Zaglaniczny (Eds.), *Nurse Anesthesia*. Philadelphia: W.B. Saunders.

105. ANSWER: **D**

Rationale: Extracellular fluid contains most of the sodium in the body. The sodium concentration is approximately 140 mEq/L, with an intercellular concentration of approximately 10 mEq/L.

Reference: Litwack, K. & Keithley, J.K. (1997). Chapter 31: Fluids, Electrolytes, and Therapy. In J. Nagelhout & K. Zaglaniczny (Eds.), *Nurse Anesthesia*. Philadelphia: W.B. Saunders.

106. ANSWER: **C**

Rationale: Signs of hypernatremia include thirst, neurologic weakness, hyperreflexia, seizures, and intracranial hemorrhage. Also commonly seen are hypovolemia and renal insufficiency.

Reference: Litwack, K. & Keithley, J.K. (1997). Chapter 31: Fluids, Electrolytes, and Therapy. In J. Nagelhout & K. Zaglaniczny (Eds.), *Nurse Anesthesia*. Philadelphia: W.B. Saunders.

107. ANSWER: **A**

Rationale: Drugs are the most common cause of hyperkalemia. Drugs that may limit potassium excretion include nonsteroidal anti-inflammatory drugs, angiotensin-converting enzyme inhibitors, cyclosporine, and potassium-sparing diuretics.

Reference: Litwack, K. & Keithley, J.K. (1997). Chapter 31: Fluids, Electrolytes, and Therapy. In J. Nagelhout & K. Zaglaniczny (Eds.), *Nurse Anesthesia*. Philadelphia: W.B. Saunders.

108. ANSWER: **B**

Rationale: Insulin deficiency will commonly result in hyperkalemia. Insulin, in a dose-dependent fashion, causes cellular uptake of potassium by increasing the activity of the sodium-potassium pump. This effect works best at high insulin levels; therefore, administration of insulin will reduce the serum potassium concentration.

Reference: Litwack, K. & Keithley, J.K. (1997). Chapter 31: Fluids, Electrolytes, and Therapy. In J. Nagelhout & K. Zaglaniczny (Eds.), *Nurse Anesthesia*. Philadelphia: W.B. Saunders.

109. ANSWER: **D**

> *Rationale:* Hemophilia A is a deficiency of factor VIII, which is known as the hemophilia factor. Treatment of the deficiency is usually with cryoprecipitate factor.
>
> *Reference:* Gerbasi, F.R. (1997). Chapter 41: Hematology and Anesthesia. In J. Nagelhout & K. Zaglaniczny (Eds.), *Nurse Anesthesia.* Philadelphia: W.B. Saunders.

110. ANSWER: **C**

> *Rationale:* The bleeding time, the most widely excepted clinical test of platelet function, measures both quality and quantity. The normal bleeding time is 3 to 8 minutes.
>
> *Reference:* Gerbasi, F.R. (1997). Chapter 41: Hematology and Anesthesia. In J. Nagelhout & K. Zaglaniczny (Eds.), *Nurse Anesthesia.* Philadelphia: W.B. Saunders.

111. ANSWER: **B**

> *Rationale:* See question 110.
>
> *Reference:* Gerbasi, F.R. (1997). Chapter 41: Hematology and Anesthesia. In J. Nagelhout & K. Zaglaniczny (Eds.), *Nurse Anesthesia.* Philadelphia: W.B. Saunders.

112. ANSWER: **A**

> *Rationale:* The majority of blood drains directly into the ventricles upon entering the heart. The atria contract to deliver the remainder to the ventricle. This component of the ventricular filling is lost during the atrial fibrillation and contributes to the reduction in stroke volume that accompanies this phenomenon.
>
> *Reference:* Morgan, R.O., Jr. (1997). Chapter 8: The Cardiovascular System. In J. Nagelhout & K. Zaglaniczny (Eds.), *Nurse Anesthesia.* Philadelphia: W.B. Saunders.

113. ANSWER: **B**

> *Rationale:* With aortic insufficiency, eccentric hypertrophy develops. This is characterized by dilated thickened chambers. It also includes slow heart rate, increased systemic vascular resistance, and occasionally hypotension and pulmonary edema.

> *Reference:* Aprile, A.E., Serwin, J.P. & Boctor, B. (1997). Chapter 38A: Cardiac Pathophysiology. In J. Nagelhout & K. Zaglaniczny (Eds.), *Nurse Anesthesia.* Philadelphia: W.B. Saunders.

114. ANSWER: **A**

> *Rationale:* In mitral stenosis, as the orifice of the valve narrows, the left atrium experiences pressure overload. This elevated atrial pressure is transmitted to the pulmonary circuit, leading to pulmonary hypertension and right-sided heart failure.
>
> *Reference:* Rojo, J. & Iacopelli, M. (1997). Chapter 39A: Respiratory Pathophysiology. In J. Nagelhout & K. Zaglaniczny (Eds.), *Nurse Anesthesia.* Philadelphia: W.B. Saunders.

115. ANSWER: **D**

> *Rationale:* In chronic mitral regurgitation, the left ventricle and atrium show volume overload, which leads to eccentric hypertrophy.
>
> *Reference:* Rojo, J. & Iacopelli, M. (1997). Chapter 39A: Respiratory Pathophysiology. In J. Nagelhout & K. Zaglaniczny (Eds.), *Nurse Anesthesia.* Philadelphia: W.B. Saunders.

116. ANSWER: **B**

> *Rationale:* After a trauma injury it is expected that there will be an increase in adrenocorticoids, glucocorticoids, and catecholamine release.
>
> *Reference:* Barton, C.R. (1997). Chapter 44: Trauma Anesthesia. In J. Nagelhout & K. Zaglaniczny (Eds.), *Nurse Anesthesia.* Philadelphia: W.B. Saunders.

117. ANSWER: **D**

> *Rationale:* The most common metabolic complication associated with total parenteral nutrition is hyperglycemia. Glucosuria also occurs. Frequent monitoring of glucose in the urine and serum is important, particularly at the start of total parenteral nutrition.
>
> *Reference:* Litwack, K. & Keithley, J.K. (1997). Chapter 31: Fluids, Electrolytes, and Therapy. In J. Nagelhout & K. Zaglaniczny (Eds.), *Nurse Anesthesia.* Philadelphia: W.B. Saunders.

118. ANSWER: **B**

> *Rationale:* The vibration of the valves immediately after closure along with the

vibration of the adjacent blood and walls of the heart travel through the chest wall and can be heard with the stethoscope.

Reference: Morgan, R.O., Jr. (1997). Chapter 8: The Cardiovascular System. In J. Nagelhout & K. Zaglaniczny (Eds.), *Nurse Anesthesia*. Philadelphia: W.B. Saunders.

119. ANSWER: A

Rationale: The second heart sound results from sudden closure of the aortic and pulmonary valves. Similar to the first heart sound, the valve closing reverberates through the tissues in the chest wall and can be heard with a stethoscope.

Reference: Morgan, R.O., Jr. (1997). Chapter 8: The Cardiovascular System. In J. Nagelhout & K. Zaglaniczny (Eds.), *Nurse Anesthesia*. Philadelphia: W.B. Saunders.

120. ANSWER: C

Rationale: The subendocardium muscle becomes infarcted before any other part of the heart muscle. Under normal conditions this layer of the muscle has difficulty obtaining adequate blood flow because of the intense compression by contraction of the heart. Any condition that compromises blood flow to the heart usually causes damage first in the subendocardium regions and then spreads outward toward the epicardium.

Reference: Aprile, A.E., Serwin, J.P. & Boctor, B. (1997). Chapter 38A: Cardiac Pathophysiology. In J. Nagelhout & K. Zaglaniczny (Eds.), *Nurse Anesthesia*. Philadelphia: W.B. Saunders.

121. ANSWER: C

Rationale: Resting coronary blood flow is approximately 225 mL/min, which is 4% to 5% of the cardiac output. During diastole, the cardiac muscle relaxes completely and no longer obstructs the blood flow through the left ventricular capillaries.

Reference: Morgan, R.O., Jr. (1997). Chapter 8: The Cardiovascular System. In J. Nagelhout & K. Zaglaniczny (Eds.), *Nurse Anesthesia*. Philadelphia: W.B. Saunders.

122. ANSWER: D

Rationale: Cardiac output is the volume of blood pumped from the heart per minute. It is the product of the heart rate and stroke volume. The cardiac output is determined by preload, afterload, heart rate, contractility, and ventricular compliance.

Reference: Morgan, R.O., Jr. (1997). Chapter 8: The Cardiovascular System. In J. Nagelhout & K. Zaglaniczny (Eds.), *Nurse Anesthesia*. Philadelphia: W.B. Saunders.

123. ANSWER: A

Rationale: The cardiac index is the cardiac output divided by the body surface area. The normal value is 2.5 to 4.0 L/min per square meter of body surface area.

Reference: Morgan, R.O., Jr. (1997). Chapter 8: The Cardiovascular System. In J. Nagelhout & K. Zaglaniczny (Eds.), *Nurse Anesthesia*. Philadelphia: W.B. Saunders.

124. ANSWER: C

Rationale: The ejection fraction (normally 0.6–0.7) is the ratio of the stroke volume to the end-diastolic volume. Severe impairment is present when the injection fraction is less than 0.4. The ejection fraction is determined by the end-diastolic volume minus the end-systolic volume divided by the end-diastolic volume.

Reference: Morgan, R.O., Jr. (1997). Chapter 8: The Cardiovascular System. In J. Nagelhout & K. Zaglaniczny (Eds.), *Nurse Anesthesia*. Philadelphia: W.B. Saunders.

125. ANSWER: B

Rationale:

$$\frac{(MAP - CVP) \times 80}{Cardiac\ output\ (L/min)}$$

The normal value is 1200 to 1500 dynes/sec/cm^5

Reference: Morgan, R.O., Jr. (1997). Chapter 8: The Cardiovascular System. In J. Nagelhout & K. Zaglaniczny (Eds.), *Nurse Anesthesia*. Philadelphia: W.B. Saunders.

126. ANSWER: B

Rationale:

$$\frac{(\overline{PA} - PCWP) \times 80}{Cardiac\ output\ (L/min)}$$

The normal value is 100 to 300 dynes/sec/cm^5

Reference: Morgan, R.O., Jr. (1997). Chapter 8: The Cardiovascular System. In J. Nagelhout & K. Zaglaniczny (Eds.), *Nurse Anesthesia.* Philadelphia: W.B. Saunders.

127. ANSWER: C

Rationale: Increased cerebrospinal fluid pressure compresses cerebral arteries, causing ischemia. The response is a natural reflex to increase arterial pressure to reperfuse the brain.

Reference: Morgan, R.O., Jr. (1997). Chapter 8: The Cardiovascular System. In J. Nagelhout & K. Zaglaniczny (Eds.), *Nurse Anesthesia.* Philadelphia: W.B. Saunders.

128. ANSWER: A

Rationale: The Bezold-Jarisch reflex induces hypotension and bradycardia and vagally influences coronary vasodilation. Reperfusion of previously ischemic myocardial tissue also elicits the reflex.

Reference: Morgan, R.O., Jr. (1997). Chapter 8: The Cardiovascular System. In J. Nagelhout & K. Zaglaniczny (Eds.), *Nurse Anesthesia.* Philadelphia: W.B. Saunders.

129. ANSWER: D

Rationale: Peripheral chemoreceptors are usually minimally active. However, occlusion of the carotid artery decreases oxygen supply and activates the reflex to increase ventilation and blood pressure while decreasing heart rate. Stimulation of the aortic bodies causes tachycardia.

Reference: Morgan, R.O., Jr. (1997). Chapter 8: The Cardiovascular System. In J. Nagelhout & K. Zaglaniczny (Eds.), *Nurse Anesthesia.* Philadelphia: W.B. Saunders.

130. ANSWER: A

Rationale: The Valsalva maneuver involves voluntary closing of the glottis while performing a forced expiration, which increases intrathoracic pressure. Venous pressure in the head and the extremities increases while venous return to the right ventricle decreases. Blood pressure decreases and heart rate increases.

Reference: Morgan, R.O., Jr. (1997). Chapter 8: The Cardiovascular System. In J. Nagelhout & K.

Zaglaniczny (Eds.), *Nurse Anesthesia.* Philadelphia: W.B. Saunders.

131. ANSWER: B

Rationale: The cardiac output is distributed to organ systems as follows: brain, 12%; heart, 4%; liver, 24%; kidneys, 20%; muscle, 23%; skin, 6%; and intestines, 8%.

Reference: Morgan, R.O., Jr. (1997). Chapter 8: The Cardiovascular System. In J. Nagelhout & K. Zaglaniczny (Eds.), *Nurse Anesthesia.* Philadelphia: W.B. Saunders.

132. ANSWER: C

Rationale: The primary effect of atrial natriuretic factor is suppression of release of antidiuretic hormone. Direct vasodilation, inhibition of aldosterone release, increase in glomerular filtration rate, and diuresis also occur.

Reference: Ouelette S.M. (1997). Chapter 11: Renal Anatomy, Physiology, and Pathophysiology, and Anesthesia. In J. Nagelhout & K. Zaglaniczny (Eds.), *Nurse Anesthesia.* Philadelphia: W.B. Saunders.

133. ANSWER: A

Rationale: The oculocardiac reflex occurs when pressure on the extraocular muscles causes bradycardia and hypotension. Traction on the medial rectus muscle, not the lateral rectus muscle, elicits the reflex. Afferent fibers run along the thalamic division of the trigeminal nerve to the gasserian ganglion nerve, and the efferent fibers travel along the vagus nerve.

Reference: Harvey, R.R. (1997). Chapter 48: Anesthesia for Ophthalmic Procedures. In J. Nagelhout & K. Zaglaniczny (Eds.), *Nurse Anesthesia.* Philadelphia: W.B. Saunders.

134. ANSWER: D

Rationale: Stroke volume is equal to the cardiac output divided by the heart rate. A normal adult averages 60 to 90 mL per beat.

Reference: Morgan, R.O., Jr. (1997). Chapter 8: The Cardiovascular System. In J. Nagelhout & K. Zaglaniczny (Eds.), *Nurse Anesthesia.* Philadelphia: W.B. Saunders.

135. ANSWER: **C**

Rationale: Bainbridge described a reflex increase in heart rate when vagal tone was high and the right atrium or central vein was distended. The response depends on pre-existing heart rate. During tachycardia it does not occur, but volume loading and a slow heart rate will elicit the reflex.

Reference: Morgan, R.O., Jr. (1997). Chapter 8: The Cardiovascular System. In J. Nagelhout & K. Zaglaniczny (Eds.), *Nurse Anesthesia.* Philadelphia: W.B. Saunders.

136. ANSWER: **B**

Rationale: The chemoreceptors are chemosensitive cells that respond to oxygen lack, carbon dioxide excess, or hydrogen ion excess. They are located in the carotid and aortic bodies.

Reference: Hall, S.M. (1997). Chapter 9: Respiratory Anatomy and Physiology. In J. Nagelhout & K. Zaglaniczny (Eds.), *Nurse Anesthesia.* Philadelphia: W.B. Saunders.

137. ANSWER: **D**

Rationale: Renin is synthesized and stored in the juxtaglomerular cells of the kidneys. It acts on angiotensin to form angiotensin I. Angiotensin I is then converted to angiotensin II in the lungs by the converting enzyme.

Reference: Ouelette S.M. (1997). Chapter 11: Renal Anatomy, Physiology, and Pathophysiology, and Anesthesia. In J. Nagelhout & K. Zaglaniczny (Eds.), *Nurse Anesthesia.* Philadelphia: W.B. Saunders.

138. ANSWER: **B**

Rationale: Besides its blood pressure–modulating properties, angiotensin II is a major influence on the reabsorption of sodium and the excretion of potassium in exchange for sodium.

Reference: Ouelette S.M. (1997). Chapter 11: Renal Anatomy, Physiology, and Pathophysiology, and Anesthesia. In J. Nagelhout & K. Zaglaniczny (Eds.), *Nurse Anesthesia.* Philadelphia: W.B. Saunders.

139. ANSWER: **A**

Rationale: Approximately 90% of all persons who have hypertension are said to have essential hypertension which means that its origin is unknown.

Reference: Alisoglu, R. (1997). Chapter 23: Cardiac Pharmacology. In J. Nagelhout & K. Zaglaniczny (Eds.), *Nurse Anesthesia.* Philadelphia: W.B. Saunders.

140. ANSWER: **A**

Rationale: Heart rate is primarily determined by the automaticity of the sino-atrial node. Neurologic influences are paramount, but hormonal influences are minimal. Neurologic influences are mediated through the autonomic nervous system.

Reference: Morgan, R.O., Jr. (1997). Chapter 8: The Cardiovascular System. In J. Nagelhout & K. Zaglaniczny (Eds.), *Nurse Anesthesia.* Philadelphia: W.B. Saunders.

141. ANSWER: **C**

Rationale: The most important difference between hemoglobin F and adult hemoglobin is its high affinity for oxygen. Hemoglobin F limits tissue oxygen delivery and hypoxic conditions due to a high oxygen binding ability.

Reference: Dobbins, P. & Hall, S.M. (1997). Chapter 14: Pediatric Anesthesia. In J. Nagelhout & K. Zaglaniczny (Eds.), *Nurse Anesthesia.* Philadelphia: W.B. Saunders.

142. ANSWER: **A**

Rationale: The hemoglobin concentration declines gradually to 10 to 11 g/dL during the first few months of life as fetal hemoglobin is replaced. It then gradually increases and is maximal at about 14 years of age.

Reference: Dobbins, P. & Hall, S.M. (1997). Chapter 14: Pediatric Anesthesia. In J. Nagelhout & K. Zaglaniczny (Eds.), *Nurse Anesthesia.* Philadelphia: W.B. Saunders.

143. ANSWER: **B**

Rationale: Congenital heart defects are classified as either increasing or decreasing pulmonary blood flow. Those exhibiting an increase in pulmonary flow include atrial septal defect, ventricular septal defect, patent ductus arteriosus, endocardial cushion defect, and aortal

pulmonary windows. Those exhibiting a decrease include tetralogy of Fallot, pulmonary atresia, tricuspid atresia, and Ebstein's anomaly.
Reference: Dobbins, P. & Hall, S.M. (1997). Chapter 14: Pediatric Anesthesia. In J. Nagelhout & K. Zaglaniczny (Eds.), *Nurse Anesthesia*. Philadelphia: W.B. Saunders.

144. ANSWER: **C**

Rationale: Halothane sensitizes the heart to the action of many sympathomimetics. If epinephrine is administered, dysrhythmias are unlikely with doses of 10 μg/kg or less.
Reference: Williams, J.R. (1997). Chapter 20: Local Anesthetics. In J. Nagelhout & K. Zaglaniczny (Eds.), *Nurse Anesthesia*. Philadelphia: W.B. Saunders.

145. ANSWER: **A**

Rationale: Infants rely on nonshivering thermogenesis to help maintain body temperature because of their high level of brown fat, which produces heat without affecting muscle metabolism.
Reference: Dobbins, P. & Hall, S.M. (1997). Chapter 14: Pediatric Anesthesia. In J. Nagelhout & K. Zaglaniczny (Eds.), *Nurse Anesthesia*. Philadelphia: W.B. Saunders.

146. ANSWER: **C**

Rationale: Patent ductus arteriosus is common in the premature infant but is usually insignificant in the newborn within the first 24 hours. It is characterized by a murmur at the left sternal border radiating to the back, bounding pulses, and increased pulmonary blood flow. Pharmacologic closure with indomethacin may be attempted before surgical intervention if the patient is severely symptomatic.
Reference: Dobbins, P. & Hall, S.M. (1997). Chapter 14: Pediatric Anesthesia. In J. Nagelhout & K. Zaglaniczny (Eds.), *Nurse Anesthesia*. Philadelphia: W.B. Saunders.

147. ANSWER: **A**

Rationale: When the lungs first expand with air at birth, pulmonary vascular resistance (PVR) falls markedly by approx-
imately 80% from prenatal levels within a few minutes of normal initiation of ventilation. As PVR falls, blood flow to the lungs in the pulmonary veins close the atrial septum over the foramen ovale.
Reference: Dobbins, P. & Hall, S.M. (1997). Chapter 14: Pediatric Anesthesia. In J. Nagelhout & K. Zaglaniczny (Eds.), *Nurse Anesthesia*. Philadelphia: W.B. Saunders.

148. ANSWER: **B**

Rationale: Neonates exposed to hypoxemia suffer pulmonary and systemic vasoconstriction, bradycardia, and a decrease in cardiac output. Because of their high metabolic rate for oxygen, hypoxemia also develops more rapidly in the neonate.
Reference: Dobbins, P. & Hall, S.M. (1997). Chapter 14: Pediatric Anesthesia. In J. Nagelhout & K. Zaglaniczny (Eds.), *Nurse Anesthesia*. Philadelphia: W.B. Saunders.

149. ANSWER: **A**

Rationale: A newborn's muscles of ventilation are subject to fatigue. This tendency is determined by the types of muscle fibers present. In preterm infants, less than 10% of the fibers in the diaphragm are type I (slow twitch, highly oxidative, fatigue resistance); in term infants, 30% are type I; and in adults, 55% are type I. A child reaches adult proportions in type I diaphragmatic fibers at approximately age 1 year.
Reference: Dobbins, P. & Hall, S.M. (1997). Chapter 14: Pediatric Anesthesia. In J. Nagelhout & K. Zaglaniczny (Eds.), *Nurse Anesthesia*. Philadelphia: W.B. Saunders.

150. ANSWER: **D**

Rationale: See question 149.
Reference: Dobbins, P. & Hall, S.M. (1997). Chapter 14: Pediatric Anesthesia. In J. Nagelhout & K. Zaglaniczny (Eds.), *Nurse Anesthesia*. Philadelphia: W.B. Saunders.

151. ANSWER: **C**

Rationale: Surfactants lower surface tension and prevent alveoli from collapsing. Lecithin is produced by type II pneumo-

cytes. At 25 to 36 weeks' gestation the lung is fairly mature and surfactant is being produced at adequate levels.
Reference: Dobbins, P. & Hall, S.M. (1997). Chapter 14: Pediatric Anesthesia. In J. Nagelhout & K. Zaglaniczny (Eds.), *Nurse Anesthesia*. Philadelphia: W.B. Saunders.

152. ANSWER: **A**

Rationale: Infants have a large head and short neck, large tongue, and narrow nasal passages. The larynx is at C4 and anterior when compared with that of adults. The airway is the narrowest at the cricoid cartilage.
Reference: Dobbins, P. & Hall, S.M. (1997). Chapter 14: Pediatric Anesthesia. In J. Nagelhout & K. Zaglaniczny (Eds.), *Nurse Anesthesia*. Philadelphia: W.B. Saunders.

153. ANSWER: **A**

Rationale: Major surgery does not especially lead to disorder. Judicious use of oxygen during surgery with arterial tensions below 140 mm Hg is generally considered safe.
Reference: Dobbins, P. & Hall, S.M. (1997). Chapter 14: Pediatric Anesthesia. In J. Nagelhout & K. Zaglaniczny (Eds.), *Nurse Anesthesia*. Philadelphia: W.B. Saunders.

154. ANSWER: **C**

Rationale: Surfactant begins to be produced at 22 weeks' gestation. It increases sharply at 35 to 36 weeks as the lung matures.
Reference: Dobbins, P. & Hall, S.M. (1997). Chapter 14: Pediatric Anesthesia. In J. Nagelhout & K. Zaglaniczny (Eds.), *Nurse Anesthesia*. Philadelphia: W.B. Saunders.

155. ANSWER: **A**

Rationale: The lecithin/sphingomyelin (L/S) ratio is an assessment of surfactant production in the lungs. Type II pneumocytes produce surfactant with an L/S ratio less than 1 at 32 weeks, 2 by 35 weeks, and 4 to 6 at term.
Reference: Dobbins, P. & Hall, S.M. (1997). Chapter 14: Pediatric Anesthesia. In J. Nagelhout & K. Zaglaniczny (Eds.), *Nurse Anesthesia*. Philadelphia: W.B. Saunders.

156. ANSWER: **B**

Rationale: Premature infants with inadequate surfactant production suffer from respiratory distress syndrome (RDS). Therefore, you would expect an increase in work of breathing, hypoxemia, and acidosis.
Reference: Dobbins, P. & Hall, S.M. (1997). Chapter 14: Pediatric Anesthesia. In J. Nagelhout & K. Zaglaniczny (Eds.), *Nurse Anesthesia*. Philadelphia: W.B. Saunders.

157. ANSWER: **D**

Rationale: The bevel of the needle should face anteriorly. The drug is injected in the epidural space with a volume of 1 to 2 mL per spinal segment anesthetized. Twelve to 15 mL is required to fill the sacral canal.
Reference: Dobbins, P. & Hall, S.M. (1997). Chapter 14: Pediatric Anesthesia. In J. Nagelhout & K. Zaglaniczny (Eds.), *Nurse Anesthesia*. Philadelphia: W.B. Saunders.

158. ANSWER: **B**

Rationale: Atropine is the preferred anticholinergic agent in children. It is more effective in blocking the cardiac vagus and causes less drying of secretions than the others.
Reference: Dobbins, P. & Hall, S.M. (1997). Chapter 14: Pediatric Anesthesia. In J. Nagelhout & K. Zaglaniczny (Eds.), *Nurse Anesthesia*. Philadelphia: W.B. Saunders.

159. ANSWER: **A**

Rationale: Tetralogy of Fallot classically includes right ventricular obstruction, ventricular septal defect, right ventricular hypertrophy, and an overriding aorta.
Reference: Dobbins, P. & Hall, S.M. (1997). Chapter 14: Pediatric Anesthesia. In J. Nagelhout & K. Zaglaniczny (Eds.), *Nurse Anesthesia*. Philadelphia: W.B. Saunders.

160. ANSWER: **D**

Rationale: Echothiophate iodide or phospholine iodide is a long-acting cholinesterase inhibitor. Therefore, with systemic absorption, patients may be at a risk for low levels of cholinesterase.
Reference: Haas, R.E. & Erway, R.L. (1997). Chapter 22: Neuromuscular Blocking Agents,

Reversal Agents, and Their Monitoring. In J. Nagelhout & K. Zaglaniczny (Eds.), *Nurse Anesthesia*. Philadelphia: W.B. Saunders.

161. ANSWER: **C**

> *Rationale:* It is not necessary to avoid nitrous oxide in children with pyloric stenosis. There is no evidence of an increased gastric pressure when nitrous oxide is included in the anesthetic technique. Because these children are at such a high risk for aspiration, a rapid sequence induction, insertion of orogastric tube, and rehydration to replace fluids are all necessary.
> *Reference:* Dobbins, P. & Hall, S.M. (1997). Chapter 14: Pediatric Anesthesia. In J. Nagelhout & K. Zaglaniczny (Eds.), *Nurse Anesthesia*. Philadelphia: W.B. Saunders.

162. ANSWER: **B**

> *Rationale:* Nausea and vomiting are very common in children. They occur after numerous operations, especially eye surgery, ENT procedures, and abdominal operations. Efforts similar to those in adults to reduce the incidence of nausea and vomiting are equally important.
> *Reference:* Marley, R. (1997). Chapter 45: Outpatient Anesthesia. In J. Nagelhout & K. Zaglaniczny (Eds.), *Nurse Anesthesia*. Philadelphia: W.B. Saunders.

163. ANSWER: **D**

> *Rationale:* Most nondepolarizing muscle relaxants including vecuronium are known to be safe in patients with malignant hyperthermia. The muscle relaxant to avoid is succinlycholine as well as all inhalation anesthetics except nitrous oxide.
> *Reference:* Karlet, M.C. (1997). Chapter 40: Musculoskeletal Pathophysiology and Anesthesia. In J. Nagelhout & K. Zaglaniczny (Eds.), *Nurse Anesthesia*. Philadelphia: W.B. Saunders.

164. ANSWER: **A**

> *Rationale:* Normal hepatic blood flow is about 1500 mL/min in adults. Twenty-five to thirty percent is from the hepatic artery and 70% to 75% is from the portal vein.

Reference: Palmer, T.J. (1997). Chapter 10: Hepatobiliary and Gastrointestinal Disturbances. In J. Nagelhout & K. Zaglaniczny (Eds.), *Nurse Anesthesia*. Philadelphia: W.B. Saunders.

165. ANSWER: **A**

> *Rationale:* The afferent pathway is via the trigeminal nerve, with the efferent pathway via the vagus nerve.
> *Reference:* Harvey, R.R. (1997). Chapter 48: Anesthesia for Ophthalmic Procedures. In J. Nagelhout & K. Zaglaniczny (Eds.), *Nurse Anesthesia*. Philadelphia: W.B. Saunders.

166. ANSWER: **B**

> *Rationale:* To maintain normal body temperature, infants and children create heat by metabolizing brown fat, crying, and moving vigorously, but, unlike adults, rarely by shivering.
> *Reference:* Dobbins, P. & Hall, S.M. (1997). Chapter 14: Pediatric Anesthesia. In J. Nagelhout & K. Zaglaniczny (Eds.), *Nurse Anesthesia*. Philadelphia: W.B. Saunders.

167. ANSWER: **D**

> *Rationale:* The kidneys at birth are characterized by a decreased glomerular filtration rate (GFR), sodium excretion, and concentrating ability. The GFR increases twofold to threefold by 3 months. Adult levels are reached at about 2 years old. About 12 months are needed to obtain normal concentrating ability in urine.
> *Reference:* Dobbins, P. & Hall, S.M. (1997). Chapter 14: Pediatric Anesthesia. In J. Nagelhout & K. Zaglaniczny (Eds.), *Nurse Anesthesia*. Philadelphia: W.B. Saunders.

168. ANSWER: **C**

> *Rationale:* Neonates and infants are more sensitive to muscle relaxants. However, doses required may be higher because of an increased volume of distribution resulting from a high extracellular fluid volume.
> *Reference:* Dobbins, P. & Hall, S.M. (1997). Chapter 14: Pediatric Anesthesia. In J. Nagelhout & K. Zaglaniczny (Eds.), *Nurse Anesthesia*. Philadelphia: W.B. Saunders.

169. ANSWER: **A**

Rationale: Laryngotracheobronchitis is differentiated from epiglottitis in that it usually occurs in children 2 years or younger and is not accompanied by high fever. Its cause is viral, and it develops gradually over 1 to 3 days.
Reference: Dobbins, P. & Hall, S.M. (1997). Chapter 14: Pediatric Anesthesia. In J. Nagelhout & K. Zaglaniczny (Eds.), *Nurse Anesthesia*. Philadelphia: W.B. Saunders.

170. ANSWER: **D**

Rationale: Laryngotracheobronchitis usually occurs in children younger than 2 years old in contrast to epiglottitis. It is most frequent in 2- to 6-year olds.
Reference: Dobbins, P. & Hall, S.M. (1997). Chapter 14: Pediatric Anesthesia. In J. Nagelhout & K. Zaglaniczny (Eds.), *Nurse Anesthesia*. Philadelphia: W.B. Saunders.

171. ANSWER: **B**

Rationale: Epiglottitis is bacterial not viral; hence, antibiotics are indicated.
Reference: Dobbins, P. & Hall, S.M. (1997). Chapter 14: Pediatric Anesthesia. In J. Nagelhout & K. Zaglaniczny (Eds.), *Nurse Anesthesia*. Philadelphia: W.B. Saunders.

172. ANSWER: **C**

Rationale: The maximum safe dose for IV dantrolene is approximately 10 mg/kg. Starting dose is 2.5 mg/kg repeated as necessary to 10 mg. Dantrolene should be supplemented every 4 to 6 hours.
Reference: Karlet, M.C. (1997). Chapter 40: Musculoskeletal Pathophysiology and Anesthesia. In J. Nagelhout & K. Zaglaniczny (Eds.), *Nurse Anesthesia*. Philadelphia: W.B. Saunders.

173. ANSWER: **A**

Rationale: Diaphragmatic hernia results from incomplete closure of the diaphragm such that intestinal contents occupy the chest. Manifestations at birth include scaphoid abdomen, profound arterial hypoxemia, pulmonary hypertension, and congenital heart disease.
Reference: Dobbins, P. & Hall, S.M. (1997). Chapter 14: Pediatric Anesthesia. In J. Nagelhout & K. Zaglaniczny (Eds.), *Nurse Anesthesia*. Philadelphia: W.B. Saunders.

174. ANSWER: **D**

Rationale: Infants with pyloric stenosis generally present at 2 to 5 weeks of age with a loss of hydrogen ions from vomiting. Alkalosis, hypokalemia, and dehydration result.
Reference: Dobbins, P. & Hall, S.M. (1997). Chapter 14: Pediatric Anesthesia. In J. Nagelhout & K. Zaglaniczny (Eds.), *Nurse Anesthesia*. Philadelphia: W.B. Saunders.

175. ANSWER: **B**

Rationale: Retinopathy of prematurity is most common in infants younger than 44 weeks after conception. Other factors may include multiple blood transfusions, apnea requiring mechanical ventilation, parenteral nutrition, and hypoxemia.
Reference: Dobbins, P. & Hall, S.M. (1997). Chapter 14: Pediatric Anesthesia. In J. Nagelhout & K. Zaglaniczny (Eds.), *Nurse Anesthesia*. Philadelphia: W.B. Saunders.

176. ANSWER: **A**

Rationale: The pressure in the tank will remain unchanged at 750 to 760 psi as long as there is any liquid left in the tank. The rest of the tank fills with vapor, thus maintaining the pressure.
Reference: Dosch, M.P. (1997). Chapter 26: Anesthesia Equipment. In J. Nagelhout & K. Zaglaniczny (Eds.), *Nurse Anesthesia*. Philadelphia: W.B. Saunders.

177. ANSWER: **C**

Rationale: Infants are much more dependent on changes in heart rate in response to environmental factors than in changes in stroke volume. As infants grow, their cardiovascular system becomes less dependent on rate and more in line functionally with that of adults. An immature baroreceptor reflex contributes to this phenomenon.
Reference: Dobbins, P. & Hall, S.M. (1997). Chapter 14: Pediatric Anesthesia. In J. Nagelhout & K. Zaglaniczny (Eds.), *Nurse Anesthesia*. Philadelphia: W.B. Saunders.

178. ANSWER: **D**

Rationale: The pediatric pulmonary system is characterized by smaller alveoli.

There is a 13-fold growth in the number of alveoli between birth and 6 years of age and a 3-fold growth between age 6 years and adulthood.

Reference: Dobbins, P. & Hall, S.M. (1997). Chapter 14: Pediatric Anesthesia. In J. Nagelhout & K. Zaglaniczny (Eds.), *Nurse Anesthesia*. Philadelphia: W.B. Saunders.

179. ANSWER: **A**

Rationale: The adrenal gland is divided into the two parts. The adrenal cortex secretes androgens and mineralocorticoids such as aldosterone and glucocorticoids such as cortisone. The medulla secretes catecholamines, epinephrine, norepinephrine, and dopamine.

Reference: Karlet, M.C. & Sebastian, L.S. (1997). Chapter 12: The Endocrine System. In J. Nagelhout & K. Zaglaniczny (Eds.), *Nurse Anesthesia*. Philadelphia: W.B. Saunders.

180. ANSWER: **B**

Rationale: Catecholamines are synthesized in chromaffin cells, which originate embryologically from the neural crest.

Reference: Karlet, M.C. & Sebastian, L.A. (1997). Chapter 12: The Endocrine System. In J. Nagelhout & K. Zaglaniczny (Eds.), *Nurse Anesthesia*. Philadelphia: W.B. Saunders.

181. ANSWER: **D**

Rationale: Hypertension and tachycardia are common signs of pheochromocytoma, which accounts for 0.1% of all cases of hypertension.

Reference: Karlet, M.C. & Sebastian, L.A. (1997). Chapter 12: The Endocrine System. In J. Nagelhout & K. Zaglaniczny (Eds.), *Nurse Anesthesia*. Philadelphia: W.B. Saunders.

182. ANSWER: **A**

Rationale: Myasthenic patients exhibited resistance to succinylcholine. A higher dose is occasionally given (for example, 2 mg/kg), but a prolonged effect should be anticipated. In addition, many of these patients are on anticholinesterase agents to increase muscle strength chronically.

Reference: Karlet, M.C. (1997). Chapter 40: Musculoskeletal Pathophysiology and Anesthesia.

In J. Nagelhout & K. Zaglaniczny (Eds.), *Nurse Anesthesia*. Philadelphia: W.B. Saunders.

183. ANSWER: **C**

Rationale: The common diastolic murmurs are associated with pulmonary regurgitation, tricuspid stenosis, aortic regurgitation, and mitral stenosis. The rest tend to produce systolic murmurs.

Reference: Aprile, A.E., Serwin, J.P. & Boctor, B. (1997). Chapter 38A: Cardiac Pathophysiology. In J. Nagelhout & K. Zaglaniczny (Eds.), *Nurse Anesthesia*. Philadelphia: W.B. Saunders.

184. ANSWER: **A**

Rationale: Systolic murmurs are produced by pulmonary stenosis, tricuspid stenosis, hypertrophic cardiomyopathy, mitral valve prolapse, mitral regurgitation, ventricular septal defect, and aortic stenosis.

Reference: Aprile, A.E., Serwin, J.P. & Boctor, B. (1997). Chapter 38A: Cardiac Pathophysiology. In J. Nagelhout & K. Zaglaniczny (Eds.), *Nurse Anesthesia*. Philadelphia: W.B. Saunders.

185. ANSWER: **B**

Rationale: A single segmental branch of the aorta is called the artery of Adamkiewicz. It supplies nearly all of the flow to the lower thoracic and lumbar segment. Injury to this artery renders this entire segment of cord at risk for ischemia.

Reference: Aprile, A.E., Serwin, J.P. & Boctor, B. (1997). Chapter 38A: Cardiac Pathophysiology. In J. Nagelhout & K. Zaglaniczny (Eds.), *Nurse Anesthesia*. Philadelphia: W.B. Saunders.

186. ANSWER: **D**

Rationale: Average cerebral blood flow is 50 mL/100 g/min; however, flow in gray matter is about 80 mL, whereas that in white matter is about 20 mL, thus the 50 mL average. Total cerebral blood flow is around 750 mL/min, which is 15% to 20% of the cardiac output.

Reference: DeVane, G.G. (1997). Chapter 37: Neurosurgical Anesthesia. In J. Nagelhout & K. Zaglaniczny (Eds.), *Nurse Anesthesia*. Philadelphia: W.B. Saunders.

187. ANSWER: **A**

Rationale: The combination of a decrease in neuronal metabolic demand with an increase in cerebral blood flow has been termed *luxury perfusion*. This occurs most commonly with the inhalation anesthetic agents.

Reference: DeVane, G.G. (1997). Chapter 37: Neurosurgical Anesthesia. In J. Nagelhout & K. Zaglaniczny (Eds.), *Nurse Anesthesia*. Philadelphia: W.B. Saunders.

188. ANSWER: **D**

Rationale: Despite improved shielding from the artificial cardiac pacemaker all of the listed steps are still recommended when caring for a patient with a pacemaker. Nerve stimulators are generally safe but should be placed on the contralateral arm as far away from the pulse generator as possible.

Reference: Palmer, T.J. & Mitton, M.P. (1997). Chapter 36: Electrocardiography and Rhythm Disturbances. In J. Nagelhout & K. Zaglaniczny (Eds.), *Nurse Anesthesia*. Philadelphia: W.B. Saunders.

189. ANSWER: **C**

Rationale: The vapor pressure of a liquid is mostly dependent on the environmental temperature in which it exists. It is independent of atmospheric pressure.

Reference: Dosch, M.P. (1997). Chapter 26: Anesthesia Equipment. In J. Nagelhout & K. Zaglaniczny (Eds.), *Nurse Anesthesia*. Philadelphia: W.B. Saunders.

190. ANSWER: **A**

Rationale: The circle system characteristics include rebreathing of exhaled gases, conservation of heat and humidity, excellent ability to scavenge gases, and good control of anesthetic depth.

Reference: Dosch, M.P. (1997). Chapter 26: Anesthesia Equipment. In J. Nagelhout & K. Zaglaniczny (Eds.), *Nurse Anesthesia*. Philadelphia: W.B. Saunders.

191. ANSWER: **A**

Rationale: The fresh gas inlet is placed between the absorber and the inspiratory valve to allow for mixing of some fresh gas with rebreathed gas. This also avoids absorption and release by soda lime before inspiration.

Reference: Dosch, M.P. (1997). Chapter 26: Anesthesia Equipment. In J. Nagelhout & K. Zaglaniczny (Eds.), *Nurse Anesthesia*. Philadelphia: W.B. Saunders.

192. ANSWER: **B**

Rationale: The most common inherited defect is hemostasis factor VIII deficiency or hemophilia A. Fresh frozen plasma is considered to have 1 unit of factor VIII activity per milliliter. Cryoprecipitate has 5 to 10 units/mL. Factor VIII concentrate has 40 units/mL. Factor VIII levels greater than 50% are optimal before surgery.

Reference: Gerbasi, F.R. (1997). Chapter 41: Hematology and Anesthesia. In J. Nagelhout & K. Zaglaniczny (Eds.), *Nurse Anesthesia*. Philadelphia: W.B. Saunders.

193. ANSWER: **B**

Rationale: The smooth endoplasmic reticulum of hepatic cells contains the oxidative cytochrome enzymes responsible for most drug metabolism in the body. These sites are sometimes referred to as microsomes.

Reference: Troop, M. (1997). Chapter 16: Pharmacokinetics. In J. Nagelhout & K. Zaglaniczny (Eds.), *Nurse Anesthesia*. Philadelphia: W.B. Saunders.

194. ANSWER: **D**

Rationale: The partial pressure of an anesthetic in the brain is always equivalent to the partial pressure in the alveoli. The alveolar membrane and blood-brain barrier do not represent obstacles to diffusion. The amount in the brain will always approximate the amount in the lungs.

Reference: Nagelhout, J.J. (1997). Chapter 17: Uptake and Distribution of Inhalation Anesthetics. In J. Nagelhout & K. Zaglaniczny (Eds.), *Nurse Anesthesia*. Philadelphia: W.B. Saunders.

195. ANSWER: **A**

Rationale: The oculocardiac reflex is trigeminovagal. The afferent pathway is by way of the ciliary ganglion to the ophthalmic division of the trigeminal nerve and through the gasserian ganglion to the main sensory nucleus of the fourth ventricle. The efferent pathway is the vagus nerve.

Reference: Harvey, R.R. (1997). Chapter 48: Anesthesia for Ophthalmic Procedures. In J. Nagelhout & K. Zaglaniczny (Eds.), *Nurse Anesthesia*. Philadelphia: W.B. Saunders.

196. ANSWER: B

Rationale: The apneustic center is located in the lower part of the pons. The function of the apneustic center is not understood, but it presumably operates in association with the pneumotaxic center to control the depth of inspiration.

Reference: Harrigan, C. (1997). Chapter 6: The Central Nervous System. In J. Nagelhout & K. Zaglaniczny (Eds.), *Nurse Anesthesia*. Philadelphia: W.B. Saunders.

197. ANSWER: D

Rationale: The spinal dorsal horn and root nerves and its analogous area in the medulla are complex sensory processing areas.

Reference: Harrigan, C. (1997). Chapter 6: The Central Nervous System. In J. Nagelhout & K. Zaglaniczny (Eds.), *Nurse Anesthesia*. Philadelphia: W.B. Saunders.

198. ANSWER: B

Rationale: The cerebral circulation comes from the internal carotid artery, the anterior and posterior communication arteries, and the vertebral arteries. Together these vessels form the circle of Willis. The external carotid supplies the face and neck but not the brain.

Reference: Harrigan, C. (1997). Chapter 6: The Central Nervous System. In J. Nagelhout & K. Zaglaniczny (Eds.), *Nurse Anesthesia*. Philadelphia: W.B. Saunders.

199. ANSWER: B

Rationale: As a specialized part of the sympathetic nervous system the adrenal medulla synthesizes and secretes the catecholamines epinephrine (80%) and norepinephrine (20%).

Reference: Karlet, M.C. & Sebastian, L.A. (1997). Chapter 12: The Endocrine System. In J. Nagelhout & K. Zaglaniczny (Eds.), *Nurse Anesthesia*. Philadelphia: W.B. Saunders.

200. ANSWER: D

Rationale: The Frank-Starling law is based on the observation that if the cardiac muscle is stretched it develops greater contractile tension. Atrial as well as ventricular muscle obeys this law.

Reference: Morgan, R.O., Jr. (1997). Chapter 8: The Cardiovascular System. In J. Nagelhout & K. Zaglaniczny (Eds.), *Nurse Anesthesia*. Philadelphia: W.B. Saunders.

201. ANSWER: C

Rationale: The phrenic nerve arises from the C3-C5 nerve roots at the lateral border of the anterior scalene muscle.

Reference: Hall, S.M. (1997). Chapter 9: Respiratory Anatomy and Physiology. In J. Nagelhout & K. Zaglaniczny (Eds.), *Nurse Anesthesia*. Philadelphia: W.B. Saunders.

202. ANSWER: B

Rationale: Aortic stenosis results in a systolic heart murmur. It is increased by leg elevation and amyl nitrate and decreased by squatting or Valsalva maneuver.

Reference: Morgan, R.O., Jr. (1997). Chapter 8: The Cardiovascular System. In J. Nagelhout & K. Zaglaniczny (Eds.), *Nurse Anesthesia*. Philadelphia: W.B. Saunders.

203. ANSWER: A

Rationale: Lack of aldosterone secretion greatly reduces sodium reabsorption and allows sodium chloride and water to be lost in great amounts. Acidosis develops because of a failure of potassium and hydrogen ions to be secreted in exchange for sodium reabsorption.

Reference: Karlet, M.C. & Sebastian, L.A. (1997). Chapter 12: The Endocrine System. In J. Nagelhout & K. Zaglaniczny (Eds.), *Nurse Anesthesia*. Philadelphia: W.B. Saunders.

204. ANSWER: C

Rationale: The postganglionic sympathetic nerves in the heart secrete the catecholamine norepinephrine.

Reference: Karlet, M.C. (1997). Chapter 40: Musculoskeletal Pathophysiology and Anesthesia. In J. Nagelhout & K. Zaglaniczny (Eds.), *Nurse Anesthesia*. Philadelphia: W.B. Saunders.

205. ANSWER: **A**

Rationale: The enzyme tyrosine hydroxylase is a rate-limiting enzyme in catecholamine synthesis. It catalyzes the step from tyrosine to dopa.
Reference: Alisoglu, R. (1997). Chapter 23: Cardiac Pharmacology. In J. Nagelhout & K. Zaglaniczny (Eds.), *Nurse Anesthesia*. Philadelphia: W.B. Saunders.

206. ANSWER: **D**

Rationale: The adrenal cortex secretes primarily cortisone, which has multiple metabolic functions for controlling proteins, carbohydrates, and fats. It also secretes aldosterone.
Reference: Karlet, M.C. & Sebastian, L.A. (1997). Chapter 12: The Endocrine System. In J. Nagelhout & K. Zaglaniczny (Eds.), *Nurse Anesthesia*. Philadelphia: W.B. Saunders.

207. ANSWER: **D**

Rationale: The patient with myxedema exhibits almost total lack of thyroid function and develops bagginess under the eyes and facial swelling. For unknown reasons an increase in fluid in the interstitial space causes puffiness of the face. The edema is of the nonpitting type.
Reference: Karlet, M.C. & Sebastian, L.A. (1997). Chapter 12: The Endocrine System. In J. Nagelhout & K. Zaglaniczny (Eds.), *Nurse Anesthesia*. Philadelphia: W.B. Saunders.

208. ANSWER: **B**

Rationale: The thyroid gland is composed of a large number of closed follicles filled with a secretory substance called colloid. The major constituent of colloid is thyroglobulin, which contains thyroid hormones within the molecule.
Reference: Karlet, M.C. & Sebastian, L.A. (1997). Chapter 12: The Endocrine System. In J. Nagelhout & K. Zaglaniczny (Eds.), *Nurse Anesthesia*. Philadelphia: W.B. Saunders.

209. ANSWER: **B**

Rationale: The tunica media exhibits muscle strength and is innovated by sympathetic and parasympathetic nerves, allowing for not only local control but also neuronal control of vascular tone.

Reference: Morgan, R.O., Jr. (1997). Chapter 8: The Cardiovascular System. In J. Nagelhout & K. Zaglaniczny (Eds.), *Nurse Anesthesia*. Philadelphia: W.B. Saunders.

210. ANSWER: **D**

Rationale: The portal vein, which carries nutrients from the gut to the liver, arises from the superior mesenteric and splenic veins, with some input from the renal veins, before it enters the liver.
Reference: Palmer, T.J. (1997). Chapter 10: Hepatobiliary and Gastrointestinal Disturbances. In J. Nagelhout & K. Zaglaniczny (Eds.), *Nurse Anesthesia*. Philadelphia: W.B. Saunders.

211. ANSWER: **D**

Rationale: The right and left coronary arteries originate from the sinuses of Valsalva in the aortic valve.
Reference: Morgan, R.O., Jr. (1997). Chapter 8: The Cardiovascular System. In J. Nagelhout & K. Zaglaniczny (Eds.), *Nurse Anesthesia*. Philadelphia: W.B. Saunders.

212. ANSWER: **C**

Rationale: The great and middle cardiac veins and the posterior left ventricle vein drain into the coronary sinus located in the right atria.
Reference: Morgan, R.O., Jr. (1997). Chapter 8: The Cardiovascular System. In J. Nagelhout & K. Zaglaniczny (Eds.), *Nurse Anesthesia*. Philadelphia: W.B. Saunders.

213. ANSWER: **D**

Rationale: Cardiac muscle relaxes during diastole, allowing free flow through the coronary circulation. The flow is greatest in early diastole and the least during late diastole. The subendocardium, especially of the left ventricle, develops much greater pressure than the epicardium. This reduces flow to these areas in comparison to the outer areas of the heart muscle.
Reference: Aprile, A.E. & Aprile, F.D. (1997). Chapter 38B: Cardiac Anesthesia. In J. Nagelhout & K. Zaglaniczny (Eds.), *Nurse Anesthesia*. Philadelphia: W.B. Saunders.

214. ANSWER: **A**

Rationale: The subendocardium of the left ventricle is most susceptible to ischemia because metabolic requirements are greater due to greater systolic shortening and blood flow is restricted during systole.

Reference: Aprile, A.E., Serwin, J.P. & Boctor, B. (1997). Chapter 38A: Cardiac Pathophysiology. In J. Nagelhout & K. Zaglaniczny (Eds.), *Nurse Anesthesia.* Philadelphia: W.B. Saunders.

215. ANSWER: C

Rationale: In general, cyanosis due to hypoxia is apparent by 6 months of age in a patient with tetralogy of Fallot. This cyanosis is due to right-to-left endocardiac shunt with decreased pulmonary blood flow and arterial hypoxia.

Reference: Dobbins, P. & Hall, S.M. (1997). Chapter 14: Pediatric Anesthesia. In J. Nagelhout & K. Zaglaniczny (Eds.), *Nurse Anesthesia.* Philadelphia: W.B. Saunders.

216. ANSWER: B

Rationale: Relative humidity is a percent expression of the actual water vapor content of a gas compared with its capacity to carry water at a given temperature. At room temperature optimal humidity is 60% to 70%.

Reference: Dosch, M.P. (1997). Chapter 26: Anesthesia Equipment. In J. Nagelhout & K. Zaglaniczny (Eds.), *Nurse Anesthesia.* Philadelphia: W.B. Saunders.

217. ANSWER: C

Rationale: A line isolation monitor is a device that continuously monitors the integrity of an isolated power system. This device will sound an alarm if a faulty piece of equipment is connected to an isolated system changing it back to a conventional grounded system.

Reference: Dosch, M.P. (1997). Chapter 26: Anesthesia Equipment. In J. Nagelhout & K. Zaglaniczny (Eds.), *Nurse Anesthesia.* Philadelphia: W.B. Saunders.

218. ANSWER: C

Rationale: Phenobarbital is one of the most potent hepatic enzyme-inducing agents. Patients who take phenobarbital have an increased ability to metabolize other hepatic eliminated drugs.

Reference: Troop, M. (1997). Chapter 16: Pharmacokinetics. In J. Nagelhout & K. Zaglaniczny (Eds.), *Nurse Anesthesia.* Philadelphia: W.B. Saunders.

219. ANSWER: C

Rationale: The inspiratory capacity equals the tidal volume plus the inspiratory reserve volume. This equals about 3500 mL in a healthy adult.

Reference: Hall, S.M. (1997). Chapter 9: Respiratory Anatomy and Physiology. In J. Nagelhout & K. Zaglaniczny (Eds.), *Nurse Anesthesia.* Philadelphia: W.B. Saunders.

220. ANSWER: C

Rationale: Presynaptic receptors are referred to as autoreceptors because they autoregulate local control for the release of neurotransmitters from that particular neuron. They are designated with the number 2; thus, $alpha_2$ receptors control norepinephrine release.

Reference: Alisoglu, R. (1997). Chapter 23: Cardiac Pharmacology. In J. Nagelhout & K. Zaglaniczny (Eds.), *Nurse Anesthesia.* Philadelphia: W.B. Saunders.

221. ANSWER: D

Rationale: The blood/gas partition coefficient of an anesthetic indicates the speed of induction and emergence. A low blood/gas coefficient would yield a rapid uptake and elimination of the inhalation drug.

Reference: Nagelhout, J.J. (1997). Chapter 17: Uptake and Distribution of Inhalation Anesthetics. In J. Nagelhout & K. Zaglaniczny (Eds.), *Nurse Anesthesia.* Philadelphia: W.B. Saunders.

222. ANSWER: D

Rationale: The classic mnemonic regarding atropine poisoning states: red as a beet, hot as a hare, dry as sand, and mad as a hatter. Atropine poisoning produces central nervous system excitation not sedation.

Reference: Alisoglu, R. (1997). Chapter 23: Cardiac Pharmacology. In J. Nagelhout & K. Zaglaniczny (Eds.), *Nurse Anesthesia.* Philadelphia: W.B. Saunders.

223. ANSWER: **A**

> ***Rationale:*** The molecules bombard the wall of a container and create a pressure known as the saturated vapor pressure. Vapor pressure is independent of atmospheric pressure and depends on the physical characteristics of the liquid and the temperature. The boiling point is that temperature at which the vapor pressure equals atmospheric pressure.
>
> *Reference:* Normille, H.J. (1997). Chapter 5: Cell Anatomy and Physiology. In J. Nagelhout & K. Zaglaniczny (Eds.), *Nurse Anesthesia*. Philadelphia: W.B. Saunders.

224. ANSWER: **D**

> ***Rationale:*** Venous capacitance exceeds other vascular beds. Eighty-four percent of the blood volume is located in blood vessels, with the greatest majority being in the veins.
>
> *Reference:* Morgan, R.O., Jr. (1997). Chapter 8: The Cardiovascular System. In J. Nagelhout & K. Zaglaniczny (Eds.), *Nurse Anesthesia*. Philadelphia: W.B. Saunders.

225. ANSWER: **D**

> ***Rationale:*** The left anterior descending artery courses downward over the anterior of the left ventricle wall and supplies this area with contributions from the circumflex artery.
>
> *Reference:* Morgan, R.O. (1997). Chapter 8: The Cardiovascular System. In J. Nagelhout & K. Zaglaniczny (Eds.), *Nurse Anesthesia*. Philadelphia: W.B. Saunders.

226. ANSWER: **B**

> ***Rationale:*** A partition coefficient is the ratio that indicates to what degree a substance separates itself when in different compartments. The blood-gas solubility coefficient is an indicator of anesthetic speed.
>
> *Reference:* Nagelhout, J.J. (1997). Chapter 17: Uptake and Distribution of Inhalation Anesthetics. In J. Nagelhout & K. Zaglaniczny (Eds.), *Nurse Anesthesia*. Philadelphia: W.B. Saunders.

CHAPTER 2

Equipment

◆ ◆ ◆

1. How should nondisposable equipment be sterilized after use on a patient with tuberculosis?

   A. The use of alcohol wash is acceptable.
   B. Disinfect with a chemical such as glutaraldehyde.
   C. Forget it and throw the equipment away.
   D. Use soap and water to clean equipment.

2. Which organization published a set of anesthesia machine requirements to increase patient safety?

   A. Food and Drug Administration (FDA)
   B. American Association of Nurse Anesthetists (AANA)
   C. Ohmeda Anesthesia Systems (OAS)
   D. American National Standards Institute (ANSI)

3. What does the American Society for Testing and Materials regulate?

   A. hospital operating rooms
   B. anesthesia gas machines
   C. anesthesia reimbursement
   D. anesthetic personnel

4. All of the following are true of pulse oximetry except:

   A. Certain substances in the blood can alter readings.
   B. It measures functional saturation.
   C. It utilizes red and infrared light wavelengths.
   D. It measures fractional saturation.

5. All of the following are true of patients with methemoglobin except:

   A. The reading will be falsely high if actual SaO_2 < 85%.
   B. The reading will be falsely low if actual SaO_2 > 85%.
   C. It has no effect on pulse oximetry.
   D. It absorbs red and infrared light.

6. The correct width of a blood pressure cuff is:

   A. 60% the circumference of the extremity
   B. 40% the circumference of the extremity
   C. 20% the circumference of the extremity
   D. 50% the circumference of the extremity

7. Falsely low readings will occur with the use of blood pressure cuffs in which of the following circumstances:

   A. quick deflation
   B. cuff is too loose
   C. extremity is above the heart
   D. cuff is tight

8. The device that prevents reverse flow of gases from the anesthesia machine to the pipeline or atmosphere is:

   A. Diameter Index Safety System
   B. check valve
   C. Pin Index Safety System
   D. pressure gauge

9. The reserve cylinders located on the anesthesia machine are size:

   A. G
   B. H
   C. E
   D. A

10. All the following are functions of the check valve except:

    A. It reduces pressure in the system.
    B. It minimizes leakage from an open cylinder to the atmosphere if one cylinder is absent.
    C. It minimizes gas transfer from a cylinder at high pressure to one with a lower pressure.
    D. It allows uninterrupted gas flow from one cylinder to another.

11. The component of the anesthesia machine that changes the pressure of an incoming gas to a pressure suitable for use in the anesthesia machine is:

    A. safety valve
    B. pressure increasing valve
    C. pressure regulator
    D. check valve

12. The system designed to prevent cylinder interchangeability is:

A. cylinder regulator system
B. Diameter Index Safety System
C. yoke
D. Pin Index Safety System

13. If two cylinders are open at the same time, the cylinder supply pressure gauge will:

A. not function
B. indicate the pressure of the cylinder with the highest pressure
C. read the pressures of the two cylinders combined
D. give an erroneous reading

14. The first-stage regulator reduces gas pressure to:

A. 15 psi
B. 60 psi
C. 20 psi
D. 50 psi

15. Normal oxygen cylinder pressure is:

A. 1500 psig
B. 659 psig
C. 2200 psig
D. 745 psig

16. Nitrous oxide cylinder pressure may be as much as:

A. 2200 psig
B. 745 psig
C. 640 psig
D. 1500 psig

17. During normal operation, the reserve cylinders should be:

A. turned off
B. left on in case of pipeline failure
C. left in partial open position
D. It doesn't matter because pipeline gas will always be preferentially used.

18. The oxygen failure safety valve is controlled by:

A. oxygen pressure
B. oxygen flow
C. oxygen supply
D. the pipeline

19. The oxygen failure safety valve:

A. alerts only to decreased supply pressure
B. prevents a hypoxic mixture of gases
C. responds to decreased oxygen flow
D. alerts to decreased supply volume only

20. The oxygen failure safety valve causes the flow of anesthetic or inert gases to cease if:

A. nitrous oxide flow exceeds oxygen flow
B. oxygen flow is less than 1 L
C. the backup cylinder is nonfunctional
D. oxygen supply pressure falls to about 25 psig

21. The second-stage regulator reduces oxygen pressure to:

A. 45 psig
B. 16 psig
C. 10 psig
D. 45–55 psig

22. The second-stage regulator is located:

A. at the hanger yoke
B. just after the flowmeter
C. just before the flowmeter
D. at the common gas outlet

23. All the following are components of the high pressure system except:

A. hanger yoke
B. oxygen flush valve
C. yoke block
D. first-stage regulator

24. The oxygen flush valve delivers O_2 at:

A. 20 L/min
B. 16 L/min
C. 45 L/min
D. 35–75 L/min

25. All the following are components of the low pressure system except:

A. common gas outlet
B. oxygen flush valve
C. vaporizers
D. pressure relief valve

26. When a volatile liquid is in a closed container, molecules escape from the liquid phase to the gaseous phase. These molecules bombard the walls of the container, which is referred to as:

    A. intimacy of gas-liquid interface
    B. latent heat of vaporization
    C. vapor pressure
    D. thermal conductivity

27. Physical characteristics fundamental to vaporizer design include all except:

    A. vapor pressure
    B. radiant conductivity
    C. latent heat of vaporization
    D. specific heat

28. Contemporary vaporizers are:

    A. noncalibrated
    B. bubble through
    C. measured flow
    D. variable bypass

29. Currently used vaporizers are the following except:

    A. nonmeasured flow
    B. temperature compensated
    C. variable bypass
    D. inside the breathing system

30. The "pumping effect" occurs most often under all the following conditions except:

    A. high dial settings
    B. low levels of liquid in anesthetic chamber
    C. low flow rates
    D. during controlled or assisted respirations

31. Intermittent back-pressure resulting in increased vaporizer concentration is known as:

    A. pumping effect
    B. flow compensation
    C. high vaporizer pressure
    D. pressurizing effect

32. The Mapelson system in which fresh gas flow is distal to the reservoir bag is the:

    A. Mapelson F
    B. Mapelson D
    C. Mapelson A
    D. Mapelson B

33. With the Mapelson D, rebreathing is prevented by:

    A. fresh gas flows equal to the minute ventilation
    B. fresh gas flows greater than two times the minute ventilation
    C. short expiratory pause
    D. fast respiratory rates

34. The Bain circuit is a modification of the:

    A. Mapelson A
    B. Mapelson E
    C. Mapelson D
    D. Mapelson F

35. All the following are true of the Bain circuit except:

    A. Fresh gas enters the circuit at the patient end.
    B. It may be used for controlled as well as spontaneous ventilation.
    C. It is a coaxial circuit.
    D. Oxygen disconnect is easily recognized.

36. The Jackson-Reese is a modification of a:

    A. Mapelson E
    B. Mapelson D
    C. Mapelson F
    D. Mapelson A

37. All the following are advantages of the circle system except:

    A. minimized pollution
    B. conservation of moisture and heat
    C. can be used with low flows
    D. unlikely disconnect

38. The end product of the soda lime reaction is:

    A. calcium carbonate
    B. carbonic acid
    C. CO_2 and water
    D. potassium carbonate

39. The primary product of the baralyme reaction is:

   A. calcium carbonate
   B. barium hydroxide
   C. CO_2 and water
   D. potassium hydroxide

40. The volatile agent that may become partially degraded by soda lime is:

   A. desflurane
   B. enflurane
   C. isoflurane
   D. sevoflurane

41. Ventilator bellows on the anesthesia machine are classified by:

   A. movement on expiration
   B. size
   C. pneumatic ability
   D. movement on inspiration

42. If the anesthesia scavenging system becomes plugged:

   A. gases will go backward toward the patient
   B. gases will be vented into the room
   C. the equivalent of PEEP will occur
   D. gases will vent to the vacuum

43. What color are air tanks designated?

   A. green
   B. yellow
   C. blue
   D. black

44. The line isolation monitor alarm indicates that:

   A. a fire is imminent
   B. the power supply is partially grounded
   C. microshocks are present in monitoring equipment
   D. power has been turned off

45. The pulmonary artery wedge pressure is an approximation of which of the following?

   A. cardiac output
   B. ejection fraction
   C. pulmonary artery systolic pressure
   D. left ventricular end-diastolic pressure

```
┌─────────────────────────────────┐
│      A N S W E R S              │
│  TO PRACTICE QUESTIONS          │
│       CHAPTER 2                 │
└─────────────────────────────────┘
```

1. ANSWER: **B**

   Rationale: The tuberculosis bacilli can be safely removed from equipment by thorough washing with soap and use of a product such as glutaraldehyde.
   Reference: Dosch, M.P. (1997). Chapter 26: Anesthesia Equipment. In J. Nagelhout & K. Zaglaniczny (Eds.), *Nurse Anesthesia*. Philadelphia: W.B. Saunders.

2. ANSWER: **D**

   Rationale: The ANSI published machine safety standards that provided guidelines for manufacturers regarding minimum performance, design characteristics, and safety requirements for anesthesia machines.
   Reference: Dosch, M.P. (1997). Chapter 26: Anesthesia Equipment. In J. Nagelhout & K. Zaglaniczny (Eds.), *Nurse Anesthesia*. Philadelphia: W.B. Saunders.

3. ANSWER: **B**

   Rationale: ASTM standards have now superseded the ANSI standards. The ASTM standards are now the ones that are met by anesthesia machine manufacturers.
   Reference: Dosch, M.P. (1997). Chapter 26: Anesthesia Equipment. In J. Nagelhout & K. Zaglaniczny (Eds.), *Nurse Anesthesia*. Philadelphia: W.B. Saunders.

4. ANSWER: **D**

   Rationale: Pulse oximetry measures functional hemoglobin saturation, which is why it can be altered when different types of abnormal hemoglobins are present.
   Reference: Sinkovich, J.A. & Kossick, M.A. (1997). Chapter 27: Clinical Monitoring in Anesthesia. In J. Nagelhout & K. Zaglaniczny (Eds.), *Nurse Anesthesia*. Philadelphia: W.B. Saunders.

5. ANSWER: **C**

   Rationale: Methemoglobin influences the accuracy because it absorbs both red and infrared light. At toxic levels the saturation tends to be 85% regardless of the actual P_{O_2}.
   Reference: Sinkovich, J.A. & Kossick, M.A. (1997). Chapter 27: Clinical Monitoring in Anesthesia. In J. Nagelhout & K. Zaglaniczny (Eds.), *Nurse Anesthesia*. Philadelphia: W.B. Saunders.

6. ANSWER: **B**

   Rationale: The American Heart Association recommends that the bladder width of the blood pressure cuff should approximate 40% of the circumference of the extremity. Its length should encircle 60%.
   Reference: Sinkovich, J.A. & Kossick, M.A. (1997). Chapter 27: Clinical Monitoring in Anesthesia. In J. Nagelhout & K. Zaglaniczny (Eds.), *Nurse Anesthesia*. Philadelphia: W.B. Saunders.

7. ANSWER: **D**

   Rationale: Falsely high estimates result when the cuff is too small or applied too loosely, when the extremity is below the heart, or when uneven compression is transmitted to the artery. Falsely low readings result from the opposite conditions.
   Reference: Sinkovich, J.A. & Kossick, M.A. (1997). Chapter 27: Clinical Monitoring in Anesthesia. In J. Nagelhout & K. Zaglaniczny (Eds.), *Nurse Anesthesia*. Philadelphia: W.B. Saunders.

8. ANSWER: **B**

   Rationale: A check valve is located downstream from the inlet. It prevents reverse flow of gases from the machine to the pipeline or to the atmosphere.
   Reference: Sinkovich, J.A. & Kossick, M.A. (1997). Chapter 27: Clinical Monitoring in Anesthesia. In J. Nagelhout & K. Zaglaniczny (Eds.), *Nurse Anesthesia*. Philadelphia: W.B. Saunders.

9. ANSWER: **C**

   Rationale: Anesthesia machines have reserve E cylinders if a pipeline supply source is not available or malfunctions.

Reference: Dosch, M.P. (1997). Chapter 26: Anesthesia Equipment. In J. Nagelhout & K. Zaglaniczny (Eds.), *Nurse Anesthesia*. Philadelphia: W.B. Saunders.

10. ANSWER: **A**

Rationale: Pressure in the system is reduced by pressure-reducing valves. The check valves mainly control the forward flow of gases through the system.
Reference: Dosch, M.P. (1997). Chapter 26: Anesthesia Equipment. In J. Nagelhout & K. Zaglaniczny (Eds.), *Nurse Anesthesia*. Philadelphia: W.B. Saunders.

11. ANSWER: **C**

Rationale: Each cylinder supply source has a pressure-reducing valve known as the cylinder pressure regulator. It reduces the high and variable storage pressure to a lower more constant pressure suitable for use.
Reference: Dosch, M.P. (1997). Chapter 26: Anesthesia Equipment. In J. Nagelhout & K. Zaglaniczny (Eds.), *Nurse Anesthesia*. Philadelphia: W.B. Saunders.

12. ANSWER: **D**

Rationale: The Pin Index Safety System is a safeguard introduced to eliminate cylinder interchanging and the possibility of accidentally placing the incorrect gas on a yoke designed for another gas.
Reference: Dosch, M.P. (1997). Chapter 26: Anesthesia Equipment. In J. Nagelhout & K. Zaglaniczny (Eds.), *Nurse Anesthesia*. Philadelphia: W.B. Saunders.

13. ANSWER: **B**

Rationale: The gauge will indicate the pressure in the cylinder having the higher pressure when two reserve cylinders of the same gas are opened at the same time.
Reference: Dosch, M.P. (1997). Chapter 26: Anesthesia Equipment. In J. Nagelhout & K. Zaglaniczny (Eds.), *Nurse Anesthesia*. Philadelphia: W.B. Saunders.

14. ANSWER: **D**

Rationale: The first-stage pressure regulator reduces the gas pressures from their high cylinder level to 45 to 50 psi. The second-

stage pressure regulators then reduce the pressure even further for specific gases.
Reference: Dosch, M.P. (1997). Chapter 26: Anesthesia Equipment. In J. Nagelhout & K. Zaglaniczny (Eds.), *Nurse Anesthesia*. Philadelphia: W.B. Saunders.

15. ANSWER: **C**

Rationale: Oxygen cylinder pressure when the tank is full reads approximately 2200 psig.
Reference: Dosch, M.P. (1997). Chapter 26: Anesthesia Equipment. In J. Nagelhout & K. Zaglaniczny (Eds.), *Nurse Anesthesia*. Philadelphia: W.B. Saunders.

16. ANSWER: **B**

Rationale: The nitrous cylinder pressure regardless of how much is in the cylinder will read approximately 745 psig.
Reference: Dosch, M.P. (1997). Chapter 26: Anesthesia Equipment. In J. Nagelhout & K. Zaglaniczny (Eds.), *Nurse Anesthesia*. Philadelphia: W.B. Saunders.

17. ANSWER: **A**

Rationale: Reserve cylinders should be kept off because they will become depleted and no reserve supply will be available if there is a pipeline failure.
Reference: Dosch, M.P. (1997). Chapter 26: Anesthesia Equipment. In J. Nagelhout & K. Zaglaniczny (Eds.), *Nurse Anesthesia*. Philadelphia: W.B. Saunders.

18. ANSWER: **A**

Rationale: Oxygen safety valves on anesthesia machines are set to sense pressure changes below adequate levels. For example, if the pressure falls below 20 psi a valve closes that changes other gas flows as well.
Reference: Dosch, M.P. (1997). Chapter 26: Anesthesia Equipment. In J. Nagelhout & K. Zaglaniczny (Eds.), *Nurse Anesthesia*. Philadelphia: W.B. Saunders.

19. ANSWER: **A**

Rationale: The failure safety valve senses oxygen pressure. It does not proportion gases and therefore may not prevent the delivery of hypoxic mixtures of anesthetic gases.

Reference: Dosch, M.P. (1997). Chapter 26: Anesthesia Equipment. In J. Nagelhout & K. Zaglaniczny (Eds.), *Nurse Anesthesia*. Philadelphia: W.B. Saunders.

20. ANSWER: **D**

Rationale: Oxygen safety valves are set to close when the pressure falls below 20 to 25 psi.
Reference: Dosch, M.P. (1997). Chapter 26: Anesthesia Equipment. In J. Nagelhout & K. Zaglaniczny (Eds.), *Nurse Anesthesia*. Philadelphia: W.B. Saunders.

21. ANSWER: **B**

Rationale: Second-stage regulators reduce oxygen pressure to 12 to 19 psi. The pressure shut-off valves have a higher threshold of 20 to 30 psi. This ensures that oxygen is the last gas flow to decrease if oxygen pressure falls.
Reference: Dosch, M.P. (1997). Chapter 26: Anesthesia Equipment. In J. Nagelhout & K. Zaglaniczny (Eds.), *Nurse Anesthesia*. Philadelphia: W.B. Saunders.

22. ANSWER: **C**

Rationale: The second-stage regulator is located downstream from the oxygen supply source. This regulator supplies a constant pressure to the oxygen flow control valves regardless of fluctuating line pressures.
Reference: Dosch, M.P. (1997). Chapter 26: Anesthesia Equipment. In J. Nagelhout & K. Zaglaniczny (Eds.), *Nurse Anesthesia*. Philadelphia: W.B. Saunders.

23. ANSWER: **B**

Rationale: The oxygen flush valve allows direct communication between the high-pressure circuit and low-pressure oxygen circuits. It can deliver 35 to 75 L/min into the breathing circuit.
Reference: Dosch, M.P. (1997). Chapter 26: Anesthesia Equipment. In J. Nagelhout & K. Zaglaniczny (Eds.), *Nurse Anesthesia*. Philadelphia: W.B. Saunders.

24. ANSWER: **D**

Rationale: Actuation of the oxygen flush valve will result in the delivery of 35 to 75 L/min of oxygen.

25. ANSWER: **B**

Rationale: The oxygen flush valve is considered a component of the intermediate pressure system because it allows communication between the low- and high-pressure apparatus.
Reference: Dosch, M.P. (1997). Chapter 26: Anesthesia Equipment. In J. Nagelhout & K. Zaglaniczny (Eds.), *Nurse Anesthesia*. Philadelphia: W.B. Saunders.

26. ANSWER: **C**

Rationale: The molecules bombarding the wall of the container create a pressure referred to as the saturated vapor pressure.
Reference: Hall, S.M. (1997). Chapter 4: Chemistry and Physics for Anesthesia. In J. Naglehout & K. Zaglaniczny (Eds.), *Nurse Anesthesia*. Philadelphia: W.B. Saunders.

27. ANSWER: **B**

Rationale: The vaporizers are constructed of metals that have a high thermal conductivity that helps maintain a uniform temperature in the system.
Reference: Hall, S.M. (1997). Chapter 4: Chemistry and Physics for Anesthesia. In J. Naglehout & K. Zaglaniczny (Eds.), *Nurse Anesthesia*. Philadelphia: W.B. Saunders.

28. ANSWER: **D**

Rationale: Modern vaporizers are classified as variable bypass. This refers to the method for regulating output concentration.
Reference: Dosch, M.P. (1997). Chapter 26: Anesthesia Equipment. In J. Nagelhout & K. Zaglaniczny (Eds.), *Nurse Anesthesia*. Philadelphia: W.B. Saunders.

29. ANSWER: **D**

Rationale: Modern vaporizers are classified as agent specific, out of circuit because they are designed to accommodate a single agent and to be located outside the breathing circuit.
Reference: Dosch, M.P. (1997). Chapter 26: Anesthesia Equipment. In J. Nagelhout & K.

Zaglaniczny (Eds.), *Nurse Anesthesia*. Philadelphia: W.B. Saunders.

30. ANSWER: **A**

Rationale: Intermittent back-pressure associated with positive-pressure ventilation or oxygen flushing can cause a higher vaporizer output than the dialed setting. This is known as the pumping effect and occurs most often at low flow rates, low dial settings, and low levels of anesthetic liquid in the vaporizer.

Reference: Dosch, M.P. (1997). Chapter 26: Anesthesia Equipment. In J. Nagelhout & K. Zaglaniczny (Eds.), *Nurse Anesthesia*. Philadelphia: W.B. Saunders.

31. ANSWER: **A**

Rationale: Intermittent back-pressure caused by positive-pressure ventilation or oxygen flushing can result in higher vaporizer concentrations than the dial settings. This is known as the "pumping effect."

Reference: Dosch M.P. (1997). Chapter 26: Anesthesia Equipment. In J. Nagelhout & K. Zaglaniczny (Eds.), *Nurse Anesthesia*. Philadelphia: W.B. Saunders.

32. ANSWER: **C**

Rationale: The Mapelson A, also known as the Magill, circuit consists of a corrugated tube, a reservoir bag, and a fresh gas inflow distal to the bag.

Reference: Donnins, P. & Hall, S.M. (1997). Chapter 14: Pediatric Anesthesia. In J. Nagelhout & K. Zaglaniczny (Eds.), *Nurse Anesthesia*. Philadelphia: W.B. Saunders.

33. ANSWER: **B**

Rationale: Rebreathing can be prevented by high fresh gas flows, two times the minute ventilation, and a long expiratory pause.

Reference: Dobbins, P. & Hall, S.M. (1997). Chapter 14: Pediatric Anesthesia. In J. Nagelhout & K. Zaglaniczny (Eds.), *Nurse Anesthesia*. Philadelphia: W.B. Saunders.

34. ANSWER: **C**

Rationale: The Bain circuit is a modification of the Mapelson D system. Rebreathing can be prevented with fresh gas flows,

two times the minute volume, similar to the Mapelson D.

Reference: Dobbins, P. & Hall, S.M. (1997). Chapter 14: Pediatric Anesthesia. In J. Nagelhout & K. Zaglaniczny (Eds.), *Nurse Anesthesia*. Philadelphia: W.B. Saunders.

35. ANSWER: **D**

Rationale: The hazards of the Bain circuit include unrecognized disconnection or kinking of the inner fresh gas hose, which may lead to hypoxia from inadequate gas flow or increased resistance.

Reference: Dobbins, P. & Hall, S.M. (1997). Chapter 14: Pediatric Anesthesia. In J. Nagelhout & K. Zaglaniczny (Eds.), *Nurse Anesthesia*. Philadelphia: W.B. Saunders.

36. ANSWER: **B**

Rationale: The Jackson-Reese is a T-piece system modification of the Mapelson D. It incorporates a relief mechanism for venting exhaled gases.

Reference: Dobbins, P. & Hall, S.M. (1997). Chapter 14: Pediatric Anesthesia. In J. Nagelhout & K. Zaglaniczny (Eds.), *Nurse Anesthesia*. Philadelphia: W.B. Saunders.

37. ANSWER: **D**

Rationale: The circle has approximately 10 connections, all of which can disconnect or leak.

Reference: Dosch, M.P. (1997). Chapter 26: Anesthesia Equipment. In J. Nagelhout & K. Zaglaniczny (Eds.), *Nurse Anesthesia*. Philadelphia: W.B. Saunders.

38. ANSWER: **A**

Rationale: Sodium carbonate and calcium hydroxide result in the production of calcium carbonate during the soda lime reaction.

Reference: Dosch, M.P. (1997). Chapter 26: Anesthesia Equipment. In J. Nagelhout & K. Zaglaniczny (Eds.), *Nurse Anesthesia*. Philadelphia: W.B. Saunders.

39. ANSWER: **A**

Rationale: Calcium carbonate is also the end product of baralyme reactions. The difference is that more water is liberated by baralyme than soda lime.

Reference: Dosch, M.P. (1997). Chapter 26: Anesthesia Equipment. In J. Nagelhout & K. Zaglaniczny (Eds.), *Nurse Anesthesia*. Philadelphia: W.B. Saunders.

40. ANSWER: **D**

Rationale: Sevoflurane appears to break down in soda lime. It produces a toxin that has been named compound A and has been shown to be problematic in animal studies.

Reference: Dosch, M.P. (1997). Chapter 26: Anesthesia Equipment. In J. Nagelhout & K. Zaglaniczny (Eds.), *Nurse Anesthesia*. Philadelphia: W.B. Saunders.

41. ANSWER: **A**

Rationale: Ascending (standing) bellows ascend during the expiratory phase; descending (hanging) bellows descend during the expiratory phase.

Reference: Dosch, M.P. (1997). Chapter 26: Anesthesia Equipment. In J. Nagelhout & K. Zaglaniczny (Eds.), *Nurse Anesthesia*. Philadelphia: W.B. Saunders.

42. ANSWER: **B**

Rationale: Obstruction of the scavenging system can cause excessive positive pressure to be transmitted to the breathing system, resulting in gases being vented into the room.

Reference: Dosch, M.P. (1997). Chapter 26: Anesthesia Equipment. In J. Nagelhout & K.

Zaglaniczny (Eds.), *Nurse Anesthesia*. Philadelphia: W.B. Saunders.

43. ANSWER: **B**

Rationale: In the United States, medical gas cylinders have a standard color. Those of oxygen are green; air, yellow; nitrous oxide, blue; and nitrogen, black.

Reference: Dosch, M.P. (1997). Chapter 26: Anesthesia Equipment. In J. Nagelhout & K. Zaglaniczny (Eds.), *Nurse Anesthesia*. Philadelphia: W.B. Saunders.

44. ANSWER: **B**

Rationale: The alarm of the line isolation monitor merely indicates that the power supply has partially reverted to a grounded system because of a single fault. Two faults are required for a shock to occur.

Reference: Dosch, M.P. (1997). Chapter 26: Anesthesia Equipment. In J. Nagelhout & K. Zaglaniczny (Eds.), *Nurse Anesthesia*. Philadelphia: W.B. Saunders.

45. ANSWER: **D**

Rationale: When the catheter is wedged and the valves in the heart are open, the catheter measures pressure in the left ventricle.

Reference: Sinkovich, J.A. & Kossick, M.A. (1997). Chapter 27: Clinical Monitoring in Anesthesia. In J. Nagelhout & K. Zaglaniczny (Eds.), *Nurse Anesthesia*. Philadelphia: W.B. Saunders.

CHAPTER 3

Basic Principles

♦ ♦ ♦

1. A solution containing a 1:200,000 concentration equals:

   A. 0.5 μg/mL
   B. 1 μg/mL
   C. 5 μg/mL
   D. 50 μg/mL

2. If a patient is on MAO therapy, which is the vasopressor of choice?

   A. mephentermine
   B. phenylephrine
   C. ephedrine
   D. metaraminol

3. What premedication might be important in the diabetic patient with peripheral neuropathy?

   A. sodium citrate to increase gastric pH
   B. metoclopramide to increase gastric emptying
   C. glycopyrrolate to decrease oral secretions
   D. cimetidine for H_2 receptor antagonism

4. Which of the following would be a possible indication of a venous air embolism?

   A. increased ET_{CO_2}
   B. decreased ET_{CO_2}
   C. increased arterial blood pressure
   D. decreased pulmonary artery pressure

5. Which of the following IV solutions is best avoided in the neurosurgical patient?

   A. balanced salt solution
   B. dextrose and water
   C. normal saline
   D. lactated Ringer's solution

6. One of the quickest ways to decrease intracranial pressure in the acute situation is:

   A. cerebrospinal fluid drainage
   B. corticosteroid administration
   C. hyperventilation
   D. loop diuretics

7. In the patient with increased intracranial pressure, what should the ideal Pa_{CO_2} level be?

   A. 30–35 mm Hg
   B. 22–29 mm Hg
   C. 25–30 mm Hg
   D. 35–40 mm Hg

8. Which inhalation agent increases pulmonary vascular resistance?

   A. halothane
   B. enflurane
   C. nitrous oxide
   D. isoflurane

9. The operation of what monitoring device uses Lambert-Beer law?

   A. pulse oximetry
   B. ET_{CO_2} monitoring
   C. pneumatic blood pressure cuff
   D. mass spectrometry

10. How do you calculate cardiac output?

    A. CO = SVR × PVR
    B. CO = SV × HR
    C. CO = HR × SVR/2
    D. CO = SV × PVR

11. How do you calculate cardiac index?

    A. CI = SV × HR
    B. CI = CO × BSA
    C. CI = CO/BSA
    D. CI = NAP − CVP × BSA

12. What is the normal value for cardiac index?

    A. 2.5–4.2 L/min/m^2
    B. 5–6 L/min
    C. 2–3 L/min
    D. 5–6 L/min/m^2

13. How do you calculate systemic vascular resistance?

    A. SVR = PVR × SV
    B. SVR = (MAP − CVP) × 80/CO
    C. SVR = MAP − CO/80
    D. cannot determine

14. What is the normal value for SVR?

    A. 100–200 L/min
    B. 900–1000 L/min/m²
    C. 5–6 dynes/sec/cm⁻⁵
    D. 1200–1500 dynes/sec/cm⁻⁵

15. All of the following are complications of central venous catheters except:

    A. erratic and inaccurate readings
    B. infection
    C. venous air embolism
    D. catheter shearing

16. Which vessel is at greatest risk of accidental puncture if a left internal jugular approach is used to place a central venous line?

    A. subclavian vein
    B. external jugular vein
    C. carotid artery
    D. subclavian artery

17. One way to decrease the risk of venous air embolism during central venous catheter placement might include:

    A. have the patient hold his or her breath during the procedure
    B. administer vasopressors to increase blood pressure
    C. place the patient in a Trendelenburg position
    D. There is no way to prevent it.

18. A patient with myasthenia gravis is at major surgical risk for:

    A. aspiration pneumonitis
    B. hypothermia
    C. postoperative ventilatory failure
    D. prolonged muscle paralysis after succinylcholine administration

19. The patient complains of an intense, searing pain upon regional anesthetic injection; what most likely occurred?

    A. patient really just felt paresthesia
    B. the needle hit bone
    C. intraneuronal injection
    D. intra-arterial injection

20. Name the induction agent of choice for a patient with cardiac tamponade:

    A. thiopental sodium
    B. propofol
    C. etomidate
    D. ketamine

21. Which lung volume is reduced under anesthesia?

    A. total lung capacity
    B. residual volume only
    C. functional residual capacity
    D. vital capacity

22. Why does functional residual capacity decrease in the supine or prone position?

    A. Compliance is reduced as abdominal contents push up against the diaphragm.
    B. Intrathoracic blood volume decreases.
    C. Pulmonary lung resistance increases as a patient's position changes.
    D. There is no change in functional residual capacity.

23. Which intravenous anesthetic directly depresses the adrenal cortex?

    A. thiopental sodium
    B. propofol
    C. etomidate
    D. ketamine

24. Numbness over the lateral aspect of the thigh may be caused by damage to what nerve?

    A. lateral femoral cutaneous nerve
    B. common peroneal nerve
    C. sciatic nerve
    D. ulnar nerve

25. Complications unique to nasotracheal intubation include all of the following except:

    A. epistaxis
    B. dislodgment of pharyngeal tonsils (adenoids)
    C. tracheoesophageal fistula
    D. maxillary sinusitis

26. Dextrose-containing solutions are avoided in neurosurgery because they:

A. decrease urinary output
B. provide inadequate intravascular volume
C. promote cerebral edema
D. increase cellular metabolism

27. How much CO_2 is dissolved in arterial blood?

A. 10 mL CO_2/dL blood
B. 5 mL CO_2/dL blood
C. 1.5 mL CO_2/dL blood
D. 2.5 mL CO_2/dL blood

28. At what postconceptual age should a premature infant be scheduled for elective/outpatient surgery?

A. 30 weeks
B. 60 weeks
C. 120 weeks
D. 60 days

29. Prematurity is defined as birth before _____ weeks of gestation?

A. 20
B. 37
C. 45
D. 47

30. What is the maintenance fluid requirement for a 5-kg patient?

A. 20 mL/h
B. 22 mL/h
C. 10 mL/h
D. 14 mL/h

31. What is the maintenance fluid requirement for a 25-kg patient?

A. 25 mL/h
B. 54 mL/h
C. 65 mL/h
D. 75 mL/h

32. What is the mainstay therapy for acute/subacute management of intracranial pressure?

A. diuretics
B. normovolemia
C. hyperventilation
D. antihypertensives

33. By what mechanism does citrate produce its anticoagulant effects?

A. increases prothombin time
B. binds to calcium
C. binds to sodium
D. decreases factor VIII

34. What preservative/anticoagulant substance found in packed red blood cells can cause toxicity?

A. calcium
B. citrate
C. phosphate
D. bicarbonate

35. Packed red blood cells should not be reconstituted in lactated Ringer's solution because:

A. The calcium in lactated Ringer's may cause clotting if mixed with red blood cells.
B. The hypertonic solution may cause hemolysis.
C. A metabolic acidosis results when they are administered together.
D. A metabolic alkalosis results when they are administered together.

36. Which blood type should be given when the patient's blood type is not known?

A. O positive
B. AB positive
C. O negative
D. none

37. Which muscles abduct the vocal cords?

A. posterior cricoarytenoids
B. vagus nerve
C. lateral cricoarytenoid
D. strap muscles

38. The larynx is composed of nine cartilages; which of the following is not a paired cartilage?

A. arytenoid
B. corniculate
C. thyroid
D. cuneiform

39. Which nerve supplies sensory innervation below the vocal cords?

A. branch of the trigeminal
B. superior laryngeal
C. phrenic nerve
D. recurrent laryngeal

40. Which of the following is not an unpaired cartilage of the larynx?

A. epiglottis
B. cricoid
C. arytenoid
D. thyroid

41. Which laryngeal muscle has motor innervation by the external branch of the superior laryngeal nerve?

A. posterior cricoarytenoid
B. cricothyroid
C. lateral cricoarytenoid
D. thyroid cartilage

42. Unilateral paralysis of the recurrent laryngeal nerve results in:

A. complete airway obstruction
B. stridor and respiratory distress
C. ipsilateral cord paralysis, hoarse voice
D. no changes

43. What is the maximum PaO_2 that can be achieved on room air?

A. 90 mm Hg
B. 96 mm Hg
C. 21 mm Hg
D. 104 mm Hg

44. What is the purpose of incentive spirometry?

A. increase residual volume
B. decrease deadspace
C. prevent atelectasis
D. increase cardiac output

45. Which of the following is not an adverse effect of succinylcholine?

A. increase in intraocular pressure
B. rapid muscle relaxation
C. hyperkalemia
D. myalgia

46. The reaction between CO_2 and soda lime is classified as:

A. neutralization
B. reduction
C. combustion
D. vaporization

47. Which nerve is most commonly injured during anesthesia?

A. sciatic nerve
B. anterior tibial nerve
C. femoral nerve
D. ulnar nerve

48. Which class of antibiotics is known to potentiate nondepolarizing muscle relaxants?

A. penicillins
B. cephalosporins
C. aminoglycosides
D. sulfonamides

49. Which of the following does not contribute to perioperative hypothermia?

A. surgical exposure
B. operating room environment
C. inhibition of thermoregulation
D. increased metabolic rate

50. Intraoperative hyperthemia would not be caused by which of the following?

A. malignant hyperthermia
B. surgical exposure
C. increased metabolic rate
D. excessive environmental warming

51. Warfarin-like drugs act as anticoagulants by:

A. inhibiting vitamin K–dependent factors
B. inhibiting the intrinsic clotting cascade
C. inhibiting the extrinsic clotting cascade
D. inhibiting platelets

52. The effects of warfarin can be reversed in an emergency by:

A. giving fresh-frozen plasma or whole blood
B. giving vitamin K (phytonadione)
C. administration of protamine sulfate
D. platelet administration

53. All of the following are possible causes of thrombocytopenia except:

A. liver disease
B. massive blood transfusion
C. renal disease
D. disseminated intravascular coagulation

54. The first sign of hemolytic transfusion reaction in the anesthetized patient may be:

A. chills
B. temperature increase
C. hypertension
D. hematuria

55. All of the following are treatments for acute hemolytic transfusion reaction except:

A. alkalinize the urine with bicarbonate
B. administration of 2 units of packed red blood cells
C. support blood pressure to maintain renal blood flow
D. administration of intravascular fluid at rate of 150 mL/h

56. The approximate blood volume of an adult is:

A. 5000 mL
B. 10,000 mL
C. 3000 mL
D. 3500 mL

57. The hematocrit of packed red blood cells is approximately:

A. 50%
B. 90%
C. 60%
D. 70%

58. Common signs of citrate intoxication from bank blood include all of the following except:

A. narrow pulse pressure
B. oozing at the surgical site
C. hypercalcemia
D. hypotension

59. The citrate in bank blood causes:

A. hypokalemia
B. hypercalcemia
C. hypocalcemia
D. hyperkalemia

60. During general anesthesia, the three common signs of a hemolytic infusion reaction include all of the following except:

A. fever
B. hematuria
C. excess bleeding and oozing at the surgical site
D. hypertension

61. After 24 hours of storage what percent of platelets are viable?

A. 20%
B. 10%
C. 5%
D. 25%

62. Common acid-base and electrolyte disturbances of massive transfusion of bank blood include all of the following except:

A. hypernatremia
B. hypocalcemia
C. hyperkalemia
D. metabolic acidosis

63. In patients with severe hyponatremia, it is safe to increase serum sodium by:

A. 1–2 mEq/h
B. 5 mEq/h
C. 10 mEq/h
D. 20 mEq/h

64. The following are all manifestations of hypokalemia seen on an ECG except:

A. tall peaked T waves
B. widened QRS
C. T-wave depression
D. prominent U waves

65. A clinical manifestation of hypokalemia is:

A. ST-segment elevation
B. hypopolarization of the cardiac cell
C. shortened PR interval
D. hyperpolarization of the cardiac cell

66. All of the following are changes that may be noted on an ECG in a patient with hyperkalemia except:

A. PR prolongation
B. flattened T waves
C. widened QRS
D. asystole

67. How many half-lives does it take to eliminated 75% of the dose of a drug?

A. 1
B. 2
C. 3
D. 4

68. Pulmonary edema may be treated with all of the following except:

A. calcium channel blockers
B. morphine
C. diuretics
D. Sodium nitroprusside

69. All of the following are indications for placement of a permanent pacemaker except:

A. first-degree heart block
B. sick sinus syndrome
C. sinus bradycardia
D. third-degree heart block

70. All of the following decrease serum potassium levels except:

A. glucagon
B. calcium chloride
C. sodium polystyrene sulfonate (Kayexalate)
D. hemodialysis

71. All of the following are symptoms of TURP syndrome except:

A. lethargy
B. dysrrythmias
C. increased visual acuity
D. seizures

72. The correct size endotracheal tube for a 4-year old is:

A. 5
B. 4
C. 5.5
D. 4.5

73. In a 3-year-old child, the endotracheal tube should be inserted to:

A. 13 cm
B. 14 cm
C. 15 cm
D. 12 cm

74. All of the following are signs and symptoms of epiglottitis except:

A. inspiratory stridor
B. high fever
C. slow onset
D. drooling

75. The child with epiglottitis should be intubated:

A. in the operating room
B. in the emergency department
C. in the patient's room
D. with fiberoptic instrumentation

76. The area of the autonomic nervous system concerned with baroreceptors is the:

A. right atrium and right ventricle
B. carotid sinus and aortic arch
C. left atrium and left ventricle
D. left ventricle and abdominal aorta

77. After burns, the plasma-to-interstitial fluid shift occurs:

A. in 1 to 2 hours
B. during the first 24 hours
C. during the first 48 hours
D. during the first 72 hours

78. Among the list of calcium salts, which one ionizes the most?

    A. calcium chloride
    B. calcium gluconate
    C. calcium oxalate
    D. calcium hydroxide

79. The facial nerve performs all of the following except:

    A. supplies the muscles of facial expression
    B. conveys secretomotor fibers to the lacrimal and salivary glands
    C. transmits taste fibers from the anterior two thirds of the tongue
    D. transmits taste fibers from the posterior one third of the tongue

80. The initial dose of dantrolene for treating a malignant hyperthermia is:

    A. 1.5 mg/kg
    B. 2.5 mg/kg
    C. 10 mg/kg
    D. 20 mg/kg

81. Identify the vital sign change most detrimental in the patient with coronary artery disease:

    A. mean arterial pressure decreases to 50 mm Hg
    B. mean arterial pressure increases to 120 mm Hg
    C. heart rate increases
    D. preload decreases

82. Coronary perfusion pressure is increased as a result of:

    A. increased diastolic blood pressure
    B. increased left ventricular end-diastolic pressure
    C. systolic hypertension
    D. tachycardia

83. Which bellows is safer when there is a disconnect?

    A. ascending
    B. descending
    C. Both are equally safe.
    D. depends on the site of the disconnect

84. What is the maximum amount of hetastarch that should be given to a patient?

    A. 10 mg/kg
    B. 20 mg/kg
    C. 10 mL/kg
    D. 20 mL/kg

85. Which statement is incorrect regarding the aged patient?

    A. The elimination half-life of pancuronium is similar to that of a 30-year old.
    B. The induction dose for thiopental is decreased.
    C. The minimal alveolar concentration of halothane is decreased.
    D. The hand-to-brain circulation time is greater than 15 seconds.

86. The volume of distribution of drugs in the elderly is:

    A. increased for water-soluble drugs
    B. decreased for lipid-soluble drugs
    C. increased for lipid-soluble drugs
    D. constant for both water- and lipid-soluble drugs

87. Diffusion hypoxia is a phenomenon associated with rapid movement of which anesthetic agent from the circulation into the lungs producing a significant dilution of oxygen?

    A. halothane
    B. sevoflurane
    C. isoflurane
    D. nitrous oxide

88. The nonionized form of a local anesthetic is:

    A. water soluble
    B. lipid soluble
    C. unable to cross the placental barrier
    D. electrically charged

89. The rapidity and extent of diffusion of a local anesthetic to its site of action depends primarily on:

A. pK_a of the drug
B. concentration of drug injected
C. lipid solubility
D. all of the above

90. It is important to monitor right radial pulse during mediastinoscopy to detect:

A. right carotid artery compression
B. innominate artery
C. right brachial artery compression
D. ascending aorta compression

91. Autonomic hyperreflexia is rarely seen in cases of cord transection below:

A. T5
B. T10
C. T12
D. L2

92. Sympathetic preganglionic cardiac accelerator nerve outflow is from which ganglia?

A. C1–C4
B. C7–T5
C. T1–T5
D. T5–T10

93. The superior laryngeal nerve provides _____ innervation to the larynx.

A. sensory
B. motor
C. sensory and motor
D. proprioceptive

94. Structurally, the larynx is composed of _____ cartilages.

A. three
B. five
C. seven
D. nine

95. Indirect-acting sympathomimetic drugs exert their effect by:

A. stimulating beta receptors
B. stimulating alpha receptors
C. causing catecholamine release
D. blocking catecholamine reuptake

96. Cardiac output in the parturient is greater at what point in pregnancy?

A. 10–12 weeks' gestation
B. immediately postpartum
C. 20 weeks' gestation
D. immediately after conception

97. The vasopressor of choice for the parturient after subarachnoid block administration is:

A. phenylephrine
B. ephedrine
C. epinephrine
D. methoxamine

98. An absolute contraindication to the administration of heparin for cardiopulmonary bypass is:

A. carotid disease
B. recent cerebrovascular accident
C. increased antithrombin III activity
D. previous streptokinase therapy

99. Elderly patients may become hypertensive and not exhibit any compensatory changes in heart rate because of:

A. diminished activity of carotid sinus reflex responses
B. reduced sympathetic afferent traffic to the medulla
C. decreased responsiveness of central nervous system–mediated compensatory mechanisms
D. increased parasympathetic efferent traffic to the sinus node

100. What are the cardiovascular effects of positive end-expiratory pressure?

A. decreased cardiac output
B. stabilized pulmonary blood flow
C. augmented venous return
D. increased lymphatic flow

101. Correct application of Sellick's maneuver includes:

A. gentle pressure applied over the crico-thyroid membrane
B. using the index finger to apply pressure over the thyroid
C. maintaining cricoid pressure during positive-pressure ventilation
D. pinching the cricoid cartilage between the thumb and index finger

102. Which of the following drugs would be contraindicated in the patient with Parkinson's disease?

A. droperidol
B. thiopental
C. fentanyl
D. midazolam

103. What are the cardiovascular effects of cocaine?

A. bradycardia
B. reduced vascular resistance
C. cardiac dysrhythmias
D. decreased cardiac output

104. The most important mechanism for the termination of action of norepinephrine is:

A. uptake into the preganglionic nerve terminals
B. reuptake into the postganglionic nerve endings
C. metabolism by catechol-O-methyl transferase
D. competition of increasing acetylcholine

105. What are the effects of cocaine on the central nervous system?

A. increased seizure threshold
B. central hypothermic activity
C. stimulation then depression
D. strong antiemetic effects

106. Clonidine is a(an)

A. adrenergic neuron blocker
B. central alpha$_2$-receptor agonist
C. direct-acting arteriolar vasodilator
D. direct-acting vasodilator

107. Which physiologic derangement will result in slower metabolism of ester local anesthetics?

A. acute renal failure
B. atypical plasma cholinesterase
C. hyperkalemia
D. diabetes insipidus

108. Duchenne muscular dystrophy has been implicated with what drug in a life-threatening drug side effect?

A. verapamil
B. cyclosporine
C. esmolol
D. succinylcholine

109. A normal (average) dibucaine number is:

A. 50
B. 60
C. 80
D. 100

110. Rebound hypertension after cessation of sodium nitroprusside drip results from:

A. vasoconstriction
B. renin release
C. central nervous system stimulation
D. catecholamine release

111. The oxygen pressure from piped-in systems leading to anesthesia machines should be in the range of:

A. 40 psi
B. 50 psi
C. 60 psi
D. 70 psi

112. Pressure sensor shut-off valves will be activated when oxygen pressure falls below:

A. 15 psi
B. 25 psi
C. 35 psi
D. 40 psi

113. The statement that the amount of gas dissolving in a liquid is proportional to the partial pressure of the gas defines:

A. Charles' law
B. Boyle's law
C. Graham's law
D. Henry's law

114. (MAP − CVP) × 80/CO measures:

A. pulmonary vascular resistance
B. mean arterial and central venous pressure per heart beat
C. systemic vascular resistance
D. systemic refraction of cardiac output

115. One of the greatest advantages to a non-rebreathing system for children is:

A. loss of heat and humidity
B. low flow rates
C. minimal resistance
D. maximal deadspace

116. Clamping of the abdominal aorta during aneurysm surgery is followed by:

A. loss of blood pressure in the right arm
B. immediate drop in systolic blood pressure
C. no change
D. immediate rise in systolic blood pressure

117. The principal catalyst for carbon dioxide absorption in soda lime and baralyme is:

A. magnesium hydroxide
B. potassium hydroxide
C. sodium hydroxide
D. calcium hydroxide

118. Current F-29 standards mandate the use of ventilator bellows that:

A. descend on inspiration
B. ascend on inspiration
C. descend on expiration
D. ascend on expiration

119. Which ventilator mode allows spontaneous respiratory effort while administering a preset tidal volume at a specified interval?

A. assisted-controlled ventilation
B. synchronized intermittent mandatory ventilation
C. controlled ventilation
D. mandatory minute ventilation

120. Diaphoresis under general anesthesia may indicate:

A. hypercapnia
B. deep anesthesia
C. hypoxia
D. hypocarbia

121. Which of the following nondepolarizing muscle relaxants has the most rapid onset?

A. succinylcholine
B. vecuronium
C. rocuronium
D. pancuronium

122. During pneumonectomy, the main bronchus is clamped. What is the most important physiologic finding?

A. decreased tidal volume
B. increased CO_2
C. decreased PaO_2
D increased peak inspiratory pressure

123. Which of the following laboratory values would not be expected in a patient with chronic renal disease?

A. blood urea nitrogen: 52 mg/dL
B. creatinine: 1.2 mg/dL
C. pH: 7.41
D. hemoglobin: 9.2 g/dL

124. An agent is removed faster from the central compartment if:

A. half-life is short with small volume of distribution
B. half-life is short with large volume of distribution
C. half-life is long with small volume of distribution
D. half-life is long with large volume of distribution

125. The concentration of which of the following differs greatest in the trachea from ambient air?

    A. oxygen
    B. carbon dioxide
    C. nitrogen
    D. water

126. In banked blood, there is an excess of all of the following except:

    A. ammonia
    B. hydrogen ions
    C. 2,3-diphosphoglycerate
    D. plasma potassium

127. If an awake patient is placed in the lateral position there will be:

    A. decreased perfusion in the down lung
    B. increased ventilation in the down lung
    C. increased ventilation in the top lung
    D. increased perfusion in the top lung

128. The following findings are symptomatic in pyloric stenosis except:

    A. metabolic acidosis
    B. hypochloremia
    C. dehydration
    D. hypokalemia

129. Which of the following represents the best criterion for extubation after effective reversal of nondepolarizing muscle relaxation?

    A. return of reflexes
    B. sustained tetanus
    C. tidal volume of 5 mL/kg
    D. head lift sustained for 5 seconds

130. The Occupational Safety and Health Administration defines acceptable limits of pollutants in the operating room as:

    A. halothane: 25 parts per million
    B. halothane: 50 parts per million
    C. nitrous oxide: 2 parts per million
    D. nitrous oxide: 25 parts per million

131. Which of the following is of concern when anesthetizing the acromegalic patient?

    A. hypercalcemia
    B. laryngeal edema
    C. probable hiatal and diaphragmatic hernia
    D. altered airway structure and landmarks

132. The Department of Transportation mandates that gas cylinders be checked at what interval?

    A. each refill
    B. semi-annually
    C. annually
    D. every 5 years

133. Which level of humidity is recommended to prevent explosion hazard in the operative suite?

    A. 50% to 60% relative humidity
    B. 50% to 60% absolute humidity
    C. greater than 60% absolute humidity
    D. 100% relative humidity

134. After extubation after parathyroidectomy, your patient experiences mild stridor and significant vocal hoarseness. You suspect:

    A. hematoma formation
    B. superior laryngeal nerve injury
    C. laryngeal bruising
    D. recurrent laryngeal nerve injury

135. Current research suggests that the pathologic process underlying the clinical syndrome of malignant hyperthermia may be:

    A. interference with sodium-potassium/ATPase pump
    B. sympathetic nervous system hypersensitivity
    C. impaired intracellular control of calcium
    D. blockade of intracellular sodium/calcium pump

136. Which of the following factors is most important when planning anesthesia for the patient undergoing portacaval shunt?

    A. distended ascitic abdomen
    B. decreased level of consciousness
    C. decreased cerebral blood flow
    D. anemia

137. Drug interactions with phenytoin and warfarin include:

    A. enhanced biotransformation of warfarin and reduced bleeding time
    B. increased sedation and prolonged anticoagulant activity
    C. reduced biotransformation of warfarin and increased bleeding time
    D. increased renal excretion of phenytoin with a reduced seizure threshold

138. Drug interactions with clonidine and propranolol would cause:

    A. hypertension
    B. hypotension
    C. tachypnea
    D. hypoglycemia

139. Identify the mechanism most likely to explain the drug interactions seen with cimetidine and many classes of drugs:

    A. alteration of gastric acidity and enhanced drug absorption
    B. competitive inhibition in the distal tubule with altered excretion
    C. great reduction in hepatic blood flow and drug clearance
    D. inhibition of the microsomal cytochrome P450 system in the liver

140. What is the effect of verapamil on blood coagulation?

    A. prolonged prothrombin time
    B. shortened partial thromboplastin time
    C. inhibition of factors II and VII
    D. increased bleeding time

141. In shock, what unique feature of dopamine makes it the drug of choice?

    A. renal tissue blood flow can be increased
    B. myocardial contractility is usually decreased
    C. myocardial oxygen consumption is decreased
    D. peripheral vascular resistance is decreased

142. The treatment for extrapyramidal effects associated with droperidol is:

    A. midazolam
    B. diphenhydramine
    C. cimetidine
    D. morphine

143. Treatment of cyanide toxicity includes all of the following except:

    A. amyl nitrite
    B. sodium nitrite
    C. sodium thiosulfate
    D. sodium thiocyanate

144. The cascade of events occurring with cyanide toxicity are due to:

    A. the development of metabolic acidosis
    B. a loss of buffering capacity
    C. decreased availability of molecular oxygen
    D. inability of the tissues to utilize oxygen

145. Which of the following drugs has been shown to directly antagonize benzodiazepine-induced sedation?

    A. naloxone
    B. naltrexone
    C. doxapram
    D. aminophylline

146. The relative affinity of an anesthetic and how it partitions itself in the body is implied in which of the following?

    A. concentration effect
    B. second gas effect
    C. blood/gas solubility
    D. pressure gradient

147. Flexion of the intubated neonate's head:

    A. may cause endobronchial intubation
    B. may cause inadvertent extubation
    C. may cause laryngospasm
    D. may expose the glottic opening

148. Which of the following class of drugs lowers intraocular pressure?

    A. alpha agonist
    B. alpha blockers
    C. beta agonist
    D. beta blockers

149. Which of the following is not a pathophysiologic change in toxemia of pregnancy?

    A. decreased glomerular filtration rate
    B. proteinuria
    C. dehydration
    D. hypertension

150. In an upright normal subject, the ventilation per unit volume is greatest in:

    A. lung bases
    B. lung apices
    C. posterior portions of the lung
    D. middle portions of the lung

151. A patient develops bronchospasm under anesthesia that is not relieved by deepening levels. The next intervention may be:

    A. administer a beta blocker
    B. give a calcium channel blocker
    C. give a beta$_2$ agonist
    D. administer intravenous corticosteroids

152. Which of the following is true regarding ventilation and perfusion in the lateral position in the anesthetized, closed-chest patient?

    A. The non dependent lung is better perfused.
    B. The dependent lung is better ventilated.
    C. The nondependent lung is better ventilated.
    D. The dependent lung has less deadspace.

153. During muscle contraction calcium combines with:

    A. troponin
    B. tropomyosin
    C. actin
    D. myofibril C

154. A heat-producing mechanism in neonates is thought to exist in what tissue known to play an important role in hibernating animals:

    A. connective
    B. brown adipose
    C. mitochondrial
    D. all of the above

155. Which of the following is usually not seen in patients with pyloric stenosis?

    A. alkalosis
    B. hypervolemia
    C. hypochloremia
    D. dehydration

156. Therapeutic magnesium levels for the treatment of preeclampsia are:

    A. 1–2 mEq/L
    B. 4–6 mEq/L
    C. 8–10 mEq/L
    D. 20–25 mEq/L

157. A significant incidence of cardiotoxicity is seen following the use of:

    A. 3% chloroprocaine
    B. 4% cocaine
    C. 0.5% mepivacaine
    D. 0.75% bupivacaine

158. The last structure the needle passes through in epidural anesthesia is the:

    A. ligamentum flavum
    B. dura mater
    C. supraspinous ligament
    D. arachnoid mater

159. A postpartum patient who develops an inverted uterus with hemorrhage should be treated with what first?

    A. blood
    B. 100% oxygen
    C. halothane by mask
    D. rapid sequence induction with ketamine

160. Which of the following intravenous solutions should be avoided in the neurosurgical patient?

    A. balanced salt solution
    B. dextrose and water
    C. lactated Ringer's solution
    D. normal saline

161. Myocardial oxygen demand is decreased by:

    A. tachycardia
    B. decreased preload
    C. increased afterload
    D. increased contractility

162. Myocardial oxygen consumption is most closely associated with:

    A. heart rate
    B. blood viscosity
    C. cardiac output
    D. stroke volume

163. Cardiovascular changes that occur with advancing age are most typically associated with:

    A. decreased blood pressure
    B. decreased cardiac reserve
    C. decreased heart rate
    D. increased cardiac output

164. Which of the following is a determinant of myocardial oxygen supply?

    A. blood oxygen content
    B. preload
    C. afterload
    D. heart rate

165. Signs and symptoms of diabetes insipidus include all of the following except:

    A. polyuria
    B. increased urine osmolarity
    C. hypernatremia
    D. serum hyperosmolarity

166. The preservative in halothane that proves stability is:

    A. absolute alcohol
    B. methylene blue
    C. thymol
    D. methylparaben

167. All of the following are contraindications to using nitrous oxide except:

    A. bowel obstruction
    B. hiatal hernia
    C. air embolism
    D. pneumothorax

168. Inhalation anesthetic agents are metabolized by the:

    A. monoamine oxidase system
    B. cholinesterase
    C. microsomal enzymes
    D. hydrolysis

169. Where is nitrous oxide metabolized?

    A. brain
    B. liver
    C. kidney
    D. intestine

170. What percentage of isoflurane is metabolized?

    A. 0.2%
    B. 2%
    C. 3%
    D. 2.4%

171. Hepatic dysfunction occurs most often after repeated administration of halothane to what group of patients?

    A. young adults
    B. pediatric patients
    C. obese middle-aged females
    D. middle-aged males

172. What is the diagnostic test for malignant hyperthermia?

    A. elevated lactate dehydrogenase
    B. elevated creatinine phosphokinase
    C. halothane-caffeine contracture test
    D. genetic test of the ryanodine receptor

173. Your patient is in the sitting position. Where would you place the transducer to measure mean arterial blood pressure to monitor perfusion pressure at the brain?

    A. It doesn't matter much where the transducer is placed.
    B. Place the transducer at the right sternal border between the third and sixth intercostal spaces.
    C. Place the transducer at the level of arterial catheter insertion site.
    D. Place the transducer at the level of the external ear canal, which is at the level of the circle of Willis.

174. Which five nerves may be injured in the lithotomy position?

    A. common peroneal, sciatic, femoral, saphenous, and obturator nerves

    B. deep peroneal, sural, posterior tibial, saphenous, and femoral nerves

    C. common peroneal, superficial peroneal, posterior tibial, sciatic, and obturator nerves

    D. sciatic, femoral, pudendal, posterior tibial, and common peroneal nerves

175. Why is an axillary roll placed under the patient in the lateral decubitus position?

    A. to prevent compression of the brachial plexus and subclavian vessels near the first rib and, thus, the thoracic outlet syndrome

    B. to allow the thorax to hang free, thus minimizing loss of functional residual capacity and obstruction to venous return

    C. to lift the thorax and relieve pressure on the axillary neurovascular bundle and to prevent reduced blood flow to the hand

    D. to prevent the patient from sliding more laterally, causing ventral circumduction of the dependent shoulder and the potential for a suprascapular nerve injury

176. What is the most frequently damaged nerve in the lower extremity?

    A. sciatic nerve

    B. common peroneal nerve

    C. femoral nerve

    D. anterior tibial nerve

177. What nerve is damaged if the inside of the knee is compressed?

    A. saphenous nerve

    B. obturator nerve

    C. anterior tibial nerve

    D. common peroneal nerve

178. The rate of induction with an inhalation anesthetic varies inversely with which property of the agent?

    A. oil/gas solubility

    B. blood/gas solubility

    C. vapor pressure of the agent

    D. none of the above

179. All of the following are ultra short-acting barbiturates except:

    A. methohexital

    B. thiamylal

    C. thiopental

    D. pentobarbital

180. The termination of action of thiopental is via:

    A. distribution to the skeletal muscles

    B. oxidation

    C. redistribution

    D. reductive enzymes

181. What drug should not be administered with a monoamine oxidase inhibitor?

    A. fentanyl

    B. morphine

    C. meperidine

    D. sufentanil

182. Use of barbiturates is contraindicated in which disease?

    A. muscular dystrophy

    B. Graves' disease

    C. porphyria

    D. scleroderma

183. Use of droperidol is contraindicated in what disease?

    A. diabetes mellitus

    B. Parkinson's disease

    C. Alzheimer's disease

    D. muscular dystrophy

184. Which antimuscarinic exhibits the least central nervous system toxicity?

    A. atropine

    B. glycopyrrolate

    C. scopolamine

    D. benztropine

185. Central nervous system toxicity due to anticholinergeric drugs can be treated with:

A. neostigmine
B. pyridostigmine
C. ecothiopate
D. physostigmine

186. What percent of neuromuscular blockade is achieved if two of four thumb twitches to train-of-four stimulation of the ulnar nerve can be elicited?

A. 50
B. 75
C. 80
D. 90

187. The final metabolic product of nitroprusside is:

A. cyanide
B. thiocyanate
C. choline
D. nitrate

188. A drug that follows first-order kinetics will be eliminated from the body at:

A. a constant amount per time
B. a constant rate per time
C. the same number of milligrams per hour
D. The elimination depends on the dose.

189. What is the classification of a 140-kg patient who must undergo emergency surgery for a bowel obstruction?

A. ASA 1E
B. ASA 3E
C. ASA 4E
D. ASA 2E

190. List three diseases an ASA 3 patient may have:

A. angina pectoris, chronic obstructive pulmonary disease, and prior myocardial infarction
B. essential hypertension, diabetes mellitus, and morbid obesity
C. anemia, congestive heart failure, and persistent angina pectoris
D. extremes of age, chronic bronchitis, and hepatic dysfunction

191. All of the following are the pharmacologic effects of droperidol except:

A. hypotension
B. extrapyramidal signs
C. antiemetic properties
D. vasoconstriction

192. What nerve is injured if the arm is malpositioned with the elbow at the side of the table?

A. sciatic nerve
B. median nerve
C. radial nerve
D. ulnar nerve

193. Elevation of kidney rest compresses which structure and leads to what response?

A. The aorta is compressed, which causes lower extremity ischemia and hypertension.
B. The inferior vena cava is compressed, which causes a marked reduction in venous return and hypotension.
C. The abdominal viscera are compressed, which causes ventilation/perfusion mismatch.
D. The common peroneal nerve is compressed, which results in loss of sensation over the dorsum of the foot.

194. Anticholinergics block which muscarinic receptor subtype?

A. M-1
B. M-2
C. M-3
D. M-1, M-2, M-3

195. Pseudocholinesterase metabolizes:

A. lidocaine
B. bupivacaine
C. procaine
D. ropivacaine

196. During the onset of neuromuscular blockade, if the fourth twitch is eliminated in the train-of-four, the percentage of blockade is:

A. 50
B. 67
C. 75
D. 90

197. The maximum amount of air that can be inhaled from the resting end-expiratory level is:

    A. tidal volume
    B. vital capacity
    C. inspiratory capacity
    D. inspiratory reserve volume

198. Muscle relaxants distribute to what body compartment?

    A. skeletal muscle
    B. intracellular fluid
    C. extracellular fluid
    D. vessel-poor organs

199. The onset of action of what antimuscarinic parallels the onset of edrophonium?

    A. atropine
    B. glycopyrrolate
    C. scopolamine
    D. All of the antimuscarinics parallel the rapid onset of edrophonium.

200. Administration of an anticholinergic drug before the anticholinesterase will minimize which effect?

    A. nicotinic receptor antagonism
    B. muscarinic receptor antagonism
    C. nicotinic receptor stimulation
    D. muscarinic receptor stimulation

201. The "concentration effect" or "overpressure" during induction of anesthesia refers to:

    A. the blood/gas coefficient of an anesthetic varies with concentration
    B. the higher the concentration administered, the faster the increase in alveolar concentration
    C. the second gas effect
    D. anesthetic overdose

202. Naltrexone (ReVia), Naloxone (Narcan), and Nalmefene (Revex) are:

    A. pure agonists
    B. partial agonists
    C. partial agonist/antagonists
    D. pure antagonists

203. The "truncal rigidity" that may occur with fentanyl can be relieved by:

    A. atropine
    B. aminophylline
    C. nitroprusside
    D. succinylcholine

204. Which fibers are not cholinergic?

    A. preganglionic sympathetic
    B. postganglionic parasympathetic
    C. postganglionic sympathetic
    D. preganglionic parasympathetic

205. Which of the following would be expected to produce the most reliable amnesia?

    A. thiopental
    B. propofol
    C. etomidate
    D. midazolam

206. Nystagmus is characteristic of which "stage" of anesthesia?

    A. stage 1
    B. stage 2
    C. stage 3
    D. stage 4

207. The enzyme primarily involved in the biotransformation of exogenous catecholamines is:

    A. monoamine oxidase
    B. cytochrome P450
    C. catechol-O-methyl transferase
    D. amidase

208. The therapeutic index by definition is:

    A. 25% lethal dose/25% effective dose
    B. 50% lethal dose/50% effective dose
    C. 75% lethal dose/75% effective dose
    D. 90% lethal dose/90% effective dose

209. Anesthetic partial pressure in the brain depends on:

A. solubility of the agent
B. anesthetic partial pressure in the alveoli
C. minimal alveolar concentration of the agent
D. second gas effect

210. *Dissociative anesthesia* is a term applied to anesthesia produced by the administration of:

A. propofol
B. scopolamine
C. ketamine
D. hypnosis

211. Dual block can be caused by:

A. a nondepolarizing relaxant
B. small amounts of depolarizing relaxants
C. very large doses of depolarizing relaxants
D. administration of both nondepolarizing and depolarizing muscle relaxants

212. The most sensitive muscles to the paralyzing effect of the neuromuscular blocking drugs are:

A. abdominal muscles
B. limb muscles
C. jaw muscles
D. eye muscles

213. The most serious systemic toxicity with local anesthetics is:

A. cardiac arrhythmias
B. liver damage
C. respiratory depression
D. convulsions

214. A drug's plasma half-life is:

A. its 50% maximal response
B. the time required for plasma drug concentration to be decreased by 50%
C. its duration of action
D. its onset of action

215. The minimal alveolar concentration value of an agent is defined as:

A. potency of an agent
B. speed of induction and emergence
C. alveolar concentration where 50% of patients do not respond to surgical stimuli
D. directly proportional to the blood/gas solubility coefficient

216. The activity of acetylcholine released from cholinergic nerve endings is terminated by:

A. hydrolysis catalyzed by acetylcholinesterase
B. presynaptic neuronal uptake through an active pump
C. presynaptic neuronal uptake by endocytosis
D. monoamine oxidase

217. Drugs crossing biomembranes generally do so by which of the following processes?

A. diffusion through aqueous ion channels
B. diffusion through membrane lipid
C. permeation by active pump mechanisms
D. pinocytosis

218. The ED50 of a drug is defined as:

A. the response elicited when one half of the therapeutic dose is administered
B. the dose that elicits a therapeutic response in 50% of patients
C. one-half of the ED100
D. the threshold dose

219. A drug having a high LD50 and a low ED50:

A. is unsafe for human use
B. has a high therapeutic index and is, therefore, very dangerous
C. has a high therapeutic index and is, therefore, relatively safe
D. has a low therapeutic index and should be used with care

220. What do the letters I.T. or Z79 indicate on an endotracheal tube?

A. the endotracheal tube has passed inspection
B. endotracheal tube material free of toxic properties
C. indicates the internal diameter of the tube
D. indicates the length of the tube

221. Pulse oximetry functioning is an example of:

A. Beer's law
B. Dalton's law
C. Charles' law
D. Reynolds' law

222. Of the following, which interferes with pulse oximetry?

A. oxyhemoglobin
B. hemoglobin F
C. hemoglobin
D. methemoglobin

223. Clinical accuracy of pulse oximetry is within:

A. 2%–3%
B. 1%
C. 5%–8%
D. 100%

224. All of the following will affect SpO_2 (oxygen saturation) accuracy except:

A. hypotension
B. hyperthermia
C. altered systemic vascular resistance
D. use of vasoactive drugs

1. ANSWER: **C**

   Rationale: Based on a system of grams per liter, a 1:200,000 concentration is equal to 5 μg/mL.

   Reference: Williams, J.R. (1997). Chapter 20: Local Anesthetics. In J. Nagelhout & K. Zaglaniczny (Eds.), *Nurse Anesthesia*. Philadelphia: W.B. Saunders.

2. ANSWER: **B**

   Rationale: Direct-acting vasopressors should be used in patients on MAO therapy. Phenylephrine is the only direct-acting drug of the listed choices.

   Reference: Alisoglu, R. (1997). Chapter 23: Cardiac Pharmacology. In J. Nagelhout & K. Zaglaniczny (Eds.), *Nurse Anesthesia*. Philadelphia: W.B. Saunders.

3. ANSWER: **B**

   Rationale: Diabetic patients often have gastric atony; thus, a gastrokinetic agent such as metoclopramide may be useful to ensure an empty stomach.

   Reference: Williams, J.R. (1997). Chapter 20: Local Anesthetics. In J. Nagelhout & K. Zaglaniczny (Eds.), *Nurse Anesthesia*. Philadelphia: W.B. Saunders.

4. ANSWER: **B**

   Rationale: Venous air embolism, such as seen in sitting procedures, may be detected by a reduced end-expired CO_2, resulting from the ventilation/perfusion mismatch.

   Reference: DeVane, G.G. (1997). Chapter 37: Neurosurgical Anesthesia. In J. Nagelhout & K. Zaglaniczny (Eds.), *Nurse Anesthesia*. Philadelphia: W.B. Saunders.

5. ANSWER: **B**

   Rationale: Glucose-containing solutions are avoided in all neurosurgical patients because they can exacerbate ischemic damage and cerebral edema.

   Reference: DeVane, G.G. (1997). Chapter 37: Neurosurgical Anesthesia. In J. Nagelhout & K. Zaglaniczny (Eds.), *Nurse Anesthesia*. Philadelphia: W.B. Saunders.

6. ANSWER: **C**

   Rationale: Hyperventilation reduces brain volume by decreasing cerebral blood flow through cerebral vasoconstriction. For every millimeter of mercury change, cerebral blood flow decreases by approximately 4%.

   Reference: DeVane, G.G. (1997). Chapter 37: Neurosurgical Anesthesia. In J. Nagelhout & K. Zaglaniczny (Eds.), *Nurse Anesthesia*. Philadelphia: W.B. Saunders.

7. ANSWER: **C**

   Rationale: Hyperventilation to the $PaCO_2$ of 25 to 30 mm Hg is the mainstay of acute and subacute treatment for intracranial hypertension.

   Reference: DeVane, G.G. (1997). Chapter 37: Neurosurgical Anesthesia. In J. Nagelhout & K. Zaglaniczny (Eds.), *Nurse Anesthesia*. Philadelphia: W.B. Saunders.

8. ANSWER: **C**

   Rationale: Most inhalation anesthetics in the absence of a pathologic process have little effect on or decrease pulmonary vascular resistance. Nitrous oxide may increase resistance, especially in patients with pulmonary hypertension.

   Reference: Kossick, M.A. (1997). Chapter 18: Inhalation Anesthetics. In J. Nagelhout & K. Zaglaniczny (Eds.), *Nurse Anesthesia*. Philadelphia: W.B. Saunders.

9. ANSWER: **A**

   Rationale: The Lambert-Beer law relates to the observation that oxygenated and reduced hemoglobin differ in their absorption of red and infrared light. Pulse oximetry monitoring is based on this principle.

Reference: Sinkovich, J.A. & Kossick, M.A. (1997). Chapter 27: Clinical Monitoring in Anesthesia. In J. Nagelhout & K. Zaglaniczny (Eds.), *Nurse Anesthesia*. Philadelphia: W.B. Saunders.

10. ANSWER: **B**

Rationale: Cardiac output is equal to stroke volume times heart rate and is expressed in liters per minute. The normal range is between 4 and 6.

Reference: Aprile, A.E. & Aprile, F.D. (1997). Chapter 38B: Cardiac Anesthesia. In J. Nagelhout & K. Zaglaniczny (Eds.), *Nurse Anesthesia*. Philadelphia: W.B. Saunders.

11. ANSWER: **C**

Rationale: Cardiac index is derived from the cardiac output divided by body surface area and is expressed as liters per minute per meter squared.

Reference: Aprile, A.E. & Aprile, F.D. (1997). Chapter 38B: Cardiac Anesthesia. In J. Nagelhout & K. Zaglaniczny (Eds.), *Nurse Anesthesia*. Philadelphia: W.B. Saunders.

12. ANSWER: **A**

Rationale: Cardiac index is derived from the cardiac output divided by body surface area and is expressed as liters per minute per meter squared.

Reference: Aprile, A.E. & Aprile, F.D. (1997). Chapter 38B: Cardiac Anesthesia. In J. Nagelhout & K. Zaglaniczny (Eds.), *Nurse Anesthesia*. Philadelphia: W.B. Saunders.

13. ANSWER: **B**

Rationale: Systemic vascular resistance is calculated from the formula

$$\frac{MAP - CVP}{CO} \times 80,$$

where MAP = mean arterial pressure, CVP = central venous pressure, and CO = cardiac output.

Reference: Aprile, A.E. & Aprile, F.D. (1997). Chapter 38B: Cardiac Anesthesia. In J. Nagelhout & K. Zaglaniczny (Eds.), *Nurse Anesthesia*. Philadelphia: W.B. Saunders.

14. ANSWER: **D**

Rationale: Normal systemic vascular resistance ranges from 1200 to 1500 dynes/sec/cm^{-5}.

Reference: Aprile, A.E. & Aprile, F.D. (1997). Chapter 38B: Cardiac Anesthesia. In J. Nagelhout & K. Zaglaniczny (Eds.), *Nurse Anesthesia*. Philadelphia: W.B. Saunders.

15. ANSWER: **A**

Rationale: When properly functioning, central venous catheters rarely give erratic and inaccurate readings; however, the other complications are always possible.

Reference: Sinkovich, J.A. & Kossick, M.A. (1997). Chapter 27: Clinical Monitoring in Anesthesia. In J. Nagelhout & K. Zaglaniczny (Eds.), *Nurse Anesthesia*. Philadelphia: W.B. Saunders.

16. ANSWER: **C**

Rationale: Puncture of the carotid artery is especially prominent in left internal jugular cannulation. Using the right internal jugular vein is safer, with less likelihood of arterial puncture.

Reference: Sinkovich, J.A. & Kossick, M.A. (1997). Chapter 27: Clinical Monitoring in Anesthesia. In J. Nagelhout & K. Zaglaniczny (Eds.), *Nurse Anesthesia*. Philadelphia: W.B. Saunders.

17. ANSWER: **C**

Rationale: Air embolism can be avoided by using the Trendelenburg position to increase venous pressure, which limits the possibility of the entrance of air through the catheter.

Reference: Sinkovich, J.A. & Kossick, M.A. (1997). Chapter 27: Clinical Monitoring in Anesthesia. In J. Nagelhout & K. Zaglaniczny (Eds.), *Nurse Anesthesia*. Philadelphia: W.B. Saunders.

18. ANSWER: **C**

Rationale: Although muscle strength frequently seems adequate early after anesthesia and surgery, many patients with myasthenia gravis experience deterioration and require ventilatory support after surgery.

Reference: Karlet, M.C. (1997). Chapter 7: The Musculoskeletal System. In J. Nagelhout & K. Zaglaniczny (Eds.), *Nurse Anesthesia*. Philadelphia: W.B. Saunders.

19. ANSWER: **C**

Rationale: Accidentally pinning a nerve against an adjacent structure increases the likelihood of intraneuronal injection. When this occurs, the injection should be stopped and the needle replaced.

Reference: Ellis, W.E. (1997). Chapter 53: Regional Anesthesia. In J. Nagelhout & K. Zaglaniczny (Eds.), *Nurse Anesthesia.* Philadelphia: W.B. Saunders.

20. ANSWER: **D**

Rationale: Ketamine, by releasing catecholamines, supports blood pressure. Patients with cardiac tamponade are decompensated, and any cardiac depressant drug may cause precipitous hypotension.

Reference: Aprile, A.E. & Aprile, F.D. (1997). Chapter 38B: Cardiac Anesthesia. In J. Nagelhout & K. Zaglaniczny (Eds.), *Nurse Anesthesia.* Philadelphia: W.B. Saunders.

21. ANSWER: **C**

Rationale: Induction of anesthesia consistently produces a 15% to 20% reduction in functional residual capacity beyond that which occurs in the supine position.

Reference: Rojo, J. & Iacopelli, M. (1997). Chapter 39A: Respiratory pathophysiology. In J. Nagelhout & K. Zaglaniczny (Eds.), *Nurse Anesthesia.* Philadelphia: W.B. Saunders.

22. ANSWER: **A**

Rationale: Loss of diaphragmatic tone allows abdominal contents to rise up against the diaphragm. The higher position of the diaphragm decreases lung volumes.

Reference: Rojo, J. & Iacopelli, M. (1997). Chapter 39A: Respiratory Pathophysiology. In J. Nagelhout & K. Zaglaniczny (Eds.), *Nurse Anesthesia.* Philadelphia: W.B. Saunders.

23. ANSWER: **C**

Rationale: Etomidate inhibits the conversion of cholesterol to cortisone by inhibiting conversion enzymes. This results in adrenal suppression.

Reference: Fallacaro, N.A. & Fallacaro, M.D. (1997). Chapter 19: Intravenous Inhalation Agents. In J. Nagelhout & K. Zaglaniczny (Eds.), *Nurse Anesthesia.* Philadelphia: W.B. Saunders.

24. ANSWER: **A**

Rationale: The lateral femoral cutaneous nerve may be entrapped in the anterior

iliac spine under the inguinal ligament, resulting in numbness in the thigh.

Reference: Monti, E.J. (1997). Chapter 32: Positioning for Anesthesia and Surgery. In J. Nagelhout & K. Zaglaniczny (Eds.), *Nurse Anesthesia.* Philadelphia: W.B. Saunders.

25. ANSWER: **C**

Rationale: Complications of nasotracheal intubation may include epistaxis, dislodgment of pharyngeal tonsils, eustachian tube obstruction, maxillary sinusitis, bacteremia, and gastric distention.

Reference: Chipas, A. (1997). Chapter 33: Airway Management. In J. Nagelhout & K. Zaglaniczny (Eds.), *Nurse Anesthesia.* Philadelphia: W.B. Saunders.

26. ANSWER: **C**

Rationale: Dextrose in water acts as a hypotonic solution, thus increasing brain water, which may result in cerebral edema and ischema.

Reference: DeVane, G.G. (1997). Chapter 37: Neurosurgical Anesthesia. In J. Nagelhout & K. Zaglaniczny (Eds.), *Nurse Anesthesia.* Philadelphia: W.B. Saunders.

27. ANSWER: **D**

Rationale: Carbon dioxide is more soluble in blood than oxygen. It dissolves in plasma as well as erythrocytes and represents approximately 2.5 mL/dL of blood.

Reference: Rojo, J. & Iacopelli, M. (1997). Chapter 39A: Respiratory pathophysiology. In J. Nagelhout & K. Zaglaniczny (Eds.), *Nurse Anesthesia.* Philadelphia: W.B. Saunders.

28. ANSWER: **B**

Rationale: Premature infants younger than 60 weeks postconception are prone to postoperative episodes of obstructive and central apnea for up to 24 hours after surgery.

Reference: Dobbins, P. & Hall, S.M. (1997). Chapter 14: Pediatric Anesthesia. In J. Nagelhout & K. Zaglaniczny (Eds.), *Nurse Anesthesia.* Philadelphia: W.B. Saunders.

29. ANSWER: **B**

Rationale: Prematurity is birth before 37 weeks' gestation. This is in contrast to "small gestational age," which may describe a full-term infant.

Reference: Dobbins, P. & Hall, S.M. (1997). Chapter 14: Pediatric Anesthesia. In J. Nagelhout & K. Zaglaniczny (Eds.), *Nurse Anesthesia*. Philadelphia: W.B. Saunders.

30. ANSWER: **A**

    Rationale: Fluid requirements can be determined by the formula: 4 mL/kg/h for the first 10 kg; 2/mL/kg/h for the next 10 kg; and 1 mL/kg/h for each remaining kilogram.

    Reference: Dobbins, P. & Hall, S.M. (1997). Chapter 14: Pediatric Anesthesia. In J. Nagelhout & K. Zaglaniczny (Eds.), *Nurse Anesthesia*. Philadelphia: W.B. Saunders.

31. ANSWER: **C**

    Rationale: By using the formula discussed in question 31, the fluid requirement for this patient is calculated to be 65 mL/h.

    Reference: Dobbins, P. & Hall, S.M. (1997). Chapter 14: Pediatric Anesthesia. In J. Nagelhout & K. Zaglaniczny (Eds.), *Nurse Anesthesia*. Philadelphia: W.B. Saunders.

32. ANSWER: **C**

    Rationale: Hyperventilation is a rapid and effective method for acute management of intracranial pressure. Carbon dioxide should be kept in the 25 to 30 mm Hg range.

    Reference: DeVane, G.G. (1997). Chapter 37: Neurosurgical Anesthesia. In J. Nagelhout & K. Zaglaniczny (Eds.), *Nurse Anesthesia*. Philadelphia: W.B. Saunders.

33. ANSWER: **B**

    Rationale: Citrate binds calcium and may result in both anticoagulation and cardiac depression with rapid transfusion. Cardiac depression results from hypocalcemia due to citrate binding.

    Reference: Gerbasi, F.R. (1997). Chapter 41: Hematology and Anesthesia. In J. Nagelhout & K. Zaglaniczny (Eds.), *Nurse Anesthesia*. Philadelphia: W.B. Saunders.

34. ANSWER: **B**

    Rationale: Citrate may produce toxicity resulting in anticoagulation and cardiac

depression when massive blood transfusions are necessary.

Reference: Gerbasi, F.R. (1997). Chapter 41: Hematology and Anesthesia. In J. Nagelhout & K. Zaglaniczny (Eds.), *Nurse Anesthesia*. Philadelphia: W.B. Saunders.

35. ANSWER: **A**

    Rationale: The calcium that is present in lactated Ringer's solution may cause clotting when mixed with packed red blood cells. Therefore, these cells should be mixed with alternative crystalloid solutions.

    Reference: Gerbasi, F.R. (1997). Chapter 14: Hematology and Anesthesia. In J. Nagelhout & K. Zaglaniczny (Eds.), *Nurse Anesthesia*. Philadelphia: W.B. Saunders.

36. ANSWER: **C**

    Rationale: O Rh-negative blood is known as the universal donor because it is the least likely to initiate a transfusion reaction.

    Reference: Gerbasi, F.R. (1997). Chapter 41: Hematology and Anesthesia. In J. Nagelhout & K. Zaglaniczny (Eds.), *Nurse Anesthesia*. Philadelphia: W.B. Saunders.

37. ANSWER: **A**

    Rationale: The posterior cricoarytenoids abduct the vocal cords whereas the lateral cricoarytenoid muscles are the principal adductors.

    Reference: Hall, S.M. (1997). Chapter 9: Respiratory Anatomy and Physiology. In J. Nagelhout & K. Zaglaniczny (Eds.), *Nurse Anesthesia*. Philadelphia: W.B. Saunders.

38. ANSWER: **C**

    Rationale: The three unpaired cartilages are the thyroid, cricoid, and epiglottis. The three paired are the arytenoid, corniculate, and cuneiform.

    Reference: Hall, S.M. (1997). Chapter 9: Respiratory Anatomy and Physiology. In J. Nagelhout & K. Zaglaniczny (Eds.), *Nurse Anesthesia*. Philadelphia: W.B. Saunders.

39. ANSWER: **D**

    Rationale: The recurrent laryngeal nerve provides sensory innervation below the

cords and motor innervation for abduction of the cords.
Reference: Hall, S.M. (1997). Chapter 9: Respiratory Anatomy and Physiology. In J. Nagelhout & K. Zaglaniczny (Eds.), *Nurse Anesthesia*. Philadelphia: W.B. Saunders.

40. ANSWER: **C**

Rationale: The three unpaired cartilages are the thyroid, cricoid, and epiglottis. The three paired are the arytenoid, corniculate, and cuneiform.
Reference: Hall, S.M. (1997). Chapter 9: Respiratory Anatomy and Physiology. In J. Nagelhout & K. Zaglaniczny (Eds.), *Nurse Anesthesia*. Philadelphia: W.B. Saunders.

41. ANSWER: **B**

Rationale: The external branch of the superior laryngeal nerve provides motor innervation to the cricothyroid muscle, which tenses the vocal cords.
Reference: Hall, S.M. (1997). Chapter 9: Respiratory Anatomy and Physiology. In J. Nagelhout & K. Zaglaniczny (Eds.), Nurse Anethesia. Philadelphia: W.B. Saunders.

42. ANSWER: **C**

Rationale: Unilateral damage to this nerve results in hoarseness. Bilateral damage to the nerve results in stridor, respiratory distress, and aphonia.
Reference: Hall, S.M. (1997). Chapter 9: Respiratory Anatomy and Physiology. In J. Nagelhout & K. Zaglaniczny (Eds.), *Nurse Anesthesia*. Philadelphia: W.B. Saunders.

43. ANSWER: **D**

Rationale: Under normal conditions there is 21% oxygen in the atmosphere; and, considering deadspace, the tension that can be achieved in the blood is 102 to 104 mm Hg.
Reference: Hall, S.M. (1997). Chapter 9: Respiratory Anatomy and Physiology. In J. Nagelhout & K. Zaglaniczny (Eds.), *Nurse Anesthesia*. Philadelphia: W.B. Saunders.

44. ANSWER: **C**

Rationale: Incentive spirometry is a form of voluntary deep breathing in which patients are given an inhaled volume

as a goal to achieve. The preoperative inspiratory capacity should be the postoperative goal.
Reference: Hall, S.M. (1997). Chapter 9: Respiratory Anatomy and Physiology. In J. Nagelhout & K. Zaglaniczny (Eds.), *Nurse Anesthesia*. Philadelphia: W.B. Saunders.

45. ANSWER: **B**

Rationale: One of the most desirable properties of succinylcholine is its rapid onset of action. It has the most rapid onset among relaxants.
Reference: Haas, R.E. & Erway, R.L. (1997). Chapter 22: Neuromuscular Blocking Agents, Reversal Agents, and Their Monitoring. In J. Nagelhout & K. Zaglaniczny (Eds.), *Nurse Anesthesia*. Philadelphia: W.B. Saunders.

46. ANSWER: **A**

Rationale: Neutralization of carbon dioxide results in the production of calcium carbonate, water, and heat.
Reference: Dosch, M.P. (1997). Chapter 26: Anesthesia Equipment. In J. Nagelhout & K. Zaglaniczny (Eds.), *Nurse Anesthesia*. Philadelphia: W.B. Saunders.

47. ANSWER: **D**

Rationale: Injury to the ulnar nerve is the most common postoperative neuropathy. The nerve is frequently injured when stretched or compressed against the posterior aspect of the medial epicondyle of the humerus.
Reference: Monti, E.J. (1997). Chapter 32: Positioning for Anesthesia and Surgery. In J. Nagelhout & K. Zaglaniczny (Eds.), *Nurse Anesthesia*. Philadelphia: W.B. Saunders.

48. ANSWER: **C**

Rationale: Aminoglycosides, by chelating calcium, may prolong the action of muscle relaxants. This a rare, yet potentially serious, drug reaction.
Reference: Haas, R.E. & Erway, R.L. (1997). Chapter 22: Neuromuscular Blocking Agents, Reversal Agents, and Their Monitoring. In J. Nagelhout & K. Zaglaniczny (Eds.), *Nurse Anesthesia*. Philadelphia: W.B. Saunders.

49. ANSWER: **D**

Rationale: Increases in metabolic rate tend to produce heat, resulting in fever.

Anesthetics by nature decrease metabolic rate.

Reference: Bowen, D.R. (1997). Chapter 34: Intraoperative Thermoregulation. In J. Nagelhout & K. Zaglaniczny (Eds.), *Nurse Anesthesia.* Philadelphia: W.B. Saunders.

50. ANSWER: **B**

    Rationale: Surgical exposure of the patient (especially of large body cavities) tends to produce hypothermia during anesthesia.

    Reference: Bowen, D.R. (1997). Chapter 34: Intraoperative Thermoregulation. In J. Nagelhout & K. Zaglaniczny (Eds.), *Nurse Anesthesia.* Philadelphia: W.B. Saunders.

51. ANSWER: **A**

    Rationale: Warfarin-like drugs inhibit vitamin K–dependent factors II, VII, IX, and X.

    Reference: Gerbasi, F.R. (1997). Chapter 41: Hematology and Anesthesia. In J. Nagelhout & K. Zaglaniczny (Eds.), *Nurse Anesthesia.* Philadelphia: W.B. Saunders.

52. ANSWER: **A**

    Rationale: Vitamin K reverses warfarin because it acts by inhibiting vitamin K–dependent clotting factors; however, this reversal is slow and can take from 2 days to 1 week. Administration of fresh-frozen plasma provides the clotting factors necessary in an emergency.

    Reference: Gerbasi, F.R. (1997). Chapter 41: Hematology and Anesthesia. In J. Nagelhout & K. Zaglaniczny (Eds.), *Nurse Anesthesia.* Philadelphia: W.B. Saunders.

53. ANSWER: **C**

    Rationale: Although renal disease may result in anemia, it does not produce a decrease in platelet count.

    Reference: Gerbasi, F.R. (1997). Chapter 41: Hematology and Anesthesia. In J. Nagelhout & K. Zaglaniczny (Eds.), *Nurse Anesthesia.* Philadelphia: W.B. Saunders.

54. ANSWER: **D**

    Rationale: The onset of red urine due to free plasma hemoglobin may be the first sign of a blood reaction.

    Reference: Gerbasi, F.R. (1997). Chapter 41: Hematology and Anesthesia. In J. Nagelhout & K. Zaglaniczny (Eds.), *Nurse Anesthesia.* Philadelphia: W.B. Saunders.

55. ANSWER: **B**

    Rationale: The administration of blood would be unnecessary to treat a transfusion reaction. The other choices are common and necessary to maintain urine output and renal blood flow.

    Reference: Gerbasi, F.R. (1997). Chapter 41: Hematology and Anesthesia. In J. Nagelhout & K. Zaglaniczny (Eds.), *Nurse Anesthesia.* Philadelphia: W.B. Saunders.

56. ANSWER: **A**

    Rationale: The blood volume of an average 70-kg adult is approximately 70 mL/kg or 5000 mL.

    Reference: Gerbasi, F.R. (1997). Chapter 41: Hematology and Anesthesia. In J. Nagelhout & K. Zaglaniczny (Eds.), *Nurse Anesthesia.* Philadelphia: W.B. Saunders.

57. ANSWER: **D**

    Rationale: Whole blood has a hematocrit of approximately 40% whereas packed red cells have a hematocrit of approximately 70%. Because the plasma has been removed, cell count increases.

    Reference: Gerbasi, F.R. (1997). Chapter 41: Hematology and Anesthesia. In J. Nagelhout & K. Zaglaniczny (Eds.), *Nurse Anesthesia.* Philadelphia: W.B. Saunders.

58. ANSWER: **C**

    Rationale: Citrate intoxication results from the ability of citrate to bind calcium, causing hypocalcemia, which results in anticoagulation and cardiovascular depression.

    Reference: Gerbasi, F.R. (1997). Chapter 41: Hematology and Anesthesia. In J. Nagelhout & K. Zaglaniczny (Eds.), *Nurse Anesthesia.* Philadelphia: W.B. Saunders.

59. ANSWER: **C**

    Rationale: Citrate binds calcium, therefore producing systemic hypocalcemia.

    Reference: Gerbasi, F.R. (1997). Chapter 41: Hematology and Anesthesia. In J. Nagelhout &

K. Zaglaniczny (Eds.), *Nurse Anesthesia.* Philadelphia: W.B. Saunders.

60. ANSWER: **D**

Rationale: Common signs of hemolytic infusion reaction are fever, chills, chest pains, bleeding, hypotension, hematuria, flushing, and nausea.
Reference: Gerbasi, F.R. (1997). Chapter 41: Hematology and Anesthesia. In J. Nagelhout & K. Zaglaniczny (Eds.), *Nurse Anesthesia.* Philadelphia: W.B. Saunders.

61. ANSWER: **B**

Rationale: Storage of platelets at 4°C for 24 hours causes loss of 90% of viable transfusate. They should be used within 6 hours of preparation.
Reference: Gerbasi, F.R. (1997). Chapter 41: Hematology and Anesthesia. In J. Nagelhout & K. Zaglaniczny (Eds.), *Nurse Anesthesia.* Philadelphia: W.B. Saunders.

62. ANSWER: **D**

Rationale: Bank blood contains increased amounts of hydrogen and thus would tend toward acidosis. This, however, is not common, and administration of bicarbonate is rarely necessary.
Reference: Gerbasi, F.R. (1997). Chapter 41: Hematology and Anesthesia. In J. Nagelhout & K. Zaglaniczny (Eds.), *Nurse Anesthesia.* Philadelphia: W.B. Saunders.

63. ANSWER: **A**

Rationale: Too rapid correction of hyponatremia may result in cerebral edema and congestive heart failure; therefore, correction should proceed cautiously and slowly. Symptoms will improve within 24 hours.
Reference: Ouellette, S.M. (1997). Chapter 11: Renal Anatomy, Physiology, and Pathophysiology, and Anesthesia. In J. Nagelhout & K. Zaglaniczny (Eds.), *Nurse Anesthesia.* Philadelphia: W.B. Saunders.

64. ANSWER: **A**

Rationale: ECG changes with hypokalemia include widened QRS complex, ST depression, T-wave depression, U-wave prominence, and first-degree atrioventricular block.

Reference: Litwack, K. & Keithley, J.K. (1997). Chapter 31: Fluids, Electrolytes, and Therapy. In J. Nagelhout & K. Zaglaniczny (Eds.), *Nurse Anesthesia.* Philadelphia: W.B. Saunders.

65. ANSWER: **D**

Rationale: Acute hypokalemia causes hyperpolarization of the cardiac cell, leading to arrhythmic activity.
Reference: Litwack, K. & Keithley, J.K. (1997). Chapter 31: Fluids, Electrolytes, and Therapy. In J. Nagelhout & K. Zaglaniczny (Eds.), *Nurse Anesthesia.* Philadelphia: W.B. Saunders.

66. ANSWER: **B**

Rationale: Hyperkalemia results in tall peaked T waves, prolonged PR interval, widened QRS, a decrease in the amplitude of the P waves, and, ultimately, cardiac arrest.
Reference: Litwack, K. & Keithley, J.K. (1997). Chapter 31: Fluids, Electrolytes, and Therapy. In J. Nagelhout & K. Zaglaniczny (Eds.), *Nurse Anesthesia.* Philadelphia: W.B. Saunders.

67. ANSWER: **B**

Rationale: Half-life is the time it takes for the drug level to fall by one half. After one half-life, 50% is eliminated; two half-lives, 75% is eliminated; three half-lives, 87.5% is eliminated; and four half-lives, 95% is eliminated.
Reference: Troop, M. (1997). Chapter 17: Pharmacokinetics. In J. Nagelhout & K. Zaglaniczny (Eds.), *Nurse Anesthesia.* Philadelphia: W.B. Saunders.

68. ANSWER: **B**

Rationale: Calcium channel blockers would cause cardiac depression and possibly contribute to pulmonary stasis by decreasing cardiac function.
Reference: Rojo, J. & Iacopelli, M. (1997). Chapter 39A: Respiratory Pathophysiology. In J. Nagelhout & K. Zaglaniczny (Eds.), *Nurse Anesthesia.* Philadelphia: W.B. Saunders.

69. ANSWER: **A**

Rationale: First-degree heart block is relatively asymptomatic and usually does not require therapy. More severe heart block may be treated with a pacemaker.

Reference: Aprile, A.E. & Aprile, F.D. (1997). Chapter 38B: Cardiac Anesthesia. In J. Nagelhout & K. Zaglaniczny (Eds.), *Nurse Anesthesia*. Philadelphia: W.B. Saunders.

70. ANSWER: **A**

Rationale: Glucagon would be contraindicated because it would lower insulin levels. Insulin increases cellular uptake of potassium and is commonly given along with the other listed treatments for hyperkalemia.
Reference: Litwack, K. & Keithley, J.K. (1997). Chapter 31: Fluids, Electrolytes, and Therapy. In J. Nagelhout & K. Zaglaniczny (Eds.), *Nurse Anesthesia*. Philadelphia: W.B. Saunders.

71. ANSWER: **C**

Rationale: TURP syndrome results from hyponatremia and hypervolemia. Symptoms include visual disturbances, muscle twitching, confusion, nausea and vomiting, restlessness, hypotension, and arrhythmias.
Reference: Ouellette, S.M. (1997). Chapter 11: Renal Anatomy, Physiology, and Pathophysiology, and Anesthesia. In J. Nagelhout & K. Zaglaniczny (Eds.), *Nurse Anesthesia*. Philadelphia: W.B. Saunders.

72. ANSWER: **A**

Rationale: Correct size is confirmed by easy passage and lack of air leak at low ventilating pressure. Using the formula 4 + the child's age/4, a 4-year-old child would equal 4 + 4/4, which is 1; thus, 4 + 1 = 5.
Reference: Dobbins, P. & Hall, S.M. (1997). Chapter 14: Pediatric Anesthesia. In J. Nagelhout & K. Zaglaniczny (Eds.), *Nurse Anesthesia*. Philadelphia: W.B. Saunders.

73. ANSWER: **B**

Rationale: Endotracheal tubes should be inserted to the midtracheal position, which in a 3-year old is approximately 14 cm.
Reference: Dobbins, P. & Hall, S.M. (1997). Chapter 14: Pediatric Anesthesia. In J. Nagelhout & K. Zaglaniczny (Eds.), *Nurse Anesthesia*. Philadelphia: W.B. Saunders.

74. ANSWER: **C**

Rationale: Epiglotittis is characterized by a rapid onset of difficulties usually occurring within a 24-hour period.
Reference: Dobbins, P. & Hall, S.M. (1997). Chapter 14: Pediatric Anesthesia. In J. Nagelhout & K. Zaglaniczny (Eds.), *Nurse Anesthesia*. Philadelphia: W.B. Saunders.

75. ANSWER: **A**

Rationale: Usually intubation in the operating room is safer because emergency tracheotomy can be easily performed. However, if acute airway management can be safely ensured in the emergency department, then intubation may proceed.
Reference: Dobbins, P. & Hall, S.M. (1997). Chapter 14: Pediatric Anesthesia. In J. Nagelhout & K. Zaglaniczny (Eds.), *Nurse Anesthesia*. Philadelphia: W.B. Saunders.

76. ANSWER: **B**

Rationale: Receptors for pressure measurement in the body are located in the aortic arch and carotid sinuses with appropriate feedback mechanisms to cause changes when necessary.
Reference: Dobbins, P. & Hall, S.M. (1997). Chapter 14: Pediatric Anesthesia. In J. Nagelhout & K. Zaglaniczny (Eds.), *Nurse Anesthesia*. Philadelphia: W.B. Saunders.

77. ANSWER: **C**

Rationale: After 48 hours, capillary integrity returns to normal and colloid solutions will remain intravascular.
Reference: Sartain-Spivak, E. (1997). Chapter 43: Anesthesia for the Burn Patient. In J. Nagelhout & K. Zaglaniczny (Eds.), *Nurse Anesthesia*. Philadelphia: W.B. Saunders.

78. ANSWER: **A**

Rationale: It has been thought that calcium chloride ionizes to a greater extent and more quickly than gluconate; however, recent studies refute this dictate.
Reference: Litwack, K. & Keithley, J.K. (1997). Chapter 31: Fluids, Electrolytes, and Therapy. In J. Nagelhout & K. Zaglaniczny (Eds.), *Nurse Anesthesia*. Philadelphia: W.B. Saunders.

79. ANSWER: **D**

Rationale: The lingual and laryngeal branches of the glossopharyngeal nerve provide sensation of the posterior third of the tongue and oral pharynx.
Reference: Haas, R.E. & Erway, R.L. (1997). Chapter 22: Neuromuscular Blocking Agents, Reversal Aents, and Their Monitoring. In J. Nagelhout & K. Zaglaniczny (Eds.), *Nurse Anesthesia.* Philadelphia: W.B. Saunders.

80. ANSWER: **B**

Rationale: The usual starting dose for treatment of malignant hyperthermia is 2.5 mg/kg, repeated as necessary to a maximum of 10 mg/kg.
Reference: Karlet, M.C. (1997). Chapter 40: Musculoskeletal Pathophysiology and Anesthesia. In J. Nagelhout & K. Zaglaniczny (Eds.), *Nurse Anesthesia.* Philadelphia: W.B. Saunders.

81. ANSWER: **C**

Rationale: Tachycardia results in the greatest increase in the work of the heart, therefore the greatest potential for a mismatch between supply and demand.
Reference: Aprile, A.E. & Aprile, F.D. (1997). Chapter 38B: Cardiac Anesthesia. In J. Nagelhout & K. Zaglaniczny (Eds.), *Nurse Anesthesia.* Philadelphia: W.B. Saunders.

82. ANSWER: **A**

Rationale: Because coronary perfusion occurs during diastole, increases in diastolic pressure result in an increase in coronary perfusion.
Reference: Aprile, A.E., Serwin, J.P. & Boctor, B. (1997). Chapter 38A: Cardiac Pathophysiology. In J. Nagelhout & K. Zaglaniczny (Eds.), *Nurse Anesthesia.* Philadelphia: W.B. Saunders.

83. ANSWER: **A**

Rationale: Ascending bellows that are found in all modern anesthesia equipment are safer because a disconnect is more easily observed when the bellows do not ascend on cycling.
Reference: Dosch, M.P. (1997). Chapter 26: Anesthesia Equipment. In J. Nagelhout & K. Zaglaniczny (Eds.), *Nurse Anesthesia.* Philadelphia: W.B. Saunders.

84. ANSWER: **D**

Rationale: Hetastarch has a long plasma half-life of 1.5 days and does not affect coagulation when used in recommended doses, which should be limited to no more than 20 mL/kg.
Reference: Litwack, K. & Keithley, J.K. (1997). Chapter 31: Fluids, Electrolytes, and Therapy. In J. Nagelhout & K. Zaglaniczny (Eds.), *Nurse Anesthesia.* Philadelphia: W.B. Saunders.

85. ANSWER: **A**

Rationale: Elimination half-life of virtually all drugs is prolonged with increasing age. This includes the muscle relaxants, which last longer in elderly patients.
Reference: Martin-Sheridan, D. (1997). Chapter 42: Geriatrics and Anesthesia Practice. In J. Nagelhout & K. Zaglaniczny (Eds.), *Nurse Anesthesia.* Philadelphia: W.B. Saunders.

86. ANSWER: **C**

Rationale: Geriatric patients have a less well-developed blood-brain barrier in cell membranes. Therefore, drugs that are lipid soluble distribute more freely, resulting in a higher distribution volume.
Reference: Martin-Sheridan, D. (1997). Chapter 42: Geriatrics and Anesthesia Practice. In J. Nagelhout & K. Zaglaniczny (Eds.), *Nurse Anesthesia.* Philadelphia: W.B. Saunders.

87. ANSWER: **D**

Rationale: Diffusion hypoxia occurs owing to the insolubility of nitrous oxide and the high concentrations administered.
Reference: Nagelhout, J.J. (1997). Chapter 17: Uptake and Distribution of Inhalation Anesthetics. In J. Nagelhout & K. Zaglaniczny (Eds.), *Nurse Anesthesia.* Philadelphia: W.B. Saunders.

88. ANSWER: **B**

Rationale: Nonionized forms of all drugs will be lipid soluble because no charge is present to repel the molecule from lipid membranes.
Reference: Williams, J.R. (1997). Chapter 20: Local Anesthetics. In J. Nagelhout & K. Zaglaniczny (Eds.), *Nurse Anesthetics.* Philadelphia: W.B. Saunders.

89. ANSWER: **D**

Rationale: Local anesthetics must diffuse through the lipid nerve membrane to reach their site of action. All of the listed factors will either increase lipid solubility or concentration in the nerve.
Reference: Williams, J.R. (1997). Chapter 20: Local Anesthetics. In J. Nagelhout & K. Zaglaniczny (Eds.), *Nurse Anesthesia.* Philadelphia: W.B. Saunders.

90. ANSWER: **B**

Rationale: Monitoring the right radial pulse will signal compression by the scope on the innominate artery and allow for repositioning to ensure adequate circulation. Blood pressure should be monitored in the left arm because of this potential compression.
Reference: Cafarelli, J.M. (1997). Chapter 39B: Thoracic Surgery. In J. Nagelhout & K. Zaglaniczny (Eds.), *Nurse Anesthesia.* Philadelphia: W.B. Saunders.

91. ANSWER: **A**

Rationale: Overactivity of the sympathetic nervous system is common with transection at T5 or above and is unusual with injuries below the T10 level.
Reference: Barton, C.R. (1997). Chapter 44: Trauma Anesthesia. In J. Nagelhout & K. Zaglaniczny (Eds.), *Nurse Anesthesia.* Philadelphia: W.B. Saunders.

92. ANSWER: **C**

Rationale: Sympathetic innervation to the heart is mediated via sympathetic fibers arising from the cord at the level T1 through T5 with T3, T4, and T5 having the greatest input.
Reference: Harrigan, C. (1997). Chapter 6: The Central Nervous System. In J. Nagelhout & K. Zaglaniczny (Eds.), *Nurse Anesthesia.* Philadelphia: W.B. Saunders.

93. ANSWER: **C**

Rationale: The superior laryngeal branch of the vagus divides into an external (motor) nerve and internal (sensory) laryngeal nerve that provides sensory supply to the larynx between the epiglottis and the vocal cords.
Reference: Chipas, A. (1997). Chapter 33: Airway Management. In J. Nagelhout & K. Zaglaniczny (Eds.), *Nurse Anesthesia.* Philadelphia: W.B. Saunders.

94. ANSWER: **D**

Rationale: The larynx is composed of nine cartilages—the thyroid, cricoid, and epiglottic and the paired cartilages arytenoid, corniculate, and cuneiform.
Reference: Chipas, A. (1997). Chapter 33: Airway Management. In J. Nagelhout & K. Zaglaniczny (Eds.), *Nurse Anesthesia.* Philadelphia: W.B. Saunders.

95. ANSWER: **C**

Rationale: Many sympathomimetic drugs act by causing endogenous release of catecholamines, which results in an adrenergic effect.
Reference: Alisoglu, R. (1997). Chapter 23: Cardiac Pharmacology. In J. Nagelhout & K. Zaglaniczny (Eds.), *Nurse Anesthesia.* Philadelphia: W.B. Saunders.

96. ANSWER: **B**

Rationale: Cardiac output reaches a maximum immediately after delivery where it can be increased as much as 60% of normal. It returns to normal within 2 weeks after delivery.
Reference: Fiedler, M.A. & Shaw, B. (1997). Chapter 13: Obstetric Anesthesia. In J. Nagelhout & K. Zaglaniczny (Eds.), *Nurse Anesthesia.* Philadelphia: W.B. Saunders.

97. ANSWER: **B**

Rationale: Ephedrine preserves uterine blood flow to a greater extent than either pure alpha-receptor vasopressors or epinephrine.
Reference: Fiedler, M.A. & Shaw, B. (1997). Chapter 13: Obstetric Anesthesia. In J. Nagelhout & K. Zaglaniczny (Eds.), *Nurse Anesthesia.* Philadelphia: W.B. Saunders.

98. ANSWER: **C**

Rationale: Heparin antithrombin III and serine proteases combine to produce the anticoagulant effect. Elevated antithrombin III would affect coagulation, and heparin should be avoided.

Reference: Aprile, A.E. & Aprile, F.D. (1997). Chapter 38B: Cardiac Anesthesia. In J. Nagelhout & K. Zaglaniczny (Eds.), *Nurse Anesthesia*. Philadelphia: W.B. Saunders.

99. ANSWER: **C**

Rationale: With aging there is a decreased responsiveness to the usual compensatory mechanisms. This occurs in the central nervous system's cardiovascular control centers, which send the inputs by means of the autonomic nervous system and alpha, beta, and muscarinic receptors.

Reference: Martin-Sheridan, D. (1997). Chapter 42: Geriatrics and Anesthesia Practice. In J. Nagelhout & K. Zaglaniczny (Eds.), *Nurse Anesthesia*. Philadelphia: W.B. Saunders.

100. ANSWER: **A**

Rationale: The decrease in cardiac output produced by positive end-expiratory pressure is due to interference with venous return and a leftward displacement of the heart that restricts filling of the left ventricle.

Reference: Cafarelli, J.M. (1997). Chapter 39B: Thoracic Surgery. In J. Nagelhout & K. Zaglaniczny (Eds.), *Nurse Anesthesia*. Philadelphia: W.B. Saunders.

101. ANSWER: **C**

Rationale: Moderate positive-pressure ventilation does not increase air entry into the stomach as long as the airway remains patent.

Reference: Chipas, A. (1997). Chapter 33: Airway Management. In J. Nagelhout & K. Zaglaniczny (Eds.), *Nurse Anesthesia*. Philadelphia: W.B. Saunders.

102. ANSWER: **A**

Rationale: Droperidol has an antidopamine effect; therefore, it is contraindicated in patients with Parkinson's disease because extrapyramidal side effects may occur.

Reference: Chick, M. (1997). Chapter 21: Opioid Agonists and Antagonists. In J. Nagelhout & K. Zaglaniczny (Eds.), *Nurse Anesthesia*. Philadelphia: W.B. Saunders.

103. ANSWER: **C**

Rationale: Because of the reuptake of catecholamines, cocaine may produce multiple cardiac dysrhythmias.

Reference: Williams, J.R. (1997). Chapter 20: Local Anesthetics. In J. Nagelhout & K. Zaglaniczny (Eds.), *Nurse Anesthesia*. Philadelphia: W.B. Saunders.

104. ANSWER: **B**

Rationale: Like other neurotransmitters the main effect of norepinephrine is terminated by active reuptake and transport into the nerve terminal.

Reference: Alisoglu, R. (1997). Chapter 23: Cardiac Pharmacology. In J. Nagelhout & K. Zaglaniczny (Eds.), *Nurse Anesthesia*. Philadelphia: W.B. Saunders.

105. ANSWER: **C**

Rationale: With chronic therapy, catecholamine levels decrease and the initial stimulation is then followed by a central nervous system depression and fatigue.

Reference: Williams, J.R. (1997). Chapter 20: Local Anesthetics. In J. Nagelhout & K. Zaglaniczny (Eds.), *Nurse Anesthesia*. Philadelphia: W.B. Saunders.

106. ANSWER: **B**

Rationale: Clonidine, by stimulating central alpha$_2$-receptors, produces a vasodepressor and sedative effect.

Reference: Alisoglu, R. (1997). Chapter 23: Cardiac Pharmacology. In J. Nagelhout & K. Zaglaniczny (Eds.), *Nurse Anesthesia*. Philadelphia: W.B. Saunders.

107. ANSWER: **B**

Rationale: Ester local anesthetic metabolism is catalyzed by cholinesterase. Therefore, patients with atypical genotypes will have prolonged metabolism.

Reference: Williams, J.R. (1997). Chapter 20: Local Anesthetics. In J. Nagelhout & K. Zaglaniczny (Eds.), *Nurse Anesthesia*. Philadelphia: W.B. Saunders.

108. ANSWER: **D**

Rationale: Several recent reports of sudden cardiac arrest after administration of succinylcholine to patients with undiagnosed Duchenne muscular dystrophy has led to a warning in children younger than 12 years old.

Reference: Haas, R.E. & Erway, R.L. (1997). Chapter 22: Neuromuscular Blocking Agents, Reversal Agents, and Their Monitoring. In J. Nagelhout & K. Zaglaniczny (Eds.), *Nurse Anesthesia.* Philadelphia: W.B. Saunders.

109. ANSWER: C

Rationale: Dibucaine inhibits normal cholinesterase. The dibucaine number reflects the amount of inhibition that in the average person equals approximately 80%.

Reference: Haas, R.E. & Erway, R.L. (1997). Chapter 22: Neuromuscular Blocking Agents, Reversal Agents, and Their Monitoring. In J. Nagelhout & K. Zaglaniczny (Eds.), *Nurse Anesthesia.* Philadelphia: W.B. Saunders.

110. ANSWER: B

Rationale: After nitroprusside drip there is a rebound release of renin, which results in a period of hypertension after termination of the infusion.

Reference: Haas, R.E. & Erway, R.L. (1997). Chapter 22: Neuromuscular Blocking Agents, Reversal Agents, and Their Monitoring. In J. Nagelhout & K. Zaglaniczny (Eds.), *Nurse Anesthesia.* Philadelphia: W.B. Saunders.

111. ANSWER: B

Rationale: Hospital piping systems provides gas to the machine at approximately 50 psi, which is the normal working pressure of most machines.

Reference: Dosch, M.P. (1997). Chapter 26: Anesthesia Equipment. In J. Nagelhout & K. Zaglaniczny (Eds.), *Nurse Anesthesia.* Philadelphia: W.B. Saunders.

112. ANSWER: B

Rationale: The pressure sensor shut-off valves decrease the supply of nitrous oxide if the oxygen supply pressure falls below approximately 25 psi.

Reference: Dosch, M.P. (1997). Chapter 26: Anesthesia Equipment. In J. Nagelhout & K. Zaglaniczny (Eds.), *Nurse Anesthesia.* Philadelphia: W.B. Saunders.

113. ANSWER: D

Rationale: Henry's law states that the concentration of any gas in solution is proportional to the partial pressure of that gas.

Reference: Hall. S.M. (1997). Chapter 4: Chemistry and Physics for Anesthesia. In J. Nagelhout & K. Zaglaniczny (Eds.), *Nurse Anesthesia.* Philadelphia: W.B. Saunders.

114. ANSWER: C

Rationale: Total systemic vascular resistance is calculated from hemodynamic variables derived with a pulmonary artery catheter. The normal systemic vascular resistance is 1200 to 1500 dynes/sec/cm^{-5}.

Reference: Morgan, R.O., Jr. (1997). Chapter 8: The Cardiovascular System. In J. Nagelhout & K. Zaglaniczny (Eds.), *Nurse Anesthesia.* Philadelphia: W.B. Saunders.

115. ANSWER: C

Rationale: Non-rebreathing systems are used for children primarily because they offer little resistance to breathing and will not as easily cause fatigue in a child's respiration.

Reference: Dobbins, P. & Hall, S.M. (1997). Chapter 14: Pediatric Anesthesia. In J. Nagelhout & K. Zaglaniczny (Eds.), *Nurse Anesthesia.* Philadelphia: W.B. Saunders.

116. ANSWER: D

Rationale: Clamping the aorta produces an acute tremendous increase in left ventricular afterload, which can result in ischemia, failure, and severe hypertension. Use of vasodilators can attenuate this problem.

Reference: McIntosh, L.S. (1997). Chapter 38C: Vascular Surgery. In J. Nagelhout & K. Zaglaniczny (Eds.), *Nurse Anesthesia.* Philadelphia: W.B. Saunders.

117. ANSWER: C

Rationale: Sodium hydroxide is a catalyst for carbon dioxide absorption in soda lime, although both substances contain more calcium hydroxide than sodium hydroxide.

Reference: Dosch, M.P. (1997). Chapter 26: Anesthesia Equipment. In J. Nagelhout & K. Zaglaniczny (Eds.), *Nurse Anesthesia.* Philadelphia: W.B. Saunders.

118. ANSWER: **D**

Rationale: Ventilators whose bellows ascend on expiration have been deemed the safest regarding disconnects and are now in use on all anesthesia equipment.
Reference: Dosch, M.P. (1997). Chapter 26: Anesthesia Equipment. In J. Nagelhout & K. Zaglaniczny (Eds.), *Nurse Anesthesia.* Philadelphia: W.B. Saunders.

119. ANSWER: **B**

Rationale: Synchronized intermittent mandatory ventilation allows the patient to initiate a breath but ensures that he or she receives an adequate tidal volume.
Reference: Dosch, M.P. (1997). Chapter 26: Anesthesia Equipment. In J. Nagelhout & K. Zaglaniczny (Eds.), *Nurse Anesthesia.* Philadelphia: W.B. Saunders.

120. ANSWER: **A**

Rationale: High carbon dioxide levels result in tachycardia, restlessness, and diaphoresis. Fortunately, with improved monitoring, this has become less of a problem in modern anesthesia practice.
Reference: Rojo, J. & Iacopelli, M. (1997). Chapter 39A: Respiratory Pathophysiology. In J. Nagelhout & K. Zaglaniczny (Eds.), *Nurse Anesthesia.* Philadelphia: W.B. Saunders.

121. ANSWER: **C**

Rationale: In equivalent dosages, rocuronium exhibits the fastest onset for intubating conditions among the nondepolarizing muscle relaxants.
Reference: Haas, R.E. & Erway, R. L. (1997). Chapter 22: Neuromuscular Blocking Agents, Reversal Agents, and Their Monitoring. In J. Nagelhout & K. Zaglaniczny (Eds.), *Nurse Anesthesia.* Philadelphia: W.B. Saunders.

122. ANSWER: **D**

Rationale: Airway resistance increases greatly when the bronchus in the diseased lung is clamped. Adjustments in respiration to ensure adequate oxygenation and carbon dioxide removal are necessary.
Reference: Cafarelli, J.M. (1997). Chapter 39B: Thoracic Surgery. In J. Nagelhout & K. Zaglaniczny (Eds.), *Nurse Anesthesia.* Philadelphia: W.B. Saunders.

123. ANSWER: **C**

Rationale: Patients with chronic renal failure do not excrete nonvolatile acids, which result in high anion gap metabolic acidosis.
Reference: Ouellette, S.M. (1997). Chapter 11: Renal Anatomy, Physiology, and Pathophysiology, and Anesthesia. In J. Nagelhout & K. Zaglaniczny (Eds.), *Nurse Anesthesia.* Philadelphia: W.B. Saunders.

124. ANSWER: **A**

Rationale: A small volume of distribution means the drug is primarily in the bloodstream and, with a short half-life, this would make it easily removed from the body.
Reference: Troop, M. (1997). Chapter 16: Pharmacokinetics. In J. Nagelhout & K. Zaglaniczny (Eds.), *Nurse Anesthesia.* Philadelphia: W.B. Saunders.

125. ANSWER: **D**

Rationale: One of the main functions of the airway is to increase the humidity of gases as they are breathed; therefore, the water vapor increases as gases are drawn into the lungs.
Reference: Hall, S.M. (1997). Chapter 9: Respiratory Anatomy and Physiology. In J. Nagelhout & K. Zaglaniczny (Eds.), *Nurse Anesthesia.* Philadelphia: W.B. Saunders.

126. ANSWER: **A**

Rationale: Ammonia increases in the blood in intact humans when there is liver damage and is released as urea is synthesized. In bank blood, ammonia levels stay relatively constant and are not affected during transfusion.
Reference: Gerbasi, F.R. (1997). Chapter 41: Hematology and Anesthesia. In J. Nagelhout & K. Zaglaniczny (Eds.), *Nurse Anesthesia.* Philadelphia: W.B. Saunders.

127. ANSWER: **B**

Rationale: Spontaneous ventilation may partially compensate for the compression on the dependent hemithorax; however, there is still a slight decrease in ventilatory capacity in the down lung.
Reference: Monti, E.J. (1997). Chapter 32: Positioning for Anesthesia and Surgery. In J.

Nagelhout & K. Zaglaniczny (Eds.), *Nurse Anesthesia*. Philadelphia: W.B. Saunders.

128. ANSWER: **A**

Rationale: Persistent vomiting in a patient with pyloric stenosis depletes sodium, potassium, chloride, and hydrogen ions, causing metabolic alkalosis.
Reference: Dobbins, P. & Hall, S.M. (1997). Chapter 14: Pediatric Anesthesia. In J. Nagelhout & K. Zaglaniczny (Eds.), *Nurse Anesthesia*. Philadelphia: W.B. Saunders.

129. ANSWER: **D**

Rationale: Although all of the answers are important, sustaining headlift for 5 seconds appears to correlate with muscle strength to a greater degree than the other parameters.
Reference: Haas, R.E. & Erway, R.L. (1997). Chapter 22: Neuromuscular Blocking Agents, Reversal Agents, and Their Monitoring. In J. Nagelhout & K. Zaglaniczny (Eds.), *Nurse Anesthesia*. Philadelphia: W.B. Saunders.

130. ANSWER: **D**

Rationale: Recommendations for nitrous oxide are based on the studies by Bruce and colleagues, who noted after exposure to 25 ppm nitrous oxide that no impairment of psychomotor tests was present.
Reference: Dosch, M.P. (1997). Chapter 26: Anesthesia Equipment. In J. Nagelhout & K. Zaglaniczny (Eds.), *Nurse Anesthesia*. Philadelphia: W.B. Saunders.

131. ANSWER: **D**

Rationale: Distortion of the facial anatomy and upper airway, including enlarged tongue and epiglottis and thickened vocal cords, is common with this disorder.
Reference: Karlet, M.C. & Sebastian, L.A. (1997). Chapter 12: The Endocrine System. In J. Nagelhout & K. Zaglaniczny (Eds.), *Nurse Anesthesia*. Philadelphia: W.B. Saunders.

132. ANSWER: **D**

Rationale: To ensure the safety of medical cylinders, inspection must be complete every 5 years. This has become a standard in the United States.

Reference: Dosch, M.P. (1997). Chapter 26: Anesthesia Equipment. In J. Nagelhout & K. Zaglaniczny (Eds.), *Nurse Anesthesia*. Philadelphia: W.B. Saunders.

133. ANSWER: **A**

Rationale: Static discharges, which are a source of ignition, are much less likely if the relative humidity is at least 50%.
Reference: Dosch, M.P. (1997). Chapter 26: Anesthesia Equipment. In J. Nagelhout & K. Zaglaniczny (Eds.), *Nurse Anesthesia*. Philadelphia: W.B. Saunders.

134. ANSWER: **D**

Rationale: A diagnosis of stridor hoarseness (unilateral with aphonia) is an indication of recurrent laryngeal nerve damage.
Reference: Chipas, A. (1997). Chapter 33: Airway Management. In J. Nagelhout & K. Zaglaniczny (Eds.), *Nurse Anesthesia*. Philadelphia: W.B. Saunders.

135. ANSWER: **C**

Rationale: Malignant hyperthermia results from an increase in myoplasmic calcium. The ryanodine receptor may be involved because control of calcium by this receptor is prominent in muscle cells.
Reference: Karlet, M.C. (1997). Chapter 40: Musculoskeletal Pathophysiology and Anesthesia. In J. Nagelhout & K. Zaglaniczny (Eds.), *Nurse Anesthesia*. Philadelphia: W.B. Saunders.

136. ANSWER: **A**

Rationale: A grossly distended abdomen makes the patient at very high risk for aspiration and desaturation if the airway is difficult, as well as for hypotension from decreased venous return.
Reference: Scarsella, J. (1997). Chapter 54B: Anesthesia for Heart Transplantation. In J. Nagelhout & K. Zaglaniczny (Eds.), *Nurse Anesthesia*. Philadelphia: W.B. Saunders.

137. ANSWER: **B**

Rationale: Increased action of both phenytoin and warfarin would be expected because the interaction involves the high protein binding and displacement of the drugs, increasing free concentration.

Reference: Troop, M. (1997). Chapter 16: Pharmacokinetics. In J. Nagelhout & K. Zaglaniczny (Eds.), *Nurse Anesthesia.* Philadelphia: W.B. Saunders.

138. ANSWER: **B**

Rationale: Both clonidine and propranolol produce a vasodepressor response, so when they are given together the possibility of hypotension is greatly increased.

Reference: Troop, M. (1997). Chapter 16: Pharmacokinetics. In J. Nagelhout & K. Zaglaniczny (Eds.), *Nurse Anesthesia.* Philadelphia: W.B. Saunders.

139. ANSWER: **D**

Rationale: Cimetidine is famous for its ability to inhibit drug-metabolizing enzymes in the liver, resulting in the decreased metabolism of other drugs relying on the liver for biotransformation.

Reference: Troop, M. (1997). Chapter 16: Pharmacokinetics. In J. Nagelhout & K. Zaglaniczny (Eds.), *Nurse Anesthesia.* Philadelphia: W.B. Saunders.

140. ANSWER: **D**

Rationale: High doses of calcium channel blockers have been reported to increase bleeding by reducing calcium coagulant ability.

Reference: Alisoglu, R. (1997). Chapter 23: Cardiac Pharmacology. In J. Nagelhout & K. Zaglaniczny (Eds.), *Nurse Anesthesia.* Philadelphia: W.B. Saunders.

141. ANSWER: **A**

Rationale: Dopamine stimulates dopamine receptors in renal arteries, resulting in vasodilation, increased blood flow, and increased glomerular filtration rate.

Reference: Barton, C.R. (1997). Chapter 44: Trauma Anesthesia. In J. Nagelhout & K. Zaglaniczny (Eds.), *Nurse Anesthesia.* Philadelphia: W.B. Saunders.

142. ANSWER: **B**

Rationale: Extrapyramidal side effects usually require no treatment; however, if they are extreme, anticholinergic ther-

apy with diphenhydramine may help relieve these symptoms.

Reference: Chick, M. (1997). Chapter 21: Opioid Agonists and Antagonists. In J. Nagelhout & K. Zaglaniczny (Eds.), *Nurse Anesthesia.* Philadelphia: W.B. Saunders.

143. ANSWER: **D**

Rationale: Sodium thiocyanate is the end product of metabolism of cyanide by thiosulfate. Thiocyanate is then excreted in the kidney as a nontoxic byproduct.

Reference: Alisoglu, R. (1997). Chapter 23: Cardiac Pharmacology. In J. Nagelhout & K. Zaglaniczny (Eds.), *Nurse Anesthesia.* Philadelphia: W.B. Saunders.

144. ANSWER: **D**

Rationale: Cyanide poisoning represents histotoxic hypoxia, which is the inability of the cell to utilize oxygen.

Reference: Alisoglu, R. (1997). Chapter 23: Cardiac Pharmacology. In J. Nagelhout & K. Zaglaniczny (Eds.), *Nurse Anesthesia.* Philadelphia: W.B. Saunders.

145. ANSWER: **D**

Rationale: Aminophylline has been shown to decrease sedation from benzodiazepines possibly by means of an effect on adenosine receptors.

Reference: Fallacaro, N. A. & Fallacaro, M.D. (1997). Chapter 19: Intravenous Inhalation Agents. In J. Nagelhout & K. Zaglaniczny (Eds.), *Nurse Anesthesia.* Philadelphia: W.B. Saunders.

146. ANSWER: **C**

Rationale: Blood/gas solubility partition coefficient is a measure of how an anesthetic compartmentalizes itself in the body.

Reference: Nagelhout, J.J. (1997). Chapter 17: Uptake and Distribution of Inhalation Anesthetics. In J. Nagelhout & K. Zaglaniczny (Eds.), *Nurse Anesthesia.* Philadelphia: W.B. Saunders.

147. ANSWER: **A**

Rationale: Flexion of a child's head may advance the tube more deeply into the chest, resulting in endobronchial intubation.

Reference: Dobbins, P. & Hall, S.M. (1997). Chapter 14: Pediatric Anesthesia. In J. Nagelhout & K. Zaglaniczny (Eds.), *Nurse Anesthesia.* Philadelphia: W.B. Saunders.

148. ANSWER: **D**

Rationale: Beta-receptor blocking drugs are commonly given to people with glaucoma. These agents appear to decrease synthesis of aqueous humor, thus reducing pressure in the eye.
Reference: Harvey, R.R. (1997). Chapter 48: Anesthesia for Ophthalmic Procedures. In J. Nagelhout & K. Zaglaniczny (Eds.), *Nurse Anesthesia.* Philadelphia: W.B. Saunders.

149. ANSWER: **D**

Rationale: Hypertension is the hallmark characteristic of this pregnancy-induced syndrome also known as preeclampsia.
Reference: Fiedler, M.A. & Shaw, B. (1997). Chapter 13: Obstetric Anesthesia. In J. Nagelhout & K. Zaglaniczny (Eds.), *Nurse Anesthesia.* Philadelphia: W.B. Saunders.

150. ANSWER: **B**

Rationale: In the upright position, the greatest amount of air exchange occurs in the upper airway due to gravity.
Reference: Monti, E.J. (1997). Chapter 32: Positioning for Anesthesia and Surgery. In J. Nagelhout & K. Zaglaniczny (Eds.), *Nurse Anesthesia.* Philadelphia: W.B. Saunders.

151. ANSWER: **C**

Rationale: Administration of a bronchodilating beta$_2$ agonist by means of the inhalation or intravenous route is the most effective acute treatment of bronchial constriction.
Reference: Hall, S.M. (1997). Chapter 9: Respiratory Anatomy and Physiology. In J. Nagelhout & K. Zaglaniczny (Eds.), *Nurse Anesthesia.* Philadelphia: W.B. Saunders.

152. ANSWER: **C**

Rationale: In the lateral position, the up lung is better ventilated owing to decreased compression of the chest wall as compared with the down lung.
Reference: Monti, E.J. (1997). Chapter 32: Positioning for Anesthesia and Surgery. In J.

Nagelhout & K. Zaglaniczny (Eds.), *Nurse Anesthesia.* Philadelphia: W.B. Saunders.

153. ANSWER: **C**

Rationale: Calcium allows actin and myosin fibers to interact, thus shortening the muscle fibers.
Reference: Karlet, M.C. (1997). Chapter 40: Musculoskeletal Pathophysiology and Anesthesia. In J. Nagelhout & K. Zaglaniczny (Eds.), *Nurse Anesthesia.* Philadelphia: W.B. Saunders.

154. ANSWER: **B**

Rationale: To maintain body temperature, neonates create heat by metabolizing brown fat, crying, and moving vigorously but, unlike adults, rarely shiver.
Reference: Bowen, D.R. (1997). Chapter 34: Intraoperative Thermoregulation. In J. Nagelhout & K. Zaglaniczny (Eds.), *Nurse Anesthesia.* Philadelphia: W.B. Saunders.

155. ANSWER: **B**

Rationale: Persistent vomiting that occurs with this syndrome results in inadequate hydration and hypovolemia.
Reference: Dobbins, P. & Hall, S.M. (1997). Chapter 14: Pediatric Anesthesia. In J. Nagelhout & K. Zaglaniczny (Eds.), *Nurse Anesthesia.* Philadelphia: W.B. Saunders.

156. ANSWER: **B**

Rationale: Therapeutic magnesium levels are maintained to treat hyperreflexia and prevent convulsions until delivery of the fetus and the placenta is possible.
Reference: Fiedler, M.A. & Shaw, B. (1997). Chapter 13: Obstetric Anesthesia. In J. Nagelhout & K. Zaglaniczny (Eds.), *Nurse Anesthesia.* Philadelphia: W.B. Saunders.

157. ANSWER: **D**

Rationale: Use of high concentrations of bupivaicaine results in initial cardiac arrest after systemic absorption rather than the expected neurotoxicity.
Reference: Williams, J.R. (1997). Chapter 20: Local Anesthetics. In J. Nagelhout & K. Zaglaniczny (Eds.), *Nurse Anesthesia.* Philadelphia: W.B. Saunders.

158. ANSWER: **A**

Rationale: With the midline approach, the needle passes through the supraspi-

nous, interspinous, and ligamentum fla-
vum to reach the epidural space.
Reference: Ellis, W.E. (1997). Chapter 53: Regional
Anesthesia. In J. Nagelhout & K. Zaglaniczny
(Eds.), *Nurse Anesthesia*. Philadelphia: W.B.
Saunders.

159. ANSWER: **B**

Rationale: Ensuring proper oxygenation is
essential therapy in any hemorrhagic
emergency.
Reference: Fiedler, M.A. & Shaw, B. (1997).
Chapter 13: Obstetric Anesthesia. In J.
Nagelhout & K. Zaglaniczny (Eds.), *Nurse
Anesthesia*. Philadelphia: W.B. Saunders.

160. ANSWER: **B**

Rationale: Dextrose and water solutions
should not be used in neurosurgical patients because of the tendency for them
to produce cerebral edema and alter glucose metabolism in the brain.
Reference: DeVane, G.G. (1997). Chapter 37:
Neurosurgical Anesthesia. In J. Nagelhout & K.
Zaglaniczny (Eds.), *Nurse Anesthesia*.
Philadelphia: W.B. Saunders.

161. ANSWER: **B**

Rationale: Decreasing preload with vaso-
dilators reduces venous return and the
amount of work the heart must do to
eject returning blood flow.
Reference: Morgan, R.O., Jr. (1997). Chapter 8:
The Cardiovascular System. In J. Nagelhout & K.
Zaglaniczny (Eds.), *Nurse Anesthesia*.
Philadelphia: W.B. Saunders.

162. ANSWER: **A**

Rationale: Increases in heart rate produce
the greatest increase in cardiac work and
must be avoided in patients with ischemic heart disease and congestive heart
failure to prevent cardiac decompensa-
tion.
Reference: Morgan, R. O., Jr. (1997). Chapter 8:
The Cardiovascular System. In J. Nagelhout & K.
Zaglaniczny (Eds.), *Nurse Anesthesia*.
Philadelphia: W.B. Saunders.

163. ANSWER: **B**

Rationale: Diminished cardiac reserve in
many elderly patients may be seen as

exaggerated drops in blood pressure dur-
ing induction of anesthesia.
Reference: Martin-Sheridan, D. (1997). Chapter 42:
Geriatrics and Anesthesia Practice. In J.
Nagelhout & K. Zaglaniczny (Eds.), *Nurse
Anesthesia*. Philadelphia: W.B. Saunders.

164. ANSWER: **A**

Rationale: Preload, afterload, and heart
rate are determinants of myocardial de-
mand, whereas perfusion and oxygen-
ation are supply parameters.
Reference: Morgan, R.O., Jr. (1997). Chapter 8:
The Cardiovascular System. In J. Nagelhout & K.
Zaglaniczny (Eds.), *Nurse Anesthesia*.
Philadelphia: W.B. Saunders.

165. ANSWER: **B**

Rationale: The vast amounts of urine pro-
duced by patients with diabetes insipidus
have relatively no solute and thus a very
minimal osmolarity.
Reference: Karlet, M.C. & Sebastian, L.A. (1997).
Chapter 12: The Endocrine System. In J.
Nagelhout & K. Zaglaniczny (Eds.), *Nurse
Anesthesia*. Philadelphia: W.B. Saunders.

166. ANSWER: **C**

Rationale: Thymol 0.01% is added to hal-
othane liquid as a stabilizer to prevent
breakdown during storage.
Reference: Kossick, M.A. (1997). Chapter 18:
Inhalation Anesthetics. In J. Nagelhout & K.
Zaglaniczny (Eds.), *Nurse Anesthesia*.
Philadelphia: W.B. Saunders.

167. ANSWER: **B**

Rationale: Hiatal hernia does not involve
a closed gas space in the body; therefore,
it would not be expanded by the admin-
istration of nitrous oxide.
Reference: Kossick, M.A. (1997). Chapter 18:
Inhalation Anesthetics. In J. Nagelhout & K.
Zaglaniczny (Eds.), *Nurse Anesthesia*.
Philadelphia: W.B. Saunders.

168. ANSWER: **C**

Rationale: Some volatile anesthetics are
metabolized in the liver by drug metabolizing enzymes known as microsomal enzymes.
Reference: Kossick, M.A. (1997). Chapter 18:
Inhalation Anesthetics. In J. Nagelhout & K.

Zaglaniczny (Eds.), *Nurse Anesthesia.*
Philadelphia: W.B. Saunders.

169. ANSWER: **D**

Rationale: Trace amounts of nitrous oxide are metabolized in the intestines by intestinal bacteria.
Reference: Kossick, M.A. (1997). Chapter 18: Inhalation Anesthetics. In J. Nagelhout & K. Zaglaniczny (Eds.), *Nurse Anesthesia.* Philadelphia: W.B. Saunders.

170. ANSWER: **A**

Rationale: Isoflurane is resistant to metabolism and thus is converted in less than 1% of the administered dose to nontoxic byproducts.
Reference: Kossick, M.A. (1997). Chapter 18: Inhalation Anesthetics. In J. Nagelhout & K. Zaglaniczny (Eds.), *Nurse Anesthesia.* Philadelphia: W.B. Saunders.

171. ANSWER: **C**

Rationale: The national halothane study indicated that obese middle-aged women are the most susceptible to halothane toxicity.
Reference: Kossick, M.A. (1997). Chapter 18: Inhalation Anesthetics. In J. Nagelhout & K. Zaglaniczny (Eds.), *Nurse Anesthesia.* Philadelphia: W.B. Saunders.

172. ANSWER: **C**

Rationale: The halothane-caffeine contracture test is the most definitive diagnostic tool for malignant hyperthermia; however, it requires a muscle biopsy.
Reference: Karlet, M.C. (1997). Chapter 40: Musculoskeletal Pathophysiology and Anesthesia. In J. Nagelhout & K. Zaglaniczny (Eds.), Nurse Anesthesia. Philadelphia: W.B. Saunders.

173. ANSWER: **D**

Rationale: Place the transducer at the brain level when controlled hypotension is planned and the head is elevated. This will allow for discrepancies in pressure caused by positioning.
Reference: DeVane, G.G. (1997). Chapter 37: Neurosurgical Anesthesia. In J. Nagelhout & K. Zaglaniczny (Eds.), *Nurse Anesthesia.* Philadelphia: W.B. Saunders.

174. ANSWER: **A**

Rationale: Nerves that supply the lower extremities are often damaged because of compression or stretching with improper positioning or padding.
Reference: Monti, E.J. (1997). Chapter 32: Positioning for Anesthesia and Surgery. In J. Nagelhout & K. Zaglaniczny (Eds.), *Nurse Anesthesia.* Philadelphia: W.B. Saunders.

175. ANSWER: **C**

Rationale: A small support should be placed just caudad to the downside axilla to prevent decreased blood flow to the hand.
Reference: Monti, E.J. (1997). Chapter 32: Positioning for Anesthesia and Surgery. In J. Nagelhout & K. Zaglaniczny (Eds.), *Nurse Anesthesia.* Philadelphia: W.B. Saunders.

176. ANSWER: **B**

Rationale: The common peroneal nerve may be injured when the head of the fibula (lateral aspect of the knee) is compressed against the leg support or insufficiently padded.
Reference: Monti, E.J. (1997). Chapter 32: Positioning for Anesthesia and Surgery. In J. Nagelhout & K. Zaglaniczny (Eds.), *Nurse Anesthesia.* Philadelphia: W.B. Saunders.

177. ANSWER: **A**

Rationale: The saphenous nerve may be injured when the medial tibial condyle is compressed by the leg supports.
Reference: Monti, E.J. (1997). Chapter 32: Positioning for Anesthesia and Surgery. In J. Nagelhout & K. Zaglaniczny (Eds.), *Nurse Anesthesia.* Philadelphia: W.B. Saunders.

178. ANSWER: **B**

Rationale: The speed of induction and emergence of an anesthetic gas is determined by its blood/gas solubility. The lower the number, the faster the anesthetic.
Reference: Nagelhout, J.J. (1997). Chapter 17: Uptake and Distribution of Inhalation Anesthetics. In J. Nagelhout & K. Zaglaniczny (Eds.), *Nurse Anesthesia.* Philadelphia: W.B. Saunders.

179. ANSWER: **D**

Rationale: Pentobarbital (Nembutal) is a short-acting drug whose duration is in the range of 4 to 8 hours.

Reference: Fallacaro, N.A. & Fallacaro, M.D. (1997). Chapter 19: Intravenous Inhalation Agents. In J. Nagelhout & K. Zaglaniczny (Eds.), *Nurse Anesthesia*. Philadelphia: W.B. Saunders.

180. ANSWER: **C**

Rationale: Patients emerge from thiopental effects due to redistribution from the brain to non-neural sites. This is true of all induction drugs.

Reference: Fallacaro, N.A. & Fallacaro, M.D. (1997). Chapter 19: Intravenous Inhalation Agents. In J. Nagelhout & K. Zaglaniczny (Eds.), *Nurse Anesthesia*. Philadelphia: W.B. Saunders.

181. ANSWER: **C**

Rationale: Meperidine metabolism is affected by MAO inhibitors, possibly resulting in seizures and death.

Reference: Chick, M. (1997). Chapter 21: Opioid Agonists and Antagonists. In J. Nagelhout & K. Zaglaniczny (Eds.), *Nurse Anesthesia*. Philadelphia: W.B. Saunders.

182. ANSWER: **C**

Rationale: Barbiturates may induce the enzyme aminolevulinic acid synthetase, resulting in a precipitation of an attack in genetically susceptible patients with porphyria.

Reference: Fallacaro, N.A. & Fallacaro, M.D. (1997). Chapter 19: Intravenous Inhalation Agents. In J. Nagelhout & K. Zaglaniczny (Eds.), *Nurse Anesthesia*. Philadelphia: W.B. Saunders.

183. ANSWER: **B**

Rationale: Droperidol blocks dopamine in the brain; therefore, it is contraindicated in patients with Parkinson's disease because of its extrapyramidal side effects.

Reference: Chick, M. (1997). Chapter 21: Opioid Agonists and Antagonists. In J. Nagelhout & K. Zaglaniczny (Eds.), *Nurse Anesthesia*. Philadelphia: W.B. Saunders.

184. ANSWER: **B**

Rationale: Glycopyrrolate is a quarternary ammonia compound and does not pass the blood-brain barrier.

Reference: Alisoglu, R. (1997). Chapter 23: Cardiac Pharmacology. In J. Nagelhout & K. Zaglaniczny (Eds.), *Nurse Anesthesia*. Philadelphia: W.B. Saunders.

185. ANSWER: **D**

Rationale: Physostigmine, unlike other anticholinesterases, passes the blood-brain barrier and will relieve central nervous system symptoms.

Reference: Alisoglu, R. (1997). Chapter 23: Cardiac Pharmacology. In J. Nagelhout & K. Zaglaniczny (Eds.), *Nurse Anesthesia*. Philadelphia: W.B. Saunders.

186. ANSWER: **C**

Rationale: Two responses out of four indicate a degree of paralysis of approximately 80%. One of four would be in the 90s, three of four would be in the high 70s, and four of four would be 70% or less.

Reference: Haas, R.E. & Erway, R.L. (1997). Chapter 22: Neuromuscular Blocking Agents, Reversal Agents, and Their Monitoring. In J. Nagelhout & K. Zaglaniczny (Eds.), *Nurse Anesthesia*. Philadelphia: W.B. Saunders.

187. ANSWER: **B**

Rationale: Nitroprusside is made up of five cyanide molecules per molecule of drug. They are released during metabolism of this agent.

Reference: Alisoglu, R. (1997). Chapter 23: Cardiac Pharmacology. In J. Nagelhout & K. Zaglaniczny (Eds.), *Nurse Anesthesia*. Philadelphia: W.B. Saunders.

188. ANSWER: **B**

Rationale: In first-order kinetics it follows that a drug will be eliminated in a constant percent per unit time, for example, 10% per hour or 50% every 3 hours, etc.

Reference: Troop, M. (1997). Chapter 16: Pharmacokinetics. In J. Nagelhout & K. Zaglaniczny (Eds.), *Nurse Anesthesia*. Philadelphia: W.B. Saunders.

189. ANSWER: **D**

Rationale: A patient this large would be considered obese and thus ASA 2. A bowel obstruction is an emergency, thus the E designation.

Reference: Kachnij, J.M. (1997). Chapter 28: Preoperative Evaluation and Preparation of the Patient. In J. Nagelhout & K. Zaglaniczny (Eds.), *Nurse Anesthesia*. Philadelphia: W.B. Saunders.

190. ANSWER: **A**

Rationale: ASA 3 signifies significant chronic disease is present. Thus answer A would indicate three disorders that are categorized as serious.

Reference: Kachnij, J.M. (1997). Chapter 28: Preoperative Evaluation and Preparation of the Patient. In J. Nagelhout & K. Zaglaniczny (Eds.), *Nurse Anesthesia*. Philadelphia: W.B. Saunders.

191. ANSWER: **D**

Rationale: Droperidol blocks alpha receptors, resulting in vasodilation in the periphery.

Reference: Chick, M. (1997). Chapter 21: Opioid Agonists and Antagonists. In J. Nagelhout & K. Zaglaniczny (Eds.), *Nurse Anesthesia*. Philadelphia: W.B. Saunders.

192. ANSWER: **D**

Rationale: The ulnar nerve is the most frequently injured nerve under anesthesia. This results from improper positioning and panic when adjusting the arms.

Reference: Monti, E.J. (1997). Chapter 32: Positioning for Anesthesia and Surgery. In J. Nagelhout & K. Zaglaniczny (Eds.), *Nurse Anesthesia*. Philadelphia: W.B. Saunders.

193. ANSWER: **B**

Rationale: A kidney rest compresses the flank area, resulting in pressure on the vena cava and hypotension.

Reference: Monti, E.J. (1997). Chapter 32: Positioning for Anesthesia and Surgery. In J. Nagelhout & K. Zaglaniczny (Eds.), *Nurse Anesthesia*. Philadelphia: W.B. Saunders.

194. ANSWER: **D**

Rationale: M-1 receptors are neuronal, M-2 are in the heart, and M-3 are in smooth muscle and glands. All three types are blocked by the common antimuscarinic medications.

Reference: Alisoglu, R. (1997). Chapter 23: Cardiac Pharmacology. In J. Nagelhout & K. Zaglaniczny (Eds.), *Nurse Anesthesia*. Philadelphia: W.B. Saunders.

195. ANSWER: **C**

Rationale: Esther-type local anesthetics are metabolized by hydrolysis with the enzyme cholinesterase.

Reference: Haas, R.E. & Erway, R.L. (1997). Chapter 22: Neuromuscular Blocking Agents, Reversal Agents, and Their Monitoring. In J. Nagelhout & K. Zaglaniczny (Eds.), *Nurse Anesthesia*. Philadelphia: W.B. Saunders.

196. ANSWER: **C**

Rationale: Loss of one twitch in the train-of-four indicates a percentage of blockade in the high 70s.

Reference: Haas, R.E. & Erway, R.L. (1997). Chapter 22: Neuromuscular Blocking Agents, Reversal Agents, and Their Monitoring. In J. Nagelhout & K. Zaglaniczny (Eds.), *Nurse Anesthesia*. Philadelphia: W.B. Saunders.

197. ANSWER: **C**

Rationale: The inspiratory capacity is made up of the inspiratory reserve volume plus the tidal volume.

Reference: Hall, S.M. (1997). Chapter 9: Respiratory Anatomy and Physiology. In J. Nagelhout & K. Zaglaniczny (Eds.), *Nurse Anesthesia*. Philadelphia: W.B. Saunders.

198. ANSWER: **C**

Rationale: Muscle relaxants are 100% water soluble in the body at all times and thus distribute to the body's extracellular water only.

Reference: Haas, R.E. & Erway, R.L. (1997). Chapter 22: Neuromuscular Blocking Agents, Reversal Agents, and Their Monitoring. In J. Nagelhout & K. Zaglaniczny (Eds.), *Nurse Anesthesia*. Philadelphia: W.B. Saunders.

199. ANSWER: **A**

Rationale: Atropine has the fastest onset among the drugs listed, which correlates with the fast onset of edrophonium.

Reference: Haas, R.E. & Erway, R.L. (1997). Chapter 22: Neuromuscular Blocking Agents, Reversal Agents, and Their Monitoring. In J. Nagelhout & K. Zaglaniczny (Eds.), *Nurse Anesthesia*. Philadelphia: W.B. Saunders.

200. ANSWER: **D**

Rationale: Excess acetylcholine generated by the anticholinesterase drug will stimulate muscarinic receptors unless they are blocked within the anticholinergic drug.

Reference: Haas, R.E. & Erway, R.L. (1997). Chapter 22: Neuromuscular Blocking Agents, Reversal Agents, and Their Monitoring. In J. Nagelhout & K. Zaglaniczny (Eds.), *Nurse Anesthesia.* Philadelphia: W.B. Saunders.

201. ANSWER: **B**

Rationale: Giving higher than necessary concentrations during initial administration of an anesthetic to speed the onset is referred to as the "concentration effect."

Reference: Nagelhout, J.J. (1997). Chapter 17: Uptake and Distribution of Inhalation Anesthetics. In J. Nagelhout & K. Zaglaniczny (Eds.), *Nurse Anesthesia.* Philadelphia: W.B. Saunders.

202. ANSWER: **D**

Rationale: These three drugs are pure opiate receptor antagonists that work on all receptor subtypes.

Reference: Chick, M. (1997). Chapter 21: Opioid Agonists and Antagonists. In J. Nagelhout & K. Zaglaniczny (Eds.), *Nurse Anesthesia.* Philadelphia: W.B. Saunders.

203. ANSWER: **D**

Rationale: A muscle relaxant will relieve the tight chest produced by rapid administration of high-potency opiates.

Reference: Chick, M. (1997). Chapter 21: Opioid Agonists and Antagonists. In J. Nagelhout & K. Zaglaniczny (Eds.), *Nurse Anesthesia.* Philadelphia: W.B. Saunders.

204. ANSWER: **C**

Rationale: Postganglionic sympathetic fibers are adrenergic as they release norepinephrine.

Reference: Morgan, R.O., Jr. (1997). Chapter 8: The Cardiovascular System. In J. Nagelhout & K. Zaglaniczny (Eds.), *Nurse Anesthesia.* Philadelphia: W.B. Saunders.

205. ANSWER: **D**

Rationale: Although all of the listed agents may produce some amnesia, the benzodiazepines are the most reliable and predictable amnestic drugs.

Reference: Fallacaro, N.A. & Fallacaro, M.D. (1997). Chapter 19: Intravenous Inhalation Agents. In J. Nagelhout & K. Zaglaniczny (Eds.), *Nurse Anesthesia.* Philadelphia: W.B. Saunders.

206. ANSWER: **B**

Rationale: Nystagmus is characteristic of the excitement stage during anesthetic administration, which is noted as stage 2.

Reference: Kossick, M.A. (1997). Chapter 18: Inhalation Anesthetics. In J. Nagelhout & K. Zaglaniczny (Eds.), *Nurse Anesthesia.* Philadelphia: W.B. Saunders.

207. ANSWER: **A**

Rationale: Biogenic amines are metabolized in the body primarily by the mitochondrial enzyme monoamine oxidase.

Reference: Karlet, M.C. & Sebastian, L.A. (1997). Chapter 12: The Endocrine System. In J. Nagelhout & K. Zaglaniczny (Eds.), *Nurse Anesthesia.* Philadelphia: W.B. Saunders.

208. ANSWER: **B**

Rationale: Therapeutic index, a measure of drug safety, is defined as LD_{50}/ED_{50}.

Reference: Troop, M. (1997). Chapter 16: Pharmacokinetics. In J. Nagelhout & K. Zaglaniczny (Eds.), *Nurse Anesthesia.* Philadelphia: W.B. Saunders.

209. ANSWER: **B**

Rationale: There is always a direct correlation between the brain and lung concentrations because anesthetics are freely diffusible through biologic membranes.

Reference: Nagelhout, J.J. (1997). Chapter 17: Uptake and Distribution of Inhalation Anesthetics. In J. Nagelhout & K. Zaglaniczny (Eds.), *Nurse Anesthesia.* Philadelphia: W.B. Saunders.

210. ANSWER: **C**

Rationale: Ketamine blocks association pathways in the brain and thus is referred to as producing dissociative anesthesia.

Reference: Fallacaro, N.A. & Fallacaro, M.D. (1997). Chapter 19: Intravenous Inhalation Agents. In J. Nagelhout & K. Zaglaniczny (Eds.), *Nurse Anesthesia.* Philadelphia: W.B. Saunders.

211. ANSWER: **C**

Rationale: Administration of large amounts, usually greater than 500 mg succinylcholine, may produce a desensitization block sometimes referred to as a dual block.

Reference: Haas, R.E. & Erway, R.L. (1997). Chapter 22: Neuromuscular Blocking Agents, Reversal Agents, and Their Monitoring. In J. Nagelhout & K. Zaglaniczny (Eds.), *Nurse Anesthesia.* Philadelphia: W.B. Saunders.

212. ANSWER: **D**

Rationale: Even the small doses of muscle relaxants may produce eyelid muscle paralysis and weakness, resulting in blurred vision

Reference: Haas, R.E. & Erway, R.L. (1997). Chapter 22: Neuromuscular Blocking Agents, Reversal Agents, and Their Monitoring. In J. Nagelhout & K. Zaglaniczny (Eds.), *Nurse Anesthesia.* Philadelphia: W.B. Saunders.

213. ANSWER: **D**

Rationale: The most common serious toxicity resulting from an overdose of a local anesthetic is central nervous system stimulation, resulting in convulsions.

Reference: Williams, J.R. (1997). Chapter 20: Local Anesthetics. In J. Nagelhout & K. Zaglaniczny (Eds.), *Nurse Anesthesia.* Philadelphia: W.B. Saunders.

214. ANSWER: **B**

Rationale: The beta half-life of a drug indicates elimination. It usually takes four to five half-lives to eliminate a drug.

Reference: Troop, M. (1997). Chapter 16: Pharmacokinetics. In J. Nagelhout & K. Zaglaniczny (Eds.), *Nurse Anesthesia.* Philadelphia: W.B. Saunders.

215. ANSWER: **C**

Rationale: The minimal alveolar concentration (MAC) is an indication of anesthetic depth and is designated as the 50% point.

Reference: Kossick, M.A. (1997). Chapter 18: Inhalation Anesthetics. In J. Nagelhout & K. Zaglaniczny (Eds.), *Nurse Anesthesia.* Philadelphia: W.B. Saunders.

216. ANSWER: **A**

Rationale: Acetylcholinesterase is the isoenzyme present in the neuromuscular junction that metabolizes acetylcholine.

Reference: Haas, R.E. & Erway, R.L. (1997). Chapter 22: Neuromuscular Blocking Agents, Reversal Agents, and Their Monitoring. In J. Nagelhout & K. Zaglaniczny (Eds.), *Nurse Anesthesia.* Philadelphia: W.B. Saunders.

217. ANSWER: **B**

Rationale: Drugs have molecules too large to move through channels; therefore, they must have lipid solubility or be actively transported to move through biologic membranes.

Reference: Troop, M. (1997). Chapter 16: Pharmacokinetics. In J. Nagelhout & K. Zaglaniczny (Eds.), *Nurse Anesthesia.* Philadelphia: W.B. Saunders.

218. ANSWER: **B**

Rationale: ED_{50} represents the effective dose to reach half-efficacy on a dose-response scale.

Reference: Troop, M. (1997). Chapter 16: Pharmacokinetics. In J. Nagelhout & K. Zaglaniczny (Eds.), *Nurse Anesthesia.* Philadelphia: W.B. Saunders.

219. ANSWER: **C**

Rationale: A high therapeutic index indicates a very safe drug because the lethal dose is much higher than the effective dose.

Reference: Troop, M. (1997). Chapter 16: Pharmacokinetics. In J. Nagelhout & K. Zaglaniczny (Eds.), *Nurse Anesthesia.* Philadelphia: W.B. Saunders.

220. ANSWER: **B**

Rationale: I. T. on an endotracheal tube means implant tested to ensure nontoxicity, and Z79 stands for the Z79 committee on anesthesia equipment of the American National Standards Institute and signifies that the material is nontoxic to tissues as well.

Reference: Dosch, M.P. (1997). Chapter 26: Anesthesia Equipment. In J. Nagelhout & K. Zaglaniczny (Eds.), *Nurse Anesthesia.* Philadelphia: W.B. Saunders.

221. ANSWER: **A**

Rationale: Beer's law states that at a constant light intensity and hemoglobin concentration the intensity of light transmitted through the sample is a log function of the oxygen saturation of hemoglobin.

Reference: Hall, S.M. (1997). Chapter 4: Chemistry and Physics for Anesthesia. In J. Nagelhout & K. Zaglaniczny (Eds.), *Nurse Anesthesia.* Philadelphia: W.B. Saunders.

222. ANSWER: **D**

Rationale: Methemoglobin absorbs both red and infrared light. At a high methemoglobin level, the saturation will be 85% regardless of the actual PO_2.

Reference: Sinkovich, J.A. & Kossick, M.A. (1997). Chapter 27: Clinical Monitoring in Anesthesia. In J. Nagelhout & K. Zaglaniczny (Eds.), *Nurse Anesthesia.* Philadelphia: W.B. Saunders.

223. ANSWER: **A**

Rationale: Clinical accuracy is typically reported to be ±2% to 3% for a range of saturations between 70% and 100%.

Reference: Sinkovich, J.A. & Kossick, M.A. (1997). Chapter 27: Clinical Monitoring in Anesthesia. In J. Nagelhout & K. Zaglaniczny (Eds.), *Nurse Anesthesia.* Philadelphia: W.B. Saunders.

224. ANSWER: **B**

Rationale: Anything that alters blood flow through the sampling site may affect accuracy. All of those listed affect circulation negatively except hyperthermia.

Reference: Sinkovich, J.A. & Kossick, M.A. (1997). Chapter 27: Clinical Monitoring in Anesthesia. In J. Nagelhout & K. Zaglaniczny (Eds.), *Nurse Anesthesia.* Philadelphia: W.B. Saunders.

CHAPTER 4

Advanced Principles

• • •

1. A patient has just experienced masseter muscle rigidity from succinylcholine. What laboratory value may confirm the diagnosis of malignant hyperthermia?

   A. muscle biopsy
   B. elevation in creatinine phosphokinase (CPK) level greater than 20,000 IU/L
   C. caffeine-contracture test
   D. elevation in serum lactic dehydrogenase (LDH) level greater than 200 IU/L

2. Of the following chemotherapy agents, which can cause pulmonary fibrosis in 5% to 10% of patients?

   A. vincristine
   B. bleomycin
   C. doxorubicin
   D. cisplatin

3. Preoperative assessment of the patient with pheochromocytoma should include:

   A. evidence of digitalis effect on ECG
   B. ACTH levels
   C. exercise tolerance
   D. adequacy of adrenergic blockade

4. Drugs to be avoided in the anesthetic management of the patient with pheochromocytoma would not include:

   A. vagolytic agents
   B. histamine-releasing drugs
   C. adrenergic antagonists
   D. beta agonists

5. What should be done first if a patient's pacemaker fails intraoperatively?

   A. place a transvenous pacer as soon as possible
   B. administer atropine for bradycardia
   C. increase the patient's inspired oxygen to 100%
   D. immediately start cardiopulmonary resuscitation

6. When should the delivery of shock waves occur during extracorporeal shock wave lithotripsy for patients with a history of arrhythmias or pacemaker use?

   A. timed with the start of the P wave
   B. timed with the beginning of the R wave
   C. timed at 20 msec after the R wave
   D. timed at 30 msec after the T wave

7. Which of the following would not be considered an indication for perioperative temporary pacing?

   A. a new bundle branch or heart block
   B. symptomatic bradyarrhythmia
   C. refractory supraventricular tachycardia
   D. asymptomatic bigeminal rhythm

8. The following are keys to anesthetic management for patients with carcinoid syndrome except:

   A. avoid histamine-releasing drugs
   B. avoid catecholamine administration
   C. maintain moderate hypercapnia
   D. avoid hypotension

9. How is adenosine administered?

   A. orally with food
   B. intramuscularly
   C. by rapid intravenous bolus
   D. sublingually

10. How is adenosine metabolized?

    A. pseudocholinesterase
    B. Hoffman elimination
    C. cytochrome P-450
    D. adenosine deaminase

11. How fast is adenosine metabolized?

    A. less than 1 minute
    B. 5 to 10 minutes
    C. approximately 20 minutes
    D. in about 1 hour

12. What is the indication for adenosine?

    A. rapid atrial fibrillation or flutter
    B. re-entrant atrioventricular tachycardias
    C. bradyarrythmias
    D. Wolff-Parkinson-White syndrome

13. All of the following are anesthetic goals for the patient with sickle cell anemia, except:

A. avoid hypotension and hypovolemia
B. maintain hematocrit less than 32%
C. avoid hypothermia and hyperthermia
D. maintain FiO_2 greater than 0.50

14. When is sickling of the red blood cell most likely to occur?

   A. under extreme hypoxemia or low flow states
   B. when the hematocrit is greater than 35%
   C. with infection
   D. can occur at any time

15. Which of the following would be the most appropriate therapy for an adult diabetic patient with a blood sugar level of 300 mg/dL?

   A. NPH insulin IV
   B. regular insulin SQ
   C. Lente insulin SQ
   D. regular insulin IV

16. What ECG leads best detect myocardial ischemia or infarction if the right atrium, sinus node, atrioventricular node, and right ventricles are involved?

   A. II, III, aVF
   B. V_1, V_5
   C. I, aVL
   D. would be difficult to determine

17. What ECG leads best detect myocardial ischemia or infarction if the anterolateral aspect of the left ventricle is involved?

   A. II, III, aVF
   B. unable to determine
   C. V_3, V_5
   D. I, aVL

18. What ECG leads best detect myocardial ischemia or infarction if the lateral aspects of the left ventricle are involved?

   A. no way to determine
   B. I, aVL
   C. II, III, aVF
   D. V_1, V_5

19. What site should be avoided when placing a pulmonary catheter?

   A. right internal jugular vein
   B. left or right femoral vein
   C. left internal jugular vein
   D. right external jugular vein

20. Which of the following is not considered a serious complication of interscalene block?

   A. pneumothorax
   B. grand mal seizure after vertebral artery injection
   C. stellate ganglion block
   D. central nervous system excitation phenomena after intravenous injection

21. Which diagnosis must be considered in patients after coronary artery bypass graft surgery presenting with unexplained low cardiac output?

   A. cardiac tamponade
   B. myocardial infarction
   C. hypovolemia
   D. superior vena cava syndrome

22. Explain why the ventricle may fill during cardiopulmonary bypass.

   A. blood draining from the left atrium
   B. leak in the cardiopulmonary bypass system
   C. blood flow from the thebesian and bronchial veins
   D. blood returning from the superior vena cava

23. What is the most frequent complication of retrobulbar block?

   A. ineffective anesthesia
   B. complete loss of vision
   C. hemorrhage
   D. seizures

24. Which factor does not decrease uterine blood flow?

   A. uterine contractions
   B. maternal hyperventilation
   C. maternal hypotension
   D. vasoconstriction of uterine vasculature

25. Which of the following is not a complication of cricothyroidotomy?

    A. pneumothorax
    B. bleeding
    C. esophageal puncture
    D. respiratory alkalosis

26. Perioperative management of gastroschisis and omphalocele centers around prevention of which of the following?

    A. hypothermia, dehydration, and infection
    B. hyperthermia, hypocapnia, and oliguria
    C. hyperthermia, overhydration, and infection
    D. hypothermia, hypercapnia, and anuria

27. Which of the following complaints would distinguish local anesthetic toxicity from hyponatremia in a patient undergoing a transurethral prostatic resection?

    A. leg cramps and diaphoresis
    B. tinnitus and slurred speech
    C. confusion and dyspnea
    D. nausea and vomiting

28. What is the maximum amount of hetastarch that should be given to a patient?

    A. 1 mL/kg
    B. 50 mL/kg
    C. 25 mL/kg
    D. 20 mL/kg

29. Postoperative problems after carotid endarterectomy include all except:

    A. myocardial infarction
    B. stroke
    C. hyperkalemia
    D. hematoma formation at the operative site

30. What is the most serious complication of supraclavicular block?

    A. hemorrhage
    B. pneumothorax
    C. local anesthetic toxicity
    D. nerve injury

31. What is the most common cause of heparin resistance?

    A. repeated doses of heparin
    B. diabetic history
    C. pseudocholinesterase breakdown
    D. antithrombin III deficiency

32. What is the treatment for heparin resistance?

    A. simply increase the dose
    B. transfuse 1 unit of packed red blood cells
    C. transfuse 2 units of fresh frozen plasma
    D. wait 24 hours before giving the next dose

33. During a Bier block, what is the minimum amount of time the tourniquet needs to be inflated?

    A. 40 minutes
    B. 1 hour
    C. 20 minutes
    D. no minimum time

34. When do signs of hypocalcemia after thyroidectomy appear?

    A. This rarely occurs after thyroidectomy.
    B. typically after 1 week postoperatively
    C. immediately
    D. most often 24 to 72 hours postoperatively

35. What anesthetic technique is relatively contraindicated for patients with multiple sclerosis?

    A. general endotracheal
    B. regional anesthesia
    C. "hypotensive" technique
    D. local sedation

36. Which of the following should be avoided when managing a patient with cystic fibrosis?

    A. use higher FiO_2 of O_2 intraoperatively
    B. adequately hydrate
    C. humidify gases
    D. pretreat with atropine

37. Which factor is least likely the cause of intraoperative bronchospasm?

    A. light anesthesia
    B. mechanical obstruction
    C. endobronchial intubation
    D. acute bronchial asthma

38. An epidural anesthetic is administered; what is typically the first sign it is working?

    A. loss of motor ability of the lower extremities
    B. peripheral vasodilation
    C. sensory analgesia
    D. increased heart rate

39. Which of the following would most likely cause oozing at the surgical site in a patient who was transfused with 12 units of packed red blood cells?

    A. hemolytic transfusion reaction
    B. low platelet count
    C. dilutional thrombocytopenia
    D. citrate toxicity

40. A patient with a history of cancer and currently being treated with bleomycin is at increased risk for what?

    A. cardiac dysrhythmias
    B. hypotension
    C. pulmonary toxicity
    D. nausea and vomiting

41. When the abdominal aorta is cross-clamped, what effect does it have on heart volumes and pressures?

    A. Both afterload and peripheral vascular resistance increase.
    B. Only afterload increases and peripheral vascular resistance decreases.
    C. Peripheral vascular resistance increases but afterload decreases.
    D. There is no physiologic difference.

42. Fetal hemoglobin (HbF) circulates in the blood until about the age of 6 months; what is the P_{50} of HgF?

    A. 21 mm Hg
    B. 26 mm Hg
    C. 19 mm Hg
    D. 32 mm Hg

43. In the anesthetic management for a neonate with a diagnosed diaphragmatic hernia, before an awake intubation, what should be done?

    A. start an arterial line
    B. topicalize the oral pharynx
    C. insert an oro/nasogastric tube to decompress the stomach
    D. can sedate the child with low doses of benzodiazepine

44. Signs and symptoms of diaphragmatic hernia include all of the following except:

    A. scaphoid abdomen
    B. pectus excavatum
    C. bowel sounds auscultated in the chest
    D. arterial hypoxemia

45. The two most important aspects in the anesthetic management of omphalocele and gastroschisis would include:

    A. monitor urinary output and arterial pressures
    B. watch for cardiac arrhythmias and metabolic alkylosis
    C. preoxygenation and verifying tube placement via fiberoptic scope
    D. maintaining body temperature and fluid replacement

46. The hypertension caused from autonomic hyperreflexia should be treated with any of the following except:

    A. calcium channel blockers
    B. sodium nitroprusside
    C. ganglion-blocking drugs
    D. alpha-adrenergic antagonists

47. An 80-year-old alcoholic undergoes open gallbladder surgery 3 days after admission under general endotracheal anesthesia. Emergence was without difficulty, and spontaneous respirations were adequate.

Twenty minutes after admittance to the postanesthesia care unit the patient becomes combative, confused, and restless. The most likely cause is:

A. delirium
B. hypoxia
C. cerebral ischemia
D. hypocarbia

48. The following are all true in the geriatric patient except:

A. decreased P_{AO_2}
B. increased $A - aDO_2$
C. increased static lung compliance
D. decreased breathing capacity

49. Activated clotting time assesses:

A. intrinsic and common pathways
B. intrinsic pathway
C. common pathway
D. extrinsic and common pathways

50. Generally accepted indications for permanent pacemaker insertion include all except:

A. second-degree heart block
B. sick sinus syndrome
C. complete heart block
D. trifascicular block

51. Regarding patients with an automatic cardiovertor-defibrillator (AICD):

A. The pulse generator should be deactivated if electrocautery is planned.
B. Magnetic resonance imaging is not contraindicated.
C. Lithotripsy may be performed safely.
D. A simple magnet is not strong enough to deactivate the device.

52. In patients with idiopathic hypertrophic subaortic stenosis (IHSS), all of the following will make obstruction to outflow worse except:

A. increased left ventricular volume
B. decreased atrial pressure
C. decreased intraventricular volume
D. increased contractility

53. In the patient with aortic stenosis, all are important except:

A. pulmonary capillary wedge pressure should be monitored to estimate left ventricular end-diastolic pressure
B. maintenance of sinus rhythm
C. maintenance of preload
D. bradycardia is not tolerated

54. In anesthetizing the patient with aortic stenosis all are true except:

A. avoid bradycardia
B. maintain adequate intravascular volume
C. maintain sinus rhythm
D. maintain decreased afterload

55. With regard to the pathophysiology of aortic stenosis:

A. angina infrequently occurs
B. concentric hypertrophy develops
C. chamber size is increased
D. ventricular compliance is increased

56. In formulating an anesthesia plan for the patient with aortic insufficiency, all are needed except:

A. increased afterload
B. prevent even modest tachycardia
C. judicious fluid administration
D. increase systemic vascular resistance

57. The anesthetic considerations for the patient with mitral stenosis include all except:

A. hypercarbia will increase pulmonary vascular resistance
B. avoid hypoxemia
C. maintain increased pulmonary vascular resistance
D. maintain slow/normal heart rate

58. Hemodynamic goals for the patient with mitral regurgitation include all except:

A. hypercarbia should be avoided
B. maintain intravascular volume
C. avoid increased pulmonary vascular resistance
D. maintain slow to normal heart rate

59. All of the following are common electro-cardiographic findings of mitral regurgitation except:

    A. atrial fibrillation
    B. left bundle branch block
    C. atrial and ventricular premature beats
    D. P mitrale

60. Which of the following produces a pan-systolic murmur?

    A. aortic insufficiency
    B. aortic stenosis
    C. mitral stenosis
    D. mitral insufficiency

61. According to the New York Heart Association classification of heart disease, which of the following are characteristic of Class II?

    A. marked limitation of physical activity
    B. slight limitation of physical activity
    C. unable to carry out physical activity without discomfort
    D. no limitations of physical activity

62. Click murmur syndrome is associated with which heart valve?

    A. mitral
    B. pulmonic
    C. aortic
    D. tricuspid

63. What is the muscle relaxant of choice in the patient with mitral regurgitation?

    A. atracurium
    B. vecuronium
    C. pancuronium
    D. mivacurium

64. The first letter of the five letter pacemaker identification codes represents:

    A. chamber(s) sensed
    B. chamber(s) paced
    C. programmable functions
    D. mode of responses

65. All of the following promote hypokalemia by shifting potassium into the cells except:

    A. insulin
    B. alkalosis
    C. beta-adrenergic receptor stimulation
    D. beta blockers

66. All the following promote hyperkalemia except:

    A. diuretics
    B. acidosis
    C. alpha-adrenergic stimulation
    D. rapid increases in plasma osmolarity

67. In an acute anginal attack, intravenous administration of nitrates works to relieve angina by:

    A. direct arterial vasodilation
    B. dilating the coronary arteries
    C. decreasing preload
    D. decreasing heart rate

68. All of the following are true of the geriatric patient except:

    A. Impairment of hepatic microsomal enzymes is not age related.
    B. They are pharmacodynamically more sensitive to benzodiazepines.
    C. Minimal alveolar concentration of inhalation agents decreases with age.
    D. The elimination half-life for opioids is increased.

69. All of the following are true of the geriatric patient except:

    A. They have difficulty with glucose load.
    B. The number of effective renal glomeruli decreases with age.
    C. They have increased serum albumin levels resulting in greater protein binding of drugs.
    D. They have a declining skeletal muscle mass and blood volume with age.

70. All of the following are safe for the patient with latex allergy except:

    A. polyvinyl chloride endotracheal tube
    B. paper tape
    C. tegaderm
    D. tourniquets

71. All of the following are early manifestations of malignant hyperthermia except:

    A. unexplained tachycardia
    B. high temperature
    C. increased end-tidal CO_2
    D. masseter muscle spasm

72. Neonatal retrolental fibroplasia is a result of oxygen toxicity above what percent of oxygen:

    A. 40%
    B. 30%
    C. 50%
    D. 70%

73. All of the following have been shown to increase the incidence of postoperative nausea and vomiting except:

    A. eye surgery
    B. narcotics
    C. isoflurane
    D. tonsillectomy

74. Which of the following is an absolute contraindication to spinal anesthesia?

    A. chronic back pain
    B. sepsis
    C. uncooperative patient
    D. prior lumbar spine surgery

75. During spinal anesthesia the local anesthetic is administered between which two meningeal layers:

    A. pia and arachnoid
    B. dura and pia
    C. dura and arachnoid
    D. dura and epidura

76. When performing subarachnoid block the first ligament penetrated is:

    A. interspinous
    B. ligamentum flavum
    C. supraspinous
    D. posterior longitudinal ligament

77. The most common local anesthetic used in hypobaric subarachnoid block is:

    A. bupivacaine
    B. lidocaine
    C. tetracaine
    D. procaine

78. To achieve hyperbaric spinal anesthesia, the local anesthetic is most often mixed with:

    A. dextrose
    B. cerebrospinal fluid
    C. 0.45% NaCl
    D. epinephrine

79. All of the following cause cephalad spread of a local anesthetic when given in the subarachnoid space except:

    A. pregnancy
    B. advanced age
    C. obesity
    D. previous spine surgery

80. The most cephalad portion of the spinal canal is:

    A. third ventricle
    B. foramen magnum
    C. fourth ventricle
    D. C1

81. The spinal cord in the adult ends at:

    A. L5
    B. L3
    C. L1
    D. L2

82. Select the false statement about the epidural space:

    A. It contains a small amount of free fluid.
    B. It is filled with adipose tissue.
    C. It is filled with connective tissue.
    D. Venous plexuses are prominent.

83. An imaginary line drawn along the back from one iliac crest to the other would cross in the middle at:

    A. L3
    B. L4
    C. L3-L4 interspace
    D. L4-L5 interspace

84. The definitive treatment of postdural puncture headache is:

    A. caffeine
    B. fluids
    C. epidural blood patch
    D. supine position

85. Stimuli generated from thermal, mechanical, or chemical tissue damage are received from:

    A. both A delta and C fibers
    B. A fibers only
    C. B fibers
    D. C fibers only

86. For carotid endarterectomy under regional anesthesia, the nerves that must be blocked are:

    A. C1–C4
    B. C2–C4
    C. C2–C6
    D. C1–C3

87. As a hyperbaric anesthetic solution spreads through the cerebrospinal fluid, a gradient occurs between sympathetic and motor blockade. This is:

    A. theoretical but no actual clinical difference
    B. motor block two segments above sensory block
    C. sensory block equivalent to motor block
    D. sympathetic block one to two segments above sensory block

88. All of the following are immediate treatments of total spinal anesthesia except:

    A. pressor support
    B. reverse Trendelenburg position
    C. positive-pressure ventilation
    D. volume infusion

89. Nausea and vomiting after administration of a spinal anesthetic is caused by:

    A. unopposed sympathetic tone
    B. local anesthetic overdose
    C. local anesthetic allergy
    D. decrease in cerebral blood flow

90. Bradycardia after a spinal anesthetic may occur due to all of the following except:

    A. decrease in cerebral blood flow
    B. blockade of the cardioaccelerator fibers
    C. Bezold-Jarisch reflex
    D. unopposed vagal tone

91. When performing digital nerve blocks, all are true except:

    A. They are easily performed.
    B. Large volumes can cause pressure injury.
    C. Vasoconstrictors allow for less anesthetic volume.
    D. The nerves run along each side of the fingers.

92. The main pathway in the formation of epinephrine begins with:

    A. norepinephrine
    B. dopamine
    C. dopa
    D. phenylalanine

93. Which of the following drugs exhibit dopamine blocking activity as part of its mechanism?

    A. ketamine
    B. clonidine
    C. cimetidine
    D. metoclopramide

94. All of the following result after aortic cross-clamping except:

    A. aerobic metabolism in the lower extremities
    B. maximal vasodilation in the lower extremities
    C. halted blood flow to the lower extremities
    D. decreased renal blood flow with infrarenal cross-clamping

95. All of the following can result from infrarenal cross-clamping except:

    A. acute renal failure
    B. acute tubular necrosis
    C. increased glomerular filtration rate
    D. decreased renal blood flow

96. An exaggerated fluctuation of blood pressure during the ventilatory cycle is:

    A. pulsus alternans
    B. pulsus paradoxus
    C. pulse pressure
    D. pulse respar

97. Amaurosis fugax is:

    A. contralateral to the ischemic side
    B. indicative of a large evolving stroke
    C. drooping of the eye secondary to optic nerve ischemia
    D. transient monocular blindness

98. The paradoxic effect of hypocapnia producing increased blood flow to ischemic regions of the brain is:

    A. inverse steal
    B. intracerebral steal
    C. luxury perfusion
    D. reverse Robin Hood phenomenon

99. The most common coexisting medical condition in the patient undergoing carotid endarterectomy is:

    A. hypertension
    B. diabetes
    C. coronary artery disease
    D. renal failure

100. With regard to cerebral blood flow select the false statement:

    A. Not all general anesthetics affect cerebral blood flow.
    B. In general, volatile agents are vasodilators.
    C. In general, intravenous anesthetics are vasoconstrictors.
    D. Ketamine causes vasodilation.

101. All of the following are characteristic of Horner's syndrome except:

    A. stenosis
    B. anhidrosis
    C. miosis
    D. ptosis

102. The initial treatment of local anesthetic toxicity is:

    A. secure the airway
    B. provide ventilation
    C. provide circulatory support
    D. control seizures

103. Hypotension in the patient taking monoamine oxidase inhibitors should be treated with:

    A. direct adrenergic agonists
    B. central-acting agents
    C. combination drugs
    D. ephedrine

104. The analgesic contraindicated in the patient receiving monoamine oxidase inhibitors is:

    A. meperidine
    B. fentanyl
    C. morphine
    D. dilaudid

105. Which of the following is not contraindicated in the patient receiving monoamine oxidase inhibitors?

    A. phenylephrine
    B. mephentermine
    C. ephedrine
    D. methamphetamine

106. Maximum safe dose of lidocaine with epinephrine is:

    A. 7 mg/kg
    B. 3 mg/kg
    C. 5 mg/kg
    D. 10 mg/kg

107. Maximum safe dose of bupivacaine is:

    A. 3 mg/kg
    B. 7 mg/kg
    C. 1 mg/kg
    D. 8 mg/kg

108. Disseminated intravascular coagulation is suggested by all of the following except:

A. thrombocytopenia
B. prolonged PT interval
C. reduced serum concentration of fibrinogen
D. decreased circulating levels of fibrin split products

109. What would be the proper placement for the ultrasound Doppler device to monitor for venous embolism?

   A. right sternal border, third intercostal space
   B. tip of the sternal notch
   C. tip of xiphoid
   D. left sternal border, fifth intercostal space

110. Which of the following should be an indication of venous air embolism?

   A. increased arterial pressure
   B. increased end-tidal carbon dioxide
   C. decreased pulmonary pressure
   D. decreased end-tidal carbon dioxide

111. The action of ritodrine is to produce:

   A. decreased pulmonary pressure
   B. bronchodilation
   C. decrease uterine tone
   D. analgesia

112. The minimum acceptable potassium level after cardiopulmonary bypass is:

   A. 5.0 mEq/L
   B. 4.0 mEq/L
   C. 3.5 mEq/L
   D. 3.0 mEq/L

113. Children with a congenital heart defect with a right-to-left shunt whom we choose to induce with an inhalational agent:

   A. may have a shorter induction time
   B. may have a longer induction time
   C. may have no change in the induction time
   D. should never be induced with an inhalational agent

114. What complication is specifically associated with left jugular venous cannulation?

   A. puncture of the thoracic duct
   B. pneumothorax
   C. difficult passage into the superior vena cava
   D. infection

115. Hydralazine, procainamide, isoniazid, and occasionally the nonbarbiturate anticonvulsants may cause:

   A. systemic lupus erythematosus
   B. poliomyositis
   C. scleroderma
   D. muscular dystrophy

116. Which does not increase turbulent flow in a tube?

   A. increased flow rate
   B. decreased viscosity
   C. change in tube diameter
   D. a 30° angle

117. Afterload reduction is beneficial during anesthesia for noncardiac surgery in patients with each of the following conditions except:

   A. aortic valve insufficiency
   B. mitral valve regurgitation
   C. tetralogy of Fallot
   D. patent ductus arteriosus

118. Where is the fistula usually located in a patient with a tracheoesophageal fistula?

   A. anterior larynx
   B. above the carina on the posterior wall of the trachea
   C. lateral wall of the lower segment of the trachea
   D. posterior larynx

119. Autonomic dysfunction may manifest all of the following except:

   A. orthostatic hypotension
   B. resting tachycardia
   C. painful myocardial ischemia
   D. loss of beat-to-beat variability in heart rate

120. Symptoms of mitral regurgitation may include all except:

A. left atrial volume overload
B. reduced left ventricular stroke volume
C. large A wave on pulmonary artery tracings
D. apical systolic murmur

121. Which of the following is true regarding management of anesthesia for the patient with aortic stenosis?

A. maintain normal or slightly elevated heart rate
B. pulmonary capillary wedge pressure overestimates the left ventricular end-diastolic pressure
C. reduction of systemic vascular resistance is desirable
D. regional anesthesia is preferable to general anesthesia

122. In reference to the oxyhemoglobin-dissociation curve, which of the following factors might elicit a P_{50} of 29 mm Hg?

A. hypothermia
B. increased 2,3-diphosphoglycerate
C. chronic anemia
D. hyperventilation

123. The pain of the labor arises primarily from nociceptors in uterine and peroneal structure. Nerve fibers transmitting pain sensation during the second stage of labor travel with the parasympathetic fibers and enter the neuraxis at:

A. T1–L1
B. C8–T9
C. S2–S4
D. L1–S2

124. The blood volume of the lungs is what percent of the total blood volume in the circulatory system?

A. 3%
B. 9%
C. 15%
D. 20%

125. What conditions can cause a leftward shift of the oxyhemoglobin-dissociation curve?

A. hyperthermia
B. hypercapnia
C. polycythemia
D. carbon monoxide

126. Which of the following physiologic changes accompanies aging?

A. decreasing alveolar oxygen tension
B. increasing alveolar oxygen tension
C. decreasing arterial oxygen tension
D. increasing arterial oxygen tension

127. Which of the following will produce a left shift in the oxyhemoglobin-dissociation curve?

A. alkalosis
B. acidosis
C. increased 2,3-diphosphoglycerate
D. anemia

128. When ventilation/perfusion ratios increase the following has probably also occurred:

A. physiologic shunting
B. physiologic deadspace
C. increased minute volume
D. increased alveolar O_2

129. Infusion of excess amounts of crystalloids during the intraoperative period may result in pulmonary edema because:

A. increased capillary hydrostatic pressure
B. increased capillary permeability
C. decreased colloid osmotic pressure
D. lymphatic insufficiency

130. Which of the following is a true statement of the usual policies regarding nasogastric tubes and pyloric stenosis?

A. Nasogastric tubes are placed intraoperatively.
B. Nasogastric tubes irritate the operative area and are not inserted postoperatively.
C. A small-bore nasogastric tube is preferable to minimize trauma on insertion.
D. Nasogastric tube is always used to aspirate gastric contents in the preinduction phase.

131. The anesthesia of choice for excision of a pheochromocytoma would most likely be:

    A. narcotic technique
    B. inhalation anesthesia
    C. regional anesthesia
    D. intravenous sedation

132. The induction and intubation of a patient with Cushing's disease should be anticipated as difficult owing to all of the following except:

    A. buffalo hump of shoulders
    B. enlarged supraclavicular fat pads
    C. pendulous abdomen, obesity
    D. polycythemia

133. The typical clinical picture of a patient with hyperadrenocorticism would include all of the following except:

    A. hypertension
    B. hypoglycemia
    C. hypokalemia
    D. hypernatremia

134. A pathophysiologic change in toxemia of pregnancy is:

    A. increased glomerular filtration rate
    B. proteinuria
    C. hypotension
    D. hypervolemia

135. The nerve fibers carrying afferent pain signals to the spinal cord during the second stage of labor are primarily conveyed through the following nerve(s):

    A. nervi erigentes
    B. pudendal nerves
    C. hypogastric nerves
    D. pelvic splanchnic nerves

136. Which of the following might indicate amniotic fluid embolism?

    A. hypertension and tachypnea
    B. hypotension and gasping respirations
    C. wheezing and cyanosis
    D. tachycardia and Kussmaul's respirations

137. Which spinal nerves contribute to the formation of the brachial plexus?

    A. C4 to C8, T1 and T2
    B. C5 to C8, T1
    C. C7 and C8, T1 to T4
    D. C8, T1 to T4

138. Which of the following would be the most appropriate intervention for the adult diabetic with a blood sugar of 500 mg/dL?

    A. regular insulin SQ
    B. Lente insulin SQ
    C. regular insulin IV
    D. NPH insulin IV

139. The two major complications most frequently associated with cerebral aneurysms are:

    A. subarachnoid hemorrhage and cerebral ischemia
    B. intracranial hypertension and vasospasm
    C. vasospasm and recurrent hemorrhage
    D. cerebrovascular accident and recurrent hemorrhage

140. All of the following are hazards of the sitting position as used in neurosurgical procedures except:

    A. cardiac arrhythmia
    B. hypotension
    C. air embolism
    D. cerebral ischemia

141. Which of the following monitors is the most sensitive in detection of venous air embolism?

    A. precordial Doppler
    B. ECG
    C. pulmonary artery catheter
    D. $EtCO_2$

142. Treatment of air embolism includes all of the following except:

    A. left lateral decubitus position
    B. elevate the head of the bed
    C. 100% oxygen
    D. aspirate from the central line

143. During management of one-lung ventilation:

    A. High F_{IO_2}s are avoided to prevent absorption atelectasis.
    B. The dependent lung should be ventilated with less than 8 mL/kg to avoid hyperinflation and possible rupture of the ventilated lung.
    C. Hyperventilation is indicated to avoid Pa_{CO_2}s of over 30 mm Hg.
    D. Positive end-expiratory pressure of 10 cm H_2O to the dependent lung is beneficial because it increases lung volumes at end-expiration (FCR), which improves ventilation/perfusion relationships in the dependent lung.

144. If severe hypoxemia develops during one lung anesthesia, which of the following is not indicated?

    A. verify tube position with a fiberoptic bronchoscope
    B. institute intermittent two-lung ventilation
    C. nondependent lung continuous positive airway pressure
    D. using a tube changer, convert to a single-lumen tube

145. Postoperatively, your patient's blood pressure is 210/110 mm Hg, and his heart rate is 112. He did not take his clonidine this morning. He is comfortable, not hypoxic, and normothermic. What agent would you choose to reduce his blood pressure?

    A. nitroglycerine
    B. hydralazine
    C. nitroprusside
    D. labetolol

146. Before the removal of the abdominal aortic clamp, the anesthetist should:

    A. increase nitroglycerine to prevent myocardial ischemia
    B. administer an amnestic due to increased incidence of recall
    C. administer fluids and blood increasing cardiac filling pressures to high normal limits
    D. prepare an epinephrine and norepinephrine drip

147. Classification of "good" left ventricle function includes all of the following except:

    A. left ventricular end-diastolic pressure > 15 mm Hg
    B. hypertension
    C. normal ventriculogram
    D. absence of signs of congestive heart failure

148. What should be an important aspect of your anesthetic plan for correction of strabismus?

    A. Development of malignant hyperthermia should be anticipated.
    B. Local anesthetic is administered with intravenous sedation.
    C. An intravenous line is not necessary because it is a short procedure.
    D. Deep extubation is mandatory because it is an open-eye case.

149. The two primary means used to protect your patient's eyes from laser injuries are:

    A. placing sterile eye cups over each eye after the patient is asleep and wrapping the face with wet towels
    B. place the appropriate optical density eyewear on the patient and cover the closed eyes with wet eyepads
    C. lubricate the eyes with a non–petroleum-based, non–water-soluble lubricant and wrap the face with reflective foil
    D. place the appropriate optical density eyewear on the patient and lubricate the patient's eyes with petroleum-based non–water-soluble ophthalmic lubricant

150. A patient is undergoing CO_2 laser microlaryngoscopic vocal cord surgery under general anesthesia. The endotracheal tube of choice would be:

    A. silicone
    B. red rubber
    C. metal
    D. polyvinyl chloride

151. A double-cuffed endotracheal tube provides the following advantage during laser surgery of the airway:

A. two targets for the surgeons
B. visual obstruction of the distal portion of the larynx
C. visual acuity of the distal larynx
D. a secure cuff if one portion is impacted by the laser beam

152. The CO_2 laser beam is seen during application because it is:

A. accompanied by a helium-neon (HeNe) beam
B. bright blue
C. coherent
D. fluorescent and can be seen with the appropriate optical density eyewear

153. Cisatracurium is classified how chemically?

A. curariform
B. benzyl isoquinoline
C. steroidal
D. succinylcholine like

154. In patients with congestive heart failure, pressure overload can cause which type of hypertrophy?

A. eccentric
B. concentric
C. restrictive
D. obstructive

155. In patients with congestive heart failure, volume overload can cause which type of hypertrophy?

A. eccentric
B. concentric
C. restrictive
D. obstructive

156. Syndrome of inappropriate antidiuretic hormone secretion (SIADH) will manifest as all except:

A. obtunded mentation
B. hypotension
C. bradycardia
D. increased serum osmolarity

157. The most important inhibitor of coagulation is:

A. alpha$_2$ macroglobulin
B. protein C
C. plasminogen
D. antithrombin III

158. What are the factors that are the primary determinants of coronary perfusion pressure?

A. local and sympathetic influences
B. aortic and left ventricular pressures
C. heart rate and mean arterial pressure
D. diastolic time and myocardial wall tension

159. Neuroleptic malignant syndrome is precipitated by the administration of what drugs?

A. antiarrhythmics and antipsychotics
B. succinylcholine and volatile anesthetics
C. nondepolarizing relaxants and anticholinesterases
D. haloperidol and phenothiazines

160. What is the maximum dose of dantrolene for malignant hyperthermia?

A. 10 mg/kg
B. 20 mg/kg
C. 100 mg/kg
D. 75 mg/kg

161. In a patient who is susceptible to malignant hyperthermia, what agents will you recommend to the surgeon who wishes to use local anesthesia for the procedure?

A. Amide local anesthetics should be avoided.
B. Both ester and amide local anesthetics are now considered safe.
C. Ester local anesthetics should be avoided.
D. Both ester and amide local anesthetics should be avoided.

162. Properties of sodium nitroprusside include which of the following?

A. decreases afterload, no effect on preload
B. decreases preload, no effect on afterload
C. decreases preload and afterload
D. no effect on preload or afterload

163. The rate-limiting step in the biosynthesis of endogenous catecholamines is:

    A. metabolism of tyrosine to dopa
    B. metabolism of dopa to dopamine
    C. metabolism of norepinephrine to epinephrine
    D. metabolism of dopamine to norepinephrine

164. Administration of protamine to a patient who has not received heparin can result in:

    A. hypercoagulation
    B. seizure
    C. anticoagulation
    D. hypertension

165. The action of dantrolene, when used to treat malignant hyperthermia, is primary at the level of the:

    A. neuromuscular junction
    B. sarcoplasmic reticulum
    C. myosin filament
    D. slow muscle units

166. What substance catalyzes the final step in acetylcholine synthesis?

    A. carbonic anhydrase
    B. adenyl cyclase
    C. choline acetyl transferase
    D. glutamic transferase

167. Where is the fistula usually located in a patient with a tracheoesophageal fistula?

    A. anterior larynx
    B. above the carina on the posterior wall of the trachea
    C. lateral wall of the lower segment of the trachea
    D. posterior larynx

168. Characteristics of beta$_2$-adrenergic receptor stimulation include all of the following except:

    A. increased urinary bladder sphincter tone
    B. increased skeletal muscle
    C. bronchodilation
    D. positive inotropic action

169. What is the earliest and most reliable sign and symptom of aspiration?

    A. bronchospasm
    B. hypoxemia
    C. tachycardia
    D. cyanosis

170. What are four side effects of the muscarinic receptor stimulating properties of anticholinesterase drugs?

    A. tachycardia, bronchoconstriction, hyperperistalsis, miosis and inability to focus for near vision
    B. bradycardia, salivation, nausea and vomiting, mydriasis
    C. bradycardia, enhanced gastric fluid secretion, hyperperistalsis, miosis
    D. tachycardia, increased salivary and bronchial secretions, bronchoconstriction, peristalsis

171. Name the metabolite of ester hydrolysis of atracurium that, although unlikely, can cause central nervous system stimulation.

    A. monoethyl glycinexylidide
    B. normeperidine
    C. laudanosine
    D. toluidine

172. Post-tetanic potentiation is evidenced with:

    A. nondepolarizing blockade only
    B. depolarizing blockade only
    C. nondepolarizing and phase II blockade
    D. depolarizing and phase II blockade

173. The drug of choice for the treatment of renal and biliary colic is:

    A. morphine
    B. codeine
    C. meperidine
    D. hydromorphone (Dilaudid)

174. Pharmacokinetics, a subspecialty of pharmacology, involves the study of all of the following areas of drug activity except:

A. biotransformation
B. mechanism of action
C. distribution
D. absorption

175. Morphine and its derivatives are of which group?

A. isoquinoline
B. phenanthrene
C. steroid-like
D. methylcarbonates

176. Droperidol produces an antiemetic effect by:

A. dopamine-receptor blockade
B. serotonin-receptor blockade
C. muscarinic-receptor blockade
D. beta-receptor stimulation

177. The initial emergence from a propofol induction is due to:

A. short beta half-life
B. short alpha half-life
C. rapid metabolism
D. redistribution to non-nervous sites

178. An inhalation agent has minimal alveolar concentration of 0.25%; lipid solubility of 330; blood/gas coefficient of 0.9. It will most likely be:

A. slow and weak
B. rapid and potent
C. rapid and weak
D. slow and potent

179. The main factor determining the time for recovery from inhalation anesthesia is the agent's:

A. oil/water solubility ratio
B. blood/gas solubility ratio
C. rate of biotransformation
D. degree of plasma protein binding

180. The enzyme that may be induced in patients with porphyria by the barbiturate drugs leading to an acute attack is:

A. ALA synthetase
B. methionine synthetase
C. monoamine oxidase
D. 11-β-hydroxylase

181. The enzyme that is thought to be inhibited by etomidate leading to a prolonged decrease in adrenocorticoid levels is:

A. ALA synthetase
B. pseudocholinesterase
C. monoamine oxidase
D. 11-β-hydroxylase

182. Which of the following does not play a role in the production of compound A by sevoflurane?

A. time of administration
B. drug concentration
C. temperature
D. enzyme induction

183. Which of the following does not play a role in the production of fluoride ion by sevoflurane?

A. time of administration
B. drug concentration
C. enzyme induction
D. type of carbon dioxide granule

184. The most effective drug as an antidote for atropine poisoning is:

A. neostigmine
B. pyridostigmine
C. physostigmine
D. edrophonium

185. Changes in cardiac output will change the uptake of which type of anesthetic agent the most?

A. soluble
B. insoluble
C. Both types are equally affected.
D. Neither type is affected.

186. Ventilation/perfusion deficits will change the uptake of which type of anesthetic agent the most?

A. soluble
B. insoluble
C. Both types are equally affected.
D. Neither type is affected.

187. The calcium channel blocking drug that is approved for the treatment of cerebral vasospasm is?

A. verapamil (Isoptin)
B. nifedipine (Procardia)
C. diltiazem (Cardizem)
D. nimodipine (Nimotop)

188. Verapamil is indicated for the treatment of which of the following arrhythmias?

A. ventricular fibrillation
B. third-degree heart block
C. ventricular tachycardia
D. atrial fibrillation

189. Variant or spasmodic angina:

A. occurs upon exertion
B. results from atherosclerotic blockage of coronary arteries
C. is resistant to diltiazem therapy
D. occurs at rest

190. A characteristic of nitroglycerin therapy is:

A. frequent bradycardia
B. myocardial depression
C. development of tolerance
D. hypertension

191. Side effects common to adrenergic bronchodilators, such as terbutaline, when administered acutely, include all of the following except:

A. hyperglycemia
B. tachycardia
C. enhanced peripheral vascular resistance
D. tremor

192. A drug with a high hepatic extraction ratio would be most likely to exhibit a low:

A. plasma protein binding
B. apparent volume of distribution
C. oral bioavailability
D. therapeutic index

193. Which of the following eicosanoids is most intimately involved in producing allergic bronchoconstriction?

A. prostaglandin E_2
B. prostacyclin
C. thromboxane
D. leukotriene C_4

194. NSAIDs can cause gastric irritation, erosions, and ulcers by blocking gastric production of:

A. histamine
B. prostaglandin E_2
C. prostaglandin F_2
D. leukotriene B_2

195. Spinal opioid analgesia appears to result primarily from activation of which of the following opioid receptors?

A. mu
B. kappa
C. sigma
D. epsilon

196. Which of the following endogenous opioids is responsible for inhibiting pain transmission at the first afferent synapse in the dorsal horn of the spinal column?

A. alpha endorphin
B. beta endorphin
C. dynorphin
D. enkephalin

197. The most common side effect observed in patients receiving nitroglycerin is:

A. lupus erythematosus syndrome
B. respiratory depression
C. postural hypotension
D. methemoglobinemia

198. The diuresis that accompanies successful treatment of congestive heart failure with digitalis glycosides is due to:

A. inhibition of antidiuretic hormone secretion
B. increased plasma levels of aldosterone
C. stimulation of renal dopamine receptors
D. enhanced renal blood flow

199. The site action of the diuretic agent furosemide is the:

A. proximal convoluted tubule
B. descending limb of the loop of Henle
C. ascending limb of the loop of Henle
D. distal convoluted tubule

200. Cinchonism, a symptom-complex consisting of tinnitus, confusion, and blurred vision, is a characteristic adverse response to which of the following agents?

A. quinidine
B. digitoxin
C. furosemide
D. verapamil

201. The effectiveness of some antihistamines in the treatment of motion sickness results from which of the following actions?

A. H_1 receptor block
B. H_2 receptor block
C. anticholinergic actions
D. local anesthetic actions

202. The beta half-life of a drug describes what phase of drug action?

A. therapeutic
B. elimination
C. distribution
D. absorption

203. The alpha half-life of a drug describes what phase of drug action?

A. therapeutic
B. elimination
C. distribution
D. absorption

204. When comparing the spectrum of activity of acetaminophen with aspirin, which of the following actions are not produced by acetaminophen?

A. hepatotoxicity
B. anti-inflammatory
C. antipyretic
D. analgesia

205. Which pharmacokinetic parameter is most closely associated with duration of action of local anesthetics?

A. pK_a
B. chemical class
C. distribution
D. protein binding

206. The main benefit of ropivacaine is:

A. its metabolic pathway
B. its intermediate duration
C. it is less cardiotoxic than bupivacaine
D. its faster onset

207. Which of the following would you not see with a phase 1 block?

A. post-tetanic facilitation
B. fasciculations
C. sustained tetanus
D. no train-of-four fade

208. Remifentanil is unique among opioids owing to its:

A. mechanism of action
B. metabolism
C. side effects
D. onset

209. The treatment for severe hypernatremia after a transurethral prostatic resection is:

A. 3% saline
B. 0.9% saline
C. diuretic
D. potassium

210. During laparoscopy, which of the following complications would you not expect to see?

A. hypocapnia
B. hypotension
C. aspiration
D. hypoxia

211. Stimulation of H_2 receptors would produce all of the following except:

A. increased heart rate
B. increased acid secretion
C. bronchoconstriction
D. inotropic effect

212. Alpha receptors stimulation would produce:

    A. vasodilation
    B. cardiac stimulation
    C. hypotension
    D. reflex bradycardia

213. Which of the following drugs should not be given to a patient with increased intracranial pressure?

    A. fentanyl
    B. propofol
    C. etomidate
    D. ketamine

214. A patient undergoing a carotid endarterectomy under local anesthesia would require which block?

    A. brachial plexus
    B. interscalene
    C. superior laryngeal
    D. cervical plexus

215. Which of the following drug classes is contraindicated in a patient with renal failure?

    A. opioids
    B. nonsteroidal anti-inflammatory drugs
    C. mannitol
    D. thiopental

216. Measuring stump pressures during carotid artery surgery reflects perfusion to the:

    A. circle of Willis
    B. opposite carotid vessel
    C. middle cerebral artery
    D. vertebral arteries

217. Blood flow to the circle of Willis arises from:

    A. internal and external carotid arteries
    B. external carotid and interior spinal artery
    C. internal carotid and anterior cerebral artery
    D. internal carotid and basilar arteries

218. In a patient with a decreasing pulse pressure you would suspect:

    A. pulmonary vasodilation
    B. congestive heart failure
    C. hypovolemia
    D. increased contractile action

219. An increase in cyclic adenosine monophosphate would result in what in cardiac cells?

    A. an increased calcium concentration
    B. a decreased calcium concentration
    C. an increased phosphate concentration
    D. a decreased phosphate concentration

220. Which of the following is contraindicated in a patient with multiple sclerosis?

    A. midazolam
    B. mild hypothermia
    C. spinal anesthesia
    D. rocuronium

221. Fluoxetine (Prozac) exerts its effect by blocking reuptake in what type of receptors?

    A. serotonin
    B. beta receptors
    C. alpha receptors
    D. GABA receptors

222. Hydralazine primarily influences which of the following parameters?

    A. preload
    B. afterload
    C. pulmonary resistance
    D. cerebral resistance

223. The most common critical incident under general anesthesia is:

    A. severe hypotension
    B. life-threatening arrhythmias
    C. machine disconnect
    D. nerve palsy

224. Appearance of an S_3 gallop in an anesthetized patient is a premonitory sign of:

    A. congestive heart failure
    B. mitral stenosis
    C. angina
    D. hypertension

225. When performing a transtracheal block the needle penetrates the:

   A. cricothyroid membrane
   B. thyroid cartilage
   C. cricoid cartilage
   D. hyoid membrane

226. Fentanyl works primarily on what type of opiate receptor?

   A. mu receptor
   B. kappa receptor
   C. delta receptor
   D. sigma receptor

1. ANSWER: **B**

   Rationale: Creatinine phosphokinase levels should be checked at 6, 12, and 24 hours after an episode of masseter muscle rigidity. If CPK levels are still grossly elevated at 12 hours, additional samples should be obtained until the levels return to normal. Studies have shown that with a level greater than 20,000 IU/L in the perioperative period a concomitant myopathy is not present. The diagnosis of malignant hyperthermia can be made with certainty.

   Reference: Karlet, M.C. (1997). Chapter 40: Musculoskeletal Pathophysiology and Anesthesia. In J. Nagelhout & K. Zaglaniczny (Eds.), *Nurse Anesthesia*. Philadelphia: W.B. Saunders.

2. ANSWER: **B**

   Rationale: Five to 10% of patients treated with bleomycin develop pulmonary toxicity. One to 2% of all patients die of this complication. It is recommended that concentrations of oxygen of 30% and colloids rather than crystalloids be administered.

   Reference: Rojo, J. & Iacopelli, M. (1997). Chapter 39A: Respiratory Pathophysiology. In J. Nagelhout & K. Zaglaniczny (Eds.), *Nurse Anesthesia*. Philadelphia: W.B. Saunders.

3. ANSWER: **D**

   Rationale: Before surgery is scheduled it is important to establish alpha blockade first, followed by appropriate beta blockers. Alpha blockade should be instituted first to ensure adequate vasodilatation before the beta blocker–induced cardiac depression.

   Reference: Karlet, M.C. & Sebastian, L.A. (1997). Chapter 12: The Endocrine System. In J. Nagelhout & K. Zaglaniczny (Eds.), *Nurse Anesthesia*. Philadelphia: W.B. Saunders.

4. ANSWER: **C**

   Rationale: Alpha and beta blockers are essential for cardiovascular control owing to the increased catecholamine levels secreted by the tumors. The other agents would stimulate cardiovascular activity and thus be contraindicated.

   Reference: Karlet, M.C. & Sebastian, L.A. (1997). Chapter 12: The Endocrine System. In J. Nagelhout & K. Zaglaniczny (Eds.), *Nurse Anesthesia*. Philadelphia: W.B. Saunders.

5. ANSWER: **C**

   Rationale: If a pacemaker fails, inspired oxygen concentration should be increased to 100% immediately. Check connectors and generator battery light. The pacemaker should be set into the asynchronous mode while reasons for the failure are assessed.

   Reference: Aprile, A.E., Serwin, J.P., & Boctor, B. (1997). Chapter 38A: Cardiac Pathophysiology. In J. Nagelhout & K. Zaglaniczny (Eds.), *Nurse Anesthesia*. Philadelphia: W.B. Saunders.

6. ANSWER: **C**

   Rationale: Synchronization of the shock waves to the R waves of the ECG decreases the incidence of arrhythmias. They are usually found to be 20 msec after the R wave to correspond to the ventricular refractory period.

   Reference: Aprile, A.E., Serwin, J.P., & Boctor, B. (1997). Chapter 38A: Cardiac Pathophysiology. In J. Nagelhout & K. Zaglaniczny (Eds.), *Nurse Anesthesia*. Philadelphia: W.B. Saunders.

7. ANSWER: **D**

   Rationale: Indications for a pacemaker include a new symptomatic bradyarrhythmia, a new bundle branch block, second- or third-degree heart block associated with myocardial infarction and refractory supraventricular tachycardia.

   Reference: Aprile, A.E., Serwin, J.P., & Boctor, B. (1997). Chapter 38A: Cardiac Pathophysiology. In J. Nagelhout & K. Zaglaniczny (Eds.), *Nurse Anesthesia*. Philadelphia: W.B. Saunders.

8. ANSWER: **C**

Rationale: The key to anesthetic management for patients with carcinoid syndrome is avoiding agents or techniques that cause the tumor to release vasoactive substances. These include hypotension, histamine-releasing drugs, surgical manipulation of the tumor, and catecholamine-releasing drugs. Octreotide or steroids may be indicated.

Reference: Palmer, T.J. (1997). Chapter 10: Hepatobiliary and Gastrointestinal Disturbances. In J. Nagelhout & K. Zaglaniczny (Eds.), *Nurse Anesthesia*. Philadelphia: W.B. Saunders.

9. ANSWER: **C**

Rationale: Adenosine is administered rapidly by intravenous push. It should be given in a central line if possible and followed by a saline flush to ensure adequate cardiac levels. Adenosine is rapidly taken up into cells with a half-life measured in seconds.

Reference: Alisoglu, R. (1997). Chapter 23: Cardiac Pharmacology. In J. Nagelhout & K. Zaglaniczny (Eds.), *Nurse Anesthesia*. Philadelphia: W.B. Saunders.

10. ANSWER: **D**

Rationale: Adenosine is metabolized by adenosine deaminase and xanthine oxidase into uric acid.

Reference: Alisoglu, R. (1997). Chapter 23: Cardiac Pharmacology. In J. Nagelhout & K. Zaglaniczny (Eds.), *Nurse Anesthesia*. Philadelphia: W.B. Saunders.

11. ANSWER: **A**

Rationale: Adenosine is rapidly taken up into cells and converted to uric acid. This process takes less than a minute, which accounts for the very short duration of action of the drug.

Reference: Alisoglu, R. (1997). Chapter 23: Cardiac Pharmacology. In J. Nagelhout & K. Zaglaniczny (Eds.), *Nurse Anesthesia*. Philadelphia: W.B. Saunders.

12. ANSWER: **B**

Rationale: Re-entrant supraventricular tachyarrhythmias will respond to adenosine therapy. If the arrhythmia involves the AV node in its pathway, adenosine can terminate it by producing the atrioventricular block.

Reference: Alisoglu, R. (1997). Chapter 23: Cardiac Pharmacology. In J. Nagelhout & K. Zaglaniczny (Eds.), *Nurse Anesthesia*. Philadelphia: W.B. Saunders.

13. ANSWER: **B**

Rationale: Conditions that might promote hemoglobin desaturation or low flow states should be avoided. These include hypothermia or hyperthermia, acidosis, hypoxia, hypotension, and hypovolemia.

Reference: Gerbasi, F. R. (1997). Chapter 41: Hematology and Anesthesia. In J. Nagelhout & K. Zaglaniczny (Eds.), *Nurse Anesthesia*. Philadelphia: W.B. Saunders.

14. ANSWER: **A**

Rationale: See question 13.

Reference: Gerbasi, F. R. (1997). Chapter 41: Hematology and Anesthesia. In J. Nagelhout & K. Zaglaniczny (Eds.), *Nurse Anesthesia*. Philadelphia: W.B. Saunders.

15. ANSWER: **D**

Rationale: Regular insulin is the only form of preparation that should be used intravenously. The intravenous route circumvents the unpredictable absorption of SQ insulin, which can be aggravated by changes in blood pressure and cutaneous blood flow that occur during anesthesia.

Reference: Karlet, M.C. & Sebastian, L.A. (1997). Chapter 12: The Endocrine System. In J. Nagelhout & K. Zaglaniczny (Eds.), *Nurse Anesthesia*. Philadelphia: W.B. Saunders.

16. ANSWER: **A**

Rationale: Leads II, III, and aVF monitor the right side of the heart supplied by the right coronary artery. Leads V_3 to V_5 monitor the anterolateral aspects of the left ventricle. Leads I and aVL monitor the lateral aspects of the left ventricle.

Reference: Palmer, T.J. & Mitton, M.P. (1997). Chapter 36: Electrocardiography and Rhythm Disturbances. In J. Nagelhout & K. Zaglaniczny (Eds.), *Nurse Anesthesia*. Philadelphia: W.B. Saunders.

17. ANSWER: **C**

   Rationale: See question 16.
   Reference: Palmer, T.J. & Mitton, M.P. (1997).
      Chapter 36: Electrocardiography and Rhythm
      Disturbances. In J. Nagelhout & K. Zaglaniczny
      (Eds.), *Nurse Anesthesia*. Philadelphia: W.B.
      Saunders.

18. ANSWER: **B**

   Rationale: See question 16.
   Reference: Palmer, T.J. & Mitton, M.P. (1997).
      Chapter 36: Electrocardiography and Rhythm
      Disturbances. In J. Nagelhout & K. Zaglaniczny
      (Eds.), *Nurse Anesthesia*. Philadelphia: W.B.
      Saunders.

19. ANSWER: **C**

   Rationale: Left internal jugular cannulation is undesirable because of potential
   for damaging the thoracic duct, difficulty
   maneuvering the catheter, and potential
   for puncture of the left carotid artery
   and embolism.
   Reference: Sinkovich, J.A. & Kossick, M.A. (1997).
      Chapter 27: Clinical Monitoring in Anesthesia.
      In J. Nagelhout & K. Zaglaniczny (Eds.), *Nurse
      Anesthesia*. Philadelphia: W.B. Saunders.

20. ANSWER: **C**

   Rationale: Stellate ganglion block may
   occur with the interscalene approach to
   the brachial plexus. Stellate ganglion
   block results in Horner's syndrome,
   which includes miosis, ptosis, and hy-
   drosis. This occurs in 30% to 50% of
   interscalene blocks.
   Reference: Ellis, W.E. (1997). Chapter 53: Regional
      Anesthesia. In J. Nagelhout & K. Zaglaniczny
      (Eds.), *Nurse Anesthesia*. Philadelphia: W.B.
      Saunders.

21. ANSWER: **A**

   Rationale: Cardiac tamponade must always be considered postoperatively when
   cardiac output is minimal. Stroke volume, due to the tamponade, is limited
   and fixed, and cardiac output and blood
   pressure become dependent on heart
   rate.
   Reference: Aprile, A.E. & Aprile, F.D. (1997).
      Chapter 38B: Cardiac Anesthesia. In J.
      Nagelhout & K. Zaglaniczny (Eds.), *Nurse
      Anesthesia*. Philadelphia: W.B. Saunders.

22. ANSWER: **C**

   Rationale: When the heart is not open,
   as in coronary bypass graft procedures, it
   may be necessary to insert a catheter
   that acts as a vent to prevent distention
   from blood returning through the thebesian or bronchial veins.
   Reference: Aprile, A.E. & Aprile, F.D. (1997).
      Chapter 38B: Cardiac Anesthesia. In J.
      Nagelhout & K. Zaglaniczny (Eds.), *Nurse
      Anesthesia*. Philadelphia: W.B. Saunders.

23. ANSWER: **C**

   Rationale: The most common complication of retrobulbar block is retrobulbar
   hemorrhage. Be careful not to perform
   this technique on patients with bleeding
   disorders or who are on anticoagulants.
   Reference: Harvey, R.R. (1997). Chapter 48:
      Anesthesia for Ophthalmic Procedures. In J.
      Nagelhout & K. Zaglaniczny (Eds.), *Nurse
      Anesthesia*. Philadelphia: W.B. Saunders.

24. ANSWER: **B**

   Rationale: Uterine blood flow is not significantly affected by respiratory gas exchange except in extreme hypocarbia
   (P_{ACO_2} less than 20 mm Hg), which can
   reduce urinary blood flow.
   Reference: Fiedler, M.A. & Shaw, B. (1997).
      Chapter 13: Obstetric Anesthesia. In J.
      Nagelhout & K. Zaglaniczny (Eds.), *Nurse
      Anesthesia*. Philadelphia: W.B. Saunders.

25. ANSWER: **D**

   Rationale: Acute complications of cricothyroidotomy include pneumothorax,
   subcutaneous emphysema, mediastinal
   emphysema, bleeding, esophageal puncture, aspiration, and respiratory acidosis.
   Reference: Chipas, A. (1997). Chapter 33: Airway
      Management. In J. Nagelhout & K. Zaglaniczny
      (Eds.), *Nurse Anesthesia*. Philadelphia: W.B.
      Saunders.

26. ANSWER: **A**

   Rationale: Gastroschisis and omphalocele
   are disorders characterized by defect in
   the abdominal wall allowing herniation
   of viscera. Perioperative management
   centers around avoiding hypothermia,
   dehydration, and infection. These prob-

lems are usually more serious in gastroschisis because the protective hernial sac is absent.

Reference: Dobbins, P. & Hall, S.M. (1997). Chapter 14: Pediatric Anesthesia. In J. Nagelhout & K. Zaglaniczny (Eds.), *Nurse Anesthesia.* Philadelphia: W.B. Saunders.

27. ANSWER: B

Rationale: Tinnitus and slurred speech would be indicative of a high central nervous system (CNS) level of local anesthetic and would be premonitory signs of CNS excitation.

Reference: Williams, J.R. (1997). Chapter 20: Local Anesthetics. In J. Nagelhout & K. Zaglaniczny (Eds.), *Nurse Anesthesia.* Philadelphia: W.B. Saunders.

28. ANSWER: D

Rationale: Hetastarch is used to expand intravascular fluid volume for the treatment of hypovolemia due to burns or hemorrhage. The usual total daily intravenous dose is 20 mL/kg.

Reference: Litwack, K. & Keithley, J.K. (1997). Chapter 31: Fluids, Electrolytes and Therapy. In J. Nagelhout & K. Zaglaniczny (Eds.), *Nurse Anesthesia.* Philadelphia: W.B. Saunders.

29. ANSWER: C

Rationale: Postoperative problems of carotid endarterectomy commonly include lability of systolic blood pressure, airway compression due to hematoma formation, loss of carotid body function, myocardial infarction, and stroke.

Reference: McIntosh, L.S. (1997). Chapter 38C: Vascular Surgery. In J. Nagelhout & K. Zaglaniczny (Eds.), *Nurse Anesthesia.* Philadelphia: W.B. Saunders.

30. ANSWER: B

Rationale: Pneumothorax and hemothorax are the most common complications of this block. Incidence of pneumothorax may be as high as 6%.

Reference: Ellis, W.E. (1997). Chapter 53: Regional Anesthesia. In J. Nagelhout & K. Zaglaniczny (Eds.), *Nurse Anesthesia.* Philadelphia: W.B. Saunders.

31. ANSWER: D

Rationale: Occasional heparin resistance results from an antithrombin III deficiency. This is the serine protease that is enhanced by heparin.

Reference: Gerbasi, F.R. (1997). Chapter 41: Hematology and Anesthesia. In J. Nagelhout & K. Zaglaniczny (Eds.), *Nurse Anesthesia.* Philadelphia: W.B. Saunders.

32. ANSWER: C

Rationale: Patients with antithrombin III deficiency will achieve adequate anticoagulation after administration of fresh frozen plasma, antithrombin III concentrate, or synthetic antithrombin III.

Reference: Gerbasi, F.R. (1997). Chapter 41: Hematology and Anesthesia. In J. Nagelhout & K. Zaglaniczny (Eds.), *Nurse Anesthesia.* Philadelphia: W.B. Saunders.

33. ANSWER: C

Rationale: The minimum time the tourniquet needs to be inflated is 20 minutes to avoid sudden absorption of anesthetic into the systemic circulation. Between 20 and 40 minutes, cyclic deflation is recommended. Beyond 40 minutes, deflation can be a single maneuver.

Reference: Ellis, W.E. (1997). Regional Anesthesia. In J. Nagelhout & K. Zaglaniczny (Eds.), *Nurse Anesthesia.* Philadelphia: W.B. Saunders.

34. ANSWER: D

Rationale: Hypoparathyroidism from unintentional removal of the parathyroid glands during thyroidectomy will cause acute hypocalcemia within 24 to 72 hours postoperatively.

Reference: Karlet, M.C. & Sebastian, L.A. (1997). Chapter 12: The Endocrine System. In J. Nagelhout & K. Zaglaniczny (Eds.), *Nurse Anesthesia.* Philadelphia: W.B. Saunders.

35. ANSWER: B

Rationale: Some reports indicated that symptoms of multiple sclerosis are exacerbated by some types of anesthesia, particularly regional anesthesia. A relapse postoperatively is not uncommon.

Reference: Karlet, M.C. (1997). Chapter 40: Muscoloskeletal Pathophysiology and Anesthesia.

In J. Nagelhout & K. Zaglaniczny (Eds.), *Nurse Anesthesia*. Philadelphia: W.B. Saunders.

36. ANSWER: D

Rationale: Treatment of patients with cystic fibrosis is primarily directed to clearing secretions from the respiratory system. Atropine's drying effect would work against this priority; therefore, it should be avoided.

Reference: Rojo, J. & Iacopelli, M. (1997). Chapter 39A: Respiratory Pathophysiology. In J. Nagelhout & K. Zaglaniczny (Eds.), *Nurse Anesthesia*. Philadelphia: W.B. Saunders.

37. ANSWER: D

Rationale: Intraoperative bronchospasm is usually due to factors other than acute exacerbation of bronchial asthma. More likely causes are mechanical obstruction or light anesthesia.

Reference: Chipas, A. (1997). Chapter 33: Airway Management. In J. Nagelhout & K. Zaglaniczny (Eds.), *Nurse Anesthesia*. Philadelphia: W.B. Saunders.

38. ANSWER: C

Rationale: Sympathetic or motor blockade would occur after a change in heart rate from a test dose of epinephrine and sensory block from the local anesthetic.

Reference: Ellis, W.E. (1997). Chapter 53: Regional Anesthesia. In J. Nagelhout & K. Zaglaniczny (Eds.), *Nurse Anesthesia*. Philadelphia: W.B. Saunders.

39. ANSWER: C

Rationale: Administration of 10 to 15 units of packed red blood cells in adult patients is likely to result in a platelet count of 100,000 cells/mL or less. This dilutional thrombocytopenia is treated with infusion of platelet concentrates.

Reference: Gerbasi, F.R. (1997). Chapter 41: Hematology and Anesthesia. In J. Nagelhout & K. Zaglaniczny (Eds.), *Nurse Anesthesia*. Philadelphia: W.B. Saunders.

40. ANSWER: C

Rationale: Pulmonary toxicity after bleomycin therapy occurs in 10% to 15% of the cases.

Reference: Rojo, J. & Iacopelli, M. (1997). Chapter 39A: Respiratory Pathophysiology. In J. Nagelhout & K. Zaglaniczny (Eds.), *Nurse Anesthesia*. Philadelphia: W.B. Saunders.

41. ANSWER: A

Rationale: Occlusion of the aorta causes hypertension in the proximal segment and hypotension in the distal segment. Cross-clamping produces an increase in afterload and peripheral resistance in proportion to the level of occlusion. Similarly, myocardial stress varies with the level of occlusion.

Reference: McIntosh, L.S. (1997). Chapter 38C: Vascular Surgery. In J. Nagelhout & K. Zaglaniczny (Eds.), *Nurse Anesthesia*. Philadelphia: W.B. Saunders.

42. ANSWER: C

Rationale: Fetal hemoglobin has a P_{50} of 19 mm Hg compared with 26 mm Hg for adult hemoglobin.

Reference: Dobbins, P. & Hall. S.M. (1997). Chapter 14: Pediatric Anesthesia. In J. Nagelhout & K. Zaglaniczny (Eds.), *Nurse Anesthesia*. Philadelphia: W.B. Saunders.

43. ANSWER: C

Rationale: A diaphragmatic hernia in a neonate is an emergency procedure. It requires awake intubation of an orogastric tube and may possibly include insertion of an arterial line to determine blood gases and pH.

Reference: Dobbins, P. & Hall, S.M. (1997). Chapter 14: Pediatric Anesthesia. In J. Nagelhout & K. Zaglaniczny (Eds.), *Nurse Anesthesia*. Philadelphia: W.B. Saunders.

44. ANSWER: B

Rationale: The signs and symptoms of diaphragmatic hernia evidence soon after birth include scaphoid abdomen, barrel-shaped chest (pectus excavatum), bowel sounds during auscultation of the chest, and profound hypoxia.

Reference: Dobbins, P. & Hall. S.M. (1997). Chapter 14: Pediatric Anesthesia. In J. Nagelhout & K. Zaglaniczny (Eds.), *Nurse Anesthesia*. Philadelphia: W.B. Saunders.

45. ANSWER: **D**

Rationale: Important aspects in surgical management include maintenance of body temperature and continuation of fluid replacement because hypovolemia is almost always an issue. Postoperative ventilation and parenteral nutrition have increased survival to approximately 75%.

Reference: Dobbins, P. & Hall, S.M. (1997). Chapter 14: Pediatric Anesthesia. In J. Nagelhout & K. Zaglaniczny (Eds.), *Nurse Anesthesia*. Philadelphia: W.B. Saunders.

46. ANSWER: **A**

Rationale: Calcium channel blockers, although antihypertensive in action, would be the least likely choice of treatment for this disorder. Doses required would be high, resulting in heart block and undesirable muscle effects.

Reference: Morgan, R.O., Jr. (1997). Chapter 8: The Cardiovascular System. In J. Nagelhout & K. Zaglaniczny (Eds.), *Nurse Anesthesia*. Philadelphia: W.B. Saunders.

47. ANSWER: **A**

Rationale: Although hypoxia must be ruled out, the more likely cause is emergence delirium. A small number of patients may awaken in an agitated state, requiring restraints or re-sedation.

Reference: Hill, F.C., Jr. & Kopecky, J.F. (1997). Chapter 47: Anesthesia for Ear, Nose, Throat, and Maxillofacial Surgery. In J. Nagelhout & K. Zaglaniczny (Eds.), *Nurse Anesthesia*. Philadelphia: W.B. Saunders.

48. ANSWER: **A**

Rationale: With age, chest wall compliance decreases. In the elderly, small airways may even close during tidal breathing. This widens the alveolar/arterial gradient for oxygen. PO_2, however, is relatively unaffected.

Reference: Martin-Sheridan, D. (1997). Chapter 42: Geriatrics and Anesthesia Practice. In J. Nagelhout & K. Zaglaniczny (Eds.), *Nurse Anesthesia*. Philadelphia: W.B. Saunders.

49. ANSWER: **A**

Rationale: Activated clotting time is a test of the intrinsic system and final common pathways. It is widely used to monitor heparin therapy especially in the operating room. Normal values are usually in the range of 90 to 120 seconds.

Reference: Gerbasi, F.R. (1997). Chapter 41: Hematology and Anesthesia. In J. Nagelhout & K. Zaglaniczny (Eds.), *Nurse Anesthesia*. Philadelphia: W.B. Saunders.

50. ANSWER: **A**

Rationale: Indications for insertion of a permanent pacemaker include sinus node dysfunction, complete heart block, symptomatic atrioventricular block, and trifascicular heart block.

Reference: Aprile, A.E. & Aprile, F.D. (1997). Chapter 38B: Cardiac Anesthesia. In J. Nagelhout & K. Zaglaniczny (Eds.), *Nurse Anesthesia*. Philadelphia: W.B. Saunders.

51. ANSWER: **A**

Rationale: Patients with an AICD should have it deactivated with a magnet before electrocautery, MRI, and lithotripsy. A simple magnet device will easily deactivate and reactivate the pacemaker.

Reference: Aprile, A.E. & Aprile, F.D. (1997). Chapter 38B: Cardiac Anesthesia. In J. Nagelhout & K. Zaglaniczny (Eds.), *Nurse Anesthesia*. Philadelphia: W.B. Saunders.

52. ANSWER: **A**

Rationale: IHSS results from asymmetric hypertrophy of the interventricular septa, leading to outflow obstruction. Factors that worsen outflow obstruction include hypotension, decreased intraventricular volume, and increased contractility.

Reference: McIntosh, L.S. (1997). Chapter 38C: Vascular Surgery. In J. Nagelhout & K. Zaglaniczny (Eds.), *Nurse Anesthesia*. Philadelphia: W.B. Saunders.

53. ANSWER: **A**

Rationale: In aortic stenosis it is important to maintain sinus rhythm and adequate preload. Hypotension should be aggressively treated. Tachycardia or bradycardia is poorly tolerated. Wedge pressure will underestimate left ventricular end-diastolic pressure; therefore, it may not be useful.

Reference: McIntosh, L.S. (1997). Chapter 38C: Vascular Surgery. In J. Nagelhout & K. Zaglaniczny (Eds.), *Nurse Anesthesia.* Philadelphia: W.B. Saunders.

54. ANSWER: **D**

Rationale: Reduction in the afterload leads to a reduced blood pressure and coronary perfusion because cardiac output is relatively fixed by the stenotic valve.

Reference: McIntosh, L.S. (1997). Chapter 38C: Vascular Surgery. In J. Nagelhout & K. Zaglaniczny (Eds.), *Nurse Anesthesia.* Philadelphia: W.B. Saunders.

55. ANSWER: **B**

Rationale: Aortic stenosis is a fixed outlet obstruction to left ventricular ejection. Ventricular compliance decreases, and end-diastolic pressure increases.

Reference: McIntosh, L.S. (1997). Chapter 38C: Vascular Surgery. In J. Nagelhout & K. Zaglaniczny (Eds.), *Nurse Anesthesia.* Philadelphia: W.B. Saunders.

56. ANSWER: **A**

Rationale: Fast, full, and forward is the phrase to remember in managing these patients. Afterload reduction augments forward flow. Volume replacement is necessary to maintain preload, and tachycardia reduces ventricular volumes.

Reference: McIntosh, L.S. (1997). Chapter 38C: Vascular Surgery. In J. Nagelhout & K. Zaglaniczny (Eds.), *Nurse Anesthesia.* Philadelphia: W.B. Saunders.

57. ANSWER: **C**

Rationale: Increases in pulmonary vascular resistance exacerbate right ventricular failure. Therefore, it is important to avoid vasoconstrictor drugs, hypoxia, hypercarbia, and acidosis, which may all increase pulmonary vascular resistance.

Reference: McIntosh, L.S. (1997). Chapter 38C: Vascular Surgery. In J. Nagelhout & K. Zaglaniczny (Eds.), *Nurse Anesthesia.* Philadelphia: W.B. Saunders.

58. ANSWER: **D**

Rationale: A slightly elevated heart rate helps to decrease ventricular volume and, thus, reduces regurgitation.

Reference: McIntosh, L.S. (1997). Chapter 38C: Vascular Surgery. In J. Nagelhout & K. Zaglaniczny (Eds.), *Nurse Anesthesia.* Philadelphia: W.B. Saunders.

59. ANSWER: **B**

Rationale: Incomplete right bundle branch block is seen in 5% of the patients. Left bundle branch block is uncommon and may indicate additional ventricular disease. Atrial arrhythmias develop over time, and P mitrale may be seen in click murmur syndrome.

Reference: McIntosh, L.S. (1997). Chapter 38C: Vascular Surgery. In J. Nagelhout & K. Zaglaniczny (Eds.), *Nurse Anesthesia.* Philadelphia: W.B. Saunders.

60. ANSWER: **D**

Rationale: Mitral insufficiency produces a pansystolic murmur. Mitral stenosis produces a presystolic murmur. Aortic insufficiency produces immediate diastolic murmur. Aortic stenosis produces a systolic ejection murmur, and floppy valve syndrome produces a late systolic murmur.

Reference: McIntosh, L.S. (1997). Chapter 38C: Vascular Surgery. In J. Nagelhout & K. Zaglaniczny (Eds.), *Nurse Anesthesia.* Philadelphia: W.B. Saunders.

61. ANSWER: **B**

Rationale: New York Heart Association classification states Class I—no limitation of activity; class II—slight limitation of activity; class III is marked limitation of activity and class IV is unable to carry out any physical activity without discomfort.

Reference: Aprile, A.E., Serwin, J.P., & Boctor, B. (1997). Chapter 38A: Cardiac Pathophysiology. In J. Nagelhout & K. Zaglaniczny (Eds.), *Nurse Anesthesia.* Philadelphia: W.B. Saunders.

62. ANSWER: **A**

Rationale: Click murmur syndrome is associated with disease of the mitral valve. It is a common finding in patients with P mitrale.

Reference: Aprile, A.E. & Aprile, F.D. (1997). Chapter 38B: Cardiac Anesthesia. In J.

Nagelhout & K. Zaglaniczny (Eds.), *Nurse Anesthesia*. Philadelphia: W.B. Saunders.

63. ANSWER: C

Rationale: A muscle relaxant that maintains or increases heart rate is preferred. Pancuronium produces slight tachycardia due to a vagolytic and sympathomimetic action.

Reference: McIntosh, L.S. (1997). Chapter 38C: Vascular Surgery. In J. Nagelhout & K. Zaglaniczny (Eds.), *Nurse Anesthesia*. Philadelphia: W.B. Saunders.

64. ANSWER: B

Rationale: Five letter pacemaker code is as follows: first letter is chamber paced; second letter is chamber sensed; third letter is mode of response; fourth letter is programmable functions; and fifth letter is for special tachyarrhythmia function.

Reference: Aprile, A.E. & Aprile, F.D. (1997). Chapter 38B: Cardiac Anesthesia. In J. Nagelhout & K. Zaglaniczny (Eds.), *Nurse Anesthesia*. Philadelphia: W.B. Saunders.

65. ANSWER: D

Rationale: Beta stimulation causes release of epinephrine, which shifts potassium intracellularly, promoting hypokalemia. Therefore, beta receptor blockers would minimize this effect.

Reference: Litwack, K. & Keithley, J.K. (1997). Chapter 31: Fluids, Electrolytes, and Therapy. In J. Nagelhout & K. Zaglaniczny (Eds.), *Nurse Anesthesia*. Philadelphia: W.B. Saunders.

66. ANSWER: A

Rationale: Diuretics cause blockade of potassium reabsorption and therefore commonly produce hypokalemia.

Reference: Litwack, K. & Keithley, J.K. (1997). Chapter 31: Fluids, Electrolytes, and Therapy. In J. Nagelhout & K. Zaglaniczny (Eds.), *Nurse Anesthesia*. Philadelphia: W.B. Saunders.

67. ANSWER: C

Rationale: Nitrates are primarily the venous dilators; therefore, reducing preload and cardiac demand is the mechanism by which they relieve angina. They may

or may not produce beneficial coronary dilation.

Reference: Alisoglu, R. (1997). Chapter 23: Cardiac Pharmacology. In J. Nagelhout & K. Zaglaniczny (Eds.), *Nurse Anesthesia*. Philadelphia: W.B. Saunders.

68. ANSWER: A

Rationale: Changes in microsomal enzymes may occur at any age and are probably not the reason for dose requirement changes in the elderly with acutely administered drugs. It would be more likely that changes in these enzymes would affect chronically administered medications.

Reference: Martin-Sheridan, D. (1997). Chapter 42: Geriatrics and Anesthesia Practice. In J. Nagelhout & K. Zaglaniczny (Eds.), *Nurse Anesthesia*. Philadelphia: W.B. Saunders.

69. ANSWER: C

Rationale: Serum protein levels decrease with age. In persons older than age 50 albumin levels fall from approximately 4.0 to 3.5 g/dL.

Reference: Martin-Sheridan, D. (1997). Chapter 42: Geriatrics and Anesthesia Practice. In J. Nagelhout & K. Zaglaniczny (Eds.), *Nurse Anesthesia*. Philadelphia: W.B. Saunders.

70. ANSWER: D

Rationale: Tourniquets frequently contain latex and therefore should not be used in patients with a latex allergy. If necessary, they can be placed over clothing material so there is no direct contact with the patient.

Reference: Sommer, B. (1997). Chapter 50: The Immune System and Anesthesiology. In J. Nagelhout & K. Zaglaniczny (Eds.), *Nurse Anesthesia*. Philadelphia: W.B. Saunders.

71. ANSWER: B

Rationale: Unexplained tachycardia, increase in tidal CO_2, and masseter muscle spasms are early warning signs of malignant hyperthermia. The high temperature that is the hallmark of the disease may be a late developing sign.

Reference: Karlet, M.C. (1997). Chapter 40: Musculoskeletal Pathophysiology and Anesthesia.

In J. Nagelhout & K. Zaglaniczny (Eds.), *Nurse Anesthesia*. Philadelphia: W.B. Saunders.

72. Answer: **A**

Rationale: Oxygen therapy in neonates with immature retinas can lead to detachment, fibrosis, and disorganized vascular proliferation. Neonates younger than 36 weeks' gestation are at greatest risk, and in those up to 44 weeks' gestation some risk is present. Arterial oxygen concentrations are better correlates than alveolar oxygen concentrations. Arterial oxygen tensions less than 140 mm Hg are considered safe.
Reference: Dobbins, P. & Hall, S.M. (1997). Chapter 14: Pediatric Anesthesia. In J. Nagelhout & K. Zaglaniczny (Eds.), *Nurse Anesthesia*. Philadelphia: W.B. Saunders.

73. Answer: **C**

Rationale: The inhalation anesthetics except for nitrous oxide do not increase the incidence of postoperative nausea and vomiting.
Reference: Marley, R. (1997). Outpatient Anesthesia. In J. Nagelhout & K. Zaglaniczny (Eds.), *Nurse Anesthesia*. Philadelphia: W.B. Saunders.

74. Answer: **B**

Rationale: Sepsis is an absolute contraindication to spinal anesthesia. Introducing infection into the cerebrospinal fluid by injecting a spinal anesthetic during sepsis must be avoided. The others, although representing some difficulty, are not absolute contraindications.
Reference: Ellis, W.E. (1997). Chapter 53: Regional Anesthesia. In J. Nagelhout & K. Zaglaniczny (Eds.), *Nurse Anesthesia*. Philadelphia: W.B. Saunders.

75. Answer: **A**

Rationale: The spinal needle punctures the dura and arachnoid layers into the subarachnoid space. Therefore, the local anesthetics are injected between the arachnoid and pia meningeal layers.
Reference: Ellis, W.E. (1997). Chapter 53: Regional Anesthesia. In J. Nagelhout & K. Zaglaniczny (Eds.), *Nurse Anesthesia*. Philadelphia: W.B. Saunders.

76. Answer: **C**

Rationale: The spinal needle punctures the supraspinous ligament first, followed by the interspinous ligamentum flavum and then the meningeal layers.
Reference: Ellis, W.E. (1997). Chapter 53: Regional Anesthesia. In J. Nagelhout & K. Zaglaniczny (Eds.), *Nurse Anesthesia*. Philadelphia: W.B. Saunders.

77. Answer: **C**

Rationale: The solution of tetracaine mixed in water will have a specific gravity slightly less than that of cerebrospinal fluid and when injected will move away from the dependent area.
Reference: Ellis, W.E. (1997). Chapter 53: Regional Anesthesia. In J. Nagelhout & K. Zaglaniczny (Eds.), *Nurse Anesthesia*. Philadelphia: W.B. Saunders.

78. Answer: **A**

Rationale: Dextrose is a useful substance for producing increased baricity. It is easy to sterilize, benign, and does not influence the local anesthetic.
Reference: Ellis, W.E. (1997). Chapter 53: Regional Anesthesia. In J. Nagelhout & K. Zaglaniczny (Eds.), *Nurse Anesthesia*. Philadelphia: W.B. Saunders.

79. Answer: **D**

Rationale: The spinal and epidural spaces become smaller and less compliant with advancing age, extending the distribution of the injected local anesthetic. A reduced dose in elderly patients is indicated.
Reference: Ellis, W.E. (1997). Chapter 53: Regional Anesthesia. In J. Nagelhout & K. Zaglaniczny (Eds.), *Nurse Anesthesia*. Philadelphia: W.B. Saunders.

80. Answer: **B**

Rationale: The spinal canal extends from the foramen magnum to the sacral hiatus.
Reference: Ellis, W.E. (1997). Chapter 53: Regional Anesthesia. In J. Nagelhout & K. Zaglaniczny (Eds.), *Nurse Anesthesia*. Philadelphia: W.B. Saunders.

81. ANSWER: **D**

Rationale: The spinal cord extends from the foramen magnum to L2.

Reference: Ellis, W.E. (1997). Chapter 53: Regional Anesthesia. In J. Nagelhout & K. Zaglaniczny (Eds.), *Nurse Anesthesia.* Philadelphia: W.B. Saunders.

82. ANSWER: **A**

Rationale: The epidural space is a potential space filled with connective and adipose tissue. Venous plexuses are prominent, but no free fluid exists in the space.

Reference: Ellis, W.E. (1997). Chapter 53: Regional Anesthesia. In J. Nagelhout & K. Zaglaniczny (Eds.), *Nurse Anesthesia.* Philadelphia: W.B. Saunders.

83. ANSWER: **B**

Rationale: A line drawn between the iliac crest usually crosses the fourth lumbar vertebra. The interspace above the line is L3–4, and the interspace below the line is L4–5.

Reference: Ellis, W.E. (1997). Chapter 53: Regional Anesthesia. In J. Nagelhout & K. Zaglaniczny (Eds.), *Nurse Anesthesia.* Philadelphia: W.B. Saunders.

84. ANSWER: **C**

Rationale: Conservative treatment is usually indicated within the first 24 hours. However, if treatment is unsuccessful, then an epidural blood patch relieves the headache in over 80% of the cases if performed after 24 hours.

Reference: Ellis, W.E. (1997). Chapter 53: Regional Anesthesia. In J. Nagelhout & K. Zaglaniczny (Eds.), *Nurse Anesthesia.* Philadelphia: W.B. Saunders.

85. ANSWER: **A**

Rationale: Stimuli generated from thermal, mechanical, or chemical damage activates nociceptors that are free afferent nerve endings of myelinated A delta and unmyelinated C fibers.

Reference: Ellis, W.E. (1997). Chapter 53: Regional Anesthesia. In J. Nagelhout & K. Zaglaniczny (Eds.), *Nurse Anesthesia.* Philadelphia: W.B. Saunders.

86. ANSWER: **B**

Rationale: Anesthesia requires sensory blockade of the cervical nerves C2 to C4, which is provided by blockade of the deep cervical plexus.

Reference: McIntosh, L.S. (1997). Chapter 38C: Vascular Surgery. In J. Nagelhout & K. Zaglaniczny (Eds.), *Nurse Anesthesia.* Philadelphia: W.B. Saunders.

87. ANSWER: **D**

Rationale: A differential block results in sympathetic blockade one to two segments above the sensory block and motor blockade one to two segments below the sensory block.

Reference: Ellis, W.E. (1997). Chapter 53: Regional Anesthesia. In J. Nagelhout & K. Zaglaniczny (Eds.), *Nurse Anesthesia.* Philadelphia: W.B. Saunders.

88. ANSWER: **B**

Rationale: The Trendelenburg position in an attempt to halt further rise of the block may do more harm than good. The level will not recede in the reverse Trendelenburg position, and cardiac output will only decrease further.

Reference: Ellis, W.E. (1997). Chapter 53: Regional Anesthesia. In J. Nagelhout & K. Zaglaniczny (Eds.), *Nurse Anesthesia.* Philadelphia: W.B. Saunders.

89. ANSWER: **D**

Rationale: Nausea and vomiting are common because of unopposed vagal tone or hypotension that decreases cerebral blood flow.

Reference: Ellis, W.E. (1997). Chapter 53: Regional Anesthesia. In J. Nagelhout & K. Zaglaniczny (Eds.), *Nurse Anesthesia.* Philadelphia: W.B. Saunders.

90. ANSWER: **A**

Rationale: Bradycardia is usually multifactorial and may include vagal tone from high sympathetic blockade of the cardioaccelerator fibers, T1 to T4, and the Bezold-Jarisch reflex, which is a slowing of the heart rate due to a drop in venous return.

Reference: Ellis, W.E. (1997). Chapter 53: Regional Anesthesia. In J. Nagelhout & K. Zaglaniczny

(Eds.), *Nurse Anesthesia*. Philadelphia: W.B. Saunders.

91. ANSWER: C

Rationale: Vasoconstrictors are never used in blocks of the fingers, toes, penis, tip of the nose, or ears because intense vasoconstriction may cause ischemia and necrosis.

Reference: Ellis, W.E. (1997). Chapter 53: Regional Anesthesia. In J. Nagelhout & K. Zaglaniczny (Eds.), *Nurse Anesthesia*. Philadelphia: W.B. Saunders.

92. ANSWER: D

Rationale: Synthesis begins with phenylalanine or tyrosine and converts to dopa, dopamine, norepinephrine, and finally epinephrine.

Reference: Morgan, R.O., Jr. (1997). Chapter 8: The Cardiovascular System. In J. Nagelhout & K. Zaglaniczny (Eds.), *Nurse Anesthesia*. Philadelphia: W.B. Saunders.

93. ANSWER: D

Rationale: Metoclopramide (Reglan) produces its antiemetic effect by blocking dopamine receptors similar to droperidol and produces its gastrokinetic action through cholinergic receptors.

Reference: Sherbinski, L. & Nagelhout, J.J. (1997). Chapter 24: Additional Drugs of Interest. In J. Nagelhout & K. Zaglaniczny (Eds.), *Nurse Anesthesia*. Philadelphia: W.B. Saunders.

94. ANSWER: A

Rationale: Because of the lack of perfusion below the clamp, metabolism switches to anaerobic pathways, resulting from a lack of oxygen availability.

Reference: McIntosh, L.S. (1997). Chapter 38C: Vascular Surgery. In J. Nagelhout & K. Zaglaniczny (Eds.), *Nurse Anesthesia*. Philadelphia: W.B. Saunders.

95. ANSWER: C

Rationale: As a result of the reduction of renal blood flow, glomerular filtration rate is greatly reduced in cases where infrarenal cross-clamping occurs.

Reference: McIntosh, L.S. (1997). Chapter 38C: Vascular Surgery. In J. Nagelhout & K.

Zaglaniczny (Eds.), *Nurse Anesthesia*. Philadelphia: W.B. Saunders.

96. ANSWER: B

Rationale: Pulsus paradoxus refers to a greater than 10 mm Hg decline in blood pressure during spontaneous ventilation. It is an early sign of cardiac failure.

Reference: Morgan, R.O., Jr. (1997). Chapter 8: The Cardiovascular System. In J. Nagelhout & K. Zaglaniczny (Eds.), *Nurse Anesthesia*. Philadelphia: W.B. Saunders.

97. ANSWER: D

Rationale: Small emboli in the ophthalmic branches cause transient monocular blindness known as amaurosis fugax. They may occur during carotid artery surgery.

Reference: Harvey, R.R. (1997). Chapter 48: Anesthesia for Ophthalmic Procedures. In J. Nagelhout & K. Zaglaniczny (Eds.), *Nurse Anesthesia*. Philadelphia: W.B. Saunders.

98. ANSWER: A

Rationale: Vasoconstriction is assumed to occur in adjacent normal arterioles, thereby causing a local increase in perfusion pressure and augmenting collateral flow to the abnormal area.

Reference: Harrigan, C. (1997). Chapter 6: The Central Nervous System. In J. Nagelhout & K. Zaglaniczny (Eds.), *Nurse Anesthesia*. Philadelphia: W.B. Saunders.

99. ANSWER: A

Rationale: Although all of the conditions are possible, hypertension is very common in patients with severe carotid artery disease, likely due to decreased baroreceptor sensitivity.

Reference: McIntosh, L.S. (1997). Chapter 38C: Vascular Surgery. In J. Nagelhout & K. Zaglaniczny (Eds.), *Nurse Anesthesia*. Philadelphia: W.B. Saunders.

100. ANSWER: A

Rationale: All general anesthetics affect cerebral blood flow to some extent. The potent inhalation agents tend to be cerebral vasodilators, which increase cerebral blood flow and may increase intracranial pressure in a patient with cerebral neuro-pathology.

Reference: Harrigan, C. (1997). Chapter 6: The Central Nervous System. In J. Nagelhout & K. Zaglaniczny (Eds.), *Nurse Anesthesia.* Philadelphia: W.B. Saunders.

101. ANSWER: **A**

Rationale: Horner's syndrome is a clinical entity characterized by ptosis, miosis, and anhidrosis. It is usually associated with diseases involving the cervical sympathetics.

Reference: Ellis, W.E. (1997). Chapter 53: Regional Anesthesia. In J. Nagelhout & K. Zaglaniczny (Eds.), *Nurse Anesthesia.* Philadelphia: W.B. Saunders.

102. ANSWER: **A**

Rationale: Maintaining a patent airway is the first and most important treatment for local anesthetic toxic reactions. Maintaining oxygenation will ensure the event will have a favorable outcome with no permanent sequelae.

Reference: Williams, J.R. (1997). Chapter 20: Local Anesthetics. In J. Nagelhout & K. Zaglaniczny (Eds.), *Nurse Anesthesia.* Philadelphia: W.B. Saunders.

103. ANSWER: **A**

Rationale: Patients on monoamine oxidase inhibitors have an altered concentration of catecholamine; therefore, a direct receptor active agonist will not involve abnormal adrenergic neurons.

Reference: Alisoglu, R. (1997). Chapter 23: Cardiac Pharmacology. In J. Nagelhout & K. Zaglaniczny (Eds.), *Nurse Anesthesia.* Philadelphia: W.B. Saunders.

104. ANSWER: **A**

Rationale: Meperidine is unique among opiates in its interaction with monoamine oxidase inhibitors. Co-administration may result in serious drug reactions, including central nervous system excitement and seizures.

Reference: Alisoglu, R. (1997). Chapter 23: Cardiac Pharmacology. In J. Nagelhout & K. Zaglaniczny (Eds.), *Nurse Anesthesia.* Philadelphia: W.B. Saunders.

105. ANSWER: **A**

Rationale: Direct-acting adrenergic agonists should be used in patients receiving monoamine oxidase inhibitors. All are indirect acting except phenylephrine.

Reference: Alisoglu, R. (1997). Chapter 23: Cardiac Pharmacology. In J. Nagelhout & K. Zaglaniczny (Eds.), *Nurse Anesthesia.* Philadelphia: W.B. Saunders.

106. ANSWER: **A**

Rationale: Lidocaine toxicity is unlikely if doses are kept below 7 mg/kg regardless of the type of block.

Reference: Williams, J.R. (1997). Chapter 20: Local Anesthetics. In J. Nagelhout & K. Zaglaniczny (Eds.), *Nurse Anesthesia.* Philadelphia: W.B. Saunders.

107. ANSWER: **A**

Rationale: Safe doses of bupivacaine regardless of block to prevent cardiac and neural toxicity should be kept below 3 mg/kg.

Reference: Williams, J.R. (1997). Chapter 20: Local Anesthetics. In J. Nagelhout & K. Zaglaniczny (Eds.), *Nurse Anesthesia.* Philadelphia: W.B. Saunders.

108. ANSWER: **D**

Rationale: Disseminated intravascular coagulation is characterized by an uncontrolled activation of the coagulation system. Thrombocytopenia, prolongation of the prothrombin time and partial thromboplastin time, and increased concentration of fibrin degradation products along with diffuse hemorrhage suggest a diagnosis. Administration of platelet concentrates and fresh frozen plasma may be indicated.

Reference: Gerbasi, F.R. (1997). Chapter 41: Hematology and Anesthesia. In J. Nagelhout & K. Zaglaniczny (Eds.), *Nurse Anesthesia.* Philadelphia: W.B. Saunders.

109. ANSWER: **A**

Rationale: The transducer is placed over the right sternal border between the third and sixth intercostal space. Proper positioning of the transducer allows for detection of air in amounts as small as 0.25 mL.

Reference: DeVane, G.G. (1997). Chapter 37: Neurosurgical Anesthesia. In J. Nagelhout & K. Zaglaniczny (Eds.), *Nurse Anesthesia.* Philadelphia: W.B. Saunders.

110. ANSWER: **D**

Rationale: Small volumes of intravascular air produce a ventilation/perfusion mismatch that is reflected in reduced end-tidal carbon dioxide.
Reference: DeVane, G.G. (1997). Chapter 37: Neurosurgical Anesthesia. In J. Nagelhout & K. Zaglaniczny (Eds.), *Nurse Anesthesia.* Philadelphia: W.B. Saunders.

111. ANSWER: **C**

Rationale: Ritodrine is a beta$_2$ stimulant that produces a tocolytic action on the uterus. The pregnant uterus responds to beta$_2$ stimulation by relaxing. Tocolytic drugs are used to delay premature labor.
Reference: Fiedler, M.A. & Shaw, B. (1997). Chapter 13: Obstetric Anesthesia. In J. Nagelhout & K. Zaglaniczny (Eds.), *Nurse Anesthesia.* Philadelphia: W.B. Saunders.

112. ANSWER: **B**

Rationale: Hyperkalemia is commonly seen after cardioplegia. It is generally allowed to spontaneously correct by redistribution and diuresis; however, if it is trending to less than 4.0 mEq/L at the end of bypass, it should be supplemented.
Reference: Aprile, A.E. & Aprile, F.D. (1997). Chapter 38B: Cardiac Anesthesia. In J. Nagelhout & K. Zaglaniczny (Eds.), *Nurse Anesthesia.* Philadelphia: W.B. Saunders.

113. ANSWER: **B**

Rationale: The presence of a right-to-left shunt slows the equilibrium between alveolar and arterial partial pressures, prolonging inhalation induction.
Reference: Dobbins, P. & Hall, S.M. (1997). Pediatric Anesthesia. In J. Nagelhout & K. Zaglaniczny (Eds.), *Nurse Anesthesia.* Philadelphia: W.B. Saunders.

114. ANSWER: **A**

Rationale: Puncture of the thoracic duct, known as a chylothorax, can occur after

subclavian as well as left internal jugular venous catheter insertion.
Reference: Sinkovich, J.A. & Kossick, M.A. (1997). Chapter 27: Clinical Monitoring in Anesthesia. In J. Nagelhout & K. Zaglaniczny (Eds.), *Nurse Anesthesia.* Philadelphia: W.B. Saunders.

115. ANSWER: **A**

Rationale: Acetylation of the listed drugs occurs at two different rates: fast and slow. Those populations with slow acetylating activity run a greater risk of complications, including drug-induced lupus.
Reference: Alisoglu, R. (1997). Chapter 23: Cardiac Pharmacology. In J. Nagelhout & K. Zaglaniczny (Eds.), *Nurse Anesthesia.* Philadelphia: W.B. Saunders.

116. ANSWER: **B**

Rationale: Four conditions that will change turbulent flow are high gas flows, sharp angles within the tube, branching in the tube, and a change in tube diameter.
Reference: Hall, S.M. (1997). Chapter 4: Chemistry and Physics for Anesthesia. In J. Nagelhout & K. Zaglaniczny (Eds.), *Nurse Anesthesia.* Philadelphia: W.B. Saunders.

117. ANSWER: **C**

Rationale: With complex shunts such as tetralogy the magnitude of the shunt flow increases if pulmonary resistance goes up or systemic resistance falls.
Reference: McIntosh, L.S. (1997). Chapter 38C: Vascular Surgery. In J. Nagelhout & K. Zaglaniczny (Eds.), *Nurse Anesthesia.* Philadelphia: W.B. Saunders.

118. ANSWER: **B**

Rationale: Approximately 85% of patients with a tracheoesophageal fistula have a communication from the distal trachea to the esophagus and a blind proximal esophageal pouch.
Reference: Dobbins, P. & Hall, S.M. (1997). Chapter 14: Pediatric Anesthesia. In J. Nagelhout & K. Zaglaniczny (Eds.), *Nurse Anesthesia.* Philadelphia: W.B. Saunders.

119. ANSWER: **C**

Rationale: Myocardial ischemia is usually not present, owing to local control of coronary artery flow. Autonomics play a minor role in myocardial perfusion.

Reference: Harrigan, C. (1997). Chapter 6: The Central Nervous System. In J. Nagelhout & K. Zaglaniczny (Eds.), *Nurse Anesthesia.* Philadelphia: W.B. Saunders.

120. ANSWER: **B**

Rationale: Regurgitation through the mitral valve reduces left ventricular afterload, which often initially enhances contractility, therefore, stroke volume. Only in the latest stages of this disease does cardiac output begin to fall.

Reference: Aprile, A.E. & Aprile, F.D. (1997). Chapter 38B: Cardiac Anesthesia. In J. Nagelhout & K. Zaglaniczny (Eds.), *Nurse Anesthesia.* Philadelphia: W.B. Saunders.

121. ANSWER: **A**

Rationale: These patients have fixed stroke volume and therefore are very rate dependent. Efforts to keep the heart rate between 60 and 90 beats per minute are optimal in most patients.

Reference: McIntosh, L.S. (1997). Chapter 38C: Vascular Surgery. In J. Nagelhout & K. Zaglaniczny (Eds.), *Nurse Anesthesia.* Philadelphia: W.B. Saunders.

122. ANSWER: **B**

Rationale: The normal P_{50} is 26.6 mm Hg. A decreased 2,3-diphosphoglycerate level would cause a leftward shift, thus increasing the P_{50} to 29 mm Hg.

Reference: Morgan, R.O., Jr. (1997). Chapter 8: The Cardiovascular System. In J. Nagelhout & K. Zaglaniczny (Eds.), *Nurse Anesthesia.* Philadelphia: W.B. Saunders.

123. ANSWER: **C**

Rationale: During the first stage of labor, pain arises from the T10 to L1 dermatomes. In the second stage of labor with stretching of the pelvis and peritoneum, sensory innervation by the pudendal nerve involves S2 to S4.

Reference: Fielder, M.A. & Shaw, B. (1997). Chapter 13: Obstetric Anesthesia. In J. Nagelhout & K. Zaglaniczny (Eds.), *Nurse Anesthesia.* Philadelphia: W.B. Saunders.

124. ANSWER: **B**

Rationale: The blood volume is distributed in approximately the following percentages: heart, 7%; lungs, 9%; and systemic circulation: arterial, 15%; capillary, 5%; and venous, 64%.

Reference: Hall, S.M. (1997). Chapter 9: Respiratory Anatomy and Physiology. In J. Nagelhout & K. Zaglaniczny (Eds.), *Nurse Anesthesia.* Philadelphia: W.B. Saunders.

125. ANSWER: **D**

Rationale: A leftward shift of the curve increases the affinity of hemoglobin for oxygen, thus reducing availability to the tissues. Carbon monoxide, cyanide, nitric acid, and ammonia shift the saturation curve to the left. Carbon monoxide is especially potent, having 200 to 300 times the affinity of oxygen for hemoglobin and forming carboxyhemoglobin.

Reference: Hall, S.M. (1997). Chapter 9: Respiratory Anatomy and Physiology. In J. Nagelhout & K. Zaglaniczny (Eds.), *Nurse Anesthesia.* Philadelphia: W.B. Saunders.

126. ANSWER: **C**

Rationale: Arterial oxygen tension decreases with age, leaving a wide range of oxygen tension in elderly patients with emphysema. Oxygen tension falls an average of 0.35 mm Hg per year.

Reference: Martin-Sheridan, D. (1997). Chapter 42: Geriatrics and Anesthesia Practice. In J. Nagelhout & K. Zaglaniczny (Eds.), *Nurse Anesthesia.* Philadelphia: W.B. Saunders.

127. ANSWER: **A**

Rationale: An increase in CO_2, acidosis, increased 2,3-diphosphoglycerate, and anemia will all shift the curve to the right, promoting oxygen release. Alkalosis will shift the curve to the left.

Reference: Morgan, R.O., Jr. (1997). Chapter 8: The Cardiovascular System. In J. Nagelhout & K. Zaglaniczny (Eds.), *Nurse Anesthesia.* Philadelphia: W.B. Saunders.

128. ANSWER: **D**

Rationale: Alveolar ventilation is divided by pulmonary-capillary perfusion to derive the ventilation/perfusion ratio.

When it increases, there is either an increased alveolar oxygen or a decreased capillary perfusion.

Reference: Rojo, J. & Iacopelli, M. (1997). Chapter 39A: Respiratory Pathophysiology. In J. Nagelhout & K. Zaglaniczny (Eds.), *Nurse Anesthesia*. Philadelphia: W.B. Saunders.

129. ANSWER: **A**

Rationale: Pulmonary edema results from transudation of fluid, first from pulmonary capillaries to interstitial spaces and then into the alveoli. This occurs because of high capillary hydrostatic pressure.

Reference: Litwack, K. & Keithley J.K. (1997). Chapter 31: Fluids, Electrolytes, and Therapy. In J. Nagelhout & K. Zaglaniczny (Eds.), *Nurse Anesthesia*. Philadelphia: W.B. Saunders.

130. ANSWER: **D**

Rationale: The stomach should be emptied with the large nasogastric or orogastric tube owing to gastric dilation and increased risk of aspiration during induction.

Reference: Dobbins, P. & Hall, S.M. (1997). Chapter 14: Pediatric Anesthesia. In J. Nagelhout & K. Zaglaniczny (Eds.), *Nurse Anesthesia*. Philadelphia: W.B. Saunders.

131. ANSWER: **B**

Rationale: Inhalation anesthesia allows rapid changes in anesthetic level in response to surgical requirements. The anesthetic level can be made deeper during hypertension but decreased during lower blood pressure scenarios.

Reference: Karlet, M.C. & Sebastian, L.A. (1997). Chapter 12: The Endocrine System. In J. Nagelhout & K. Zaglaniczny (Eds.), *Nurse Anesthesia*. Philadelphia: W.B. Saunders.

132. ANSWER: **C**

Rationale: These patients frequently are obese, and airway management can be a problem. Awake intubation is indicated when appropriate.

Reference: Karlet, M.C. & Sebastian, L.A. (1997). Chapter 12: The Endocrine System. In J. Nagelhout & K. Zaglaniczny (Eds.), *Nurse Anesthesia*. Philadelphia: W.B. Saunders.

133. ANSWER: **B**

Rationale: Hyperadrenocorticism, otherwise known as Cushing's disease, is caused by overproduction of ACTH with an excess adrenocorticosteroid. The patient usually exhibits hyperglycemia, owing to the stimulatory effect on glucose caused by the ACTH excess.

Reference: Karlet, M.C. & Sebastian, L.A. (1997). Chapter 12: The Endocrine System. In J. Nagelhout & K. Zaglaniczny (Eds.), *Nurse Anesthesia*. Philadelphia: W.B. Saunders.

134. ANSWER: **B**

Rationale: Toxemia, now known as pregnancy-induced hypertension, is associated with renal changes, including a loss of protein in the urine, resulting in decreased colloid osmotic pressure.

Reference: Fielder, M.A. & Shaw, B. (1997). Chapter 13: Obstetric Anesthesia. In J. Nagelhout & K. Zaglaniczny (Eds.), *Nurse Anesthesia*. Philadelphia: W.B. Saunders.

135. ANSWER: **B**

Rationale: Pudendal nerves arising from S2 to S4 carry the sensory input during the second stage of labor.

Reference: Fielder, M.A. & Shaw, B. (1997). Chapter 13: Obstetric Anesthesia. In J. Nagelhout & K. Zaglaniczny (Eds.), *Nurse Anesthesia*. Philadelphia: W.B. Saunders.

136. ANSWER: **B**

Rationale: Entry of amniotic fluid into the pulmonary circulation results in a sudden onset of profound hypotension, respiratory distress, and hypoxia.

Reference: Fielder, M.A. & Shaw, B. (1997). Chapter 13: Obstetric Anesthesia. In J. Nagelhout & K. Zaglaniczny (Eds.), *Nurse Anesthesia*. Philadelphia: W.B. Saunders.

137. ANSWER: **B**

Rationale: The brachial plexus supplying the major nerves to the arm arises from spinal levels C5 through T1.

Reference: Ellis, W.E. (1997). Chapter 53: Regional Anesthesia. In J. Nagelhout & K. Zaglaniczny (Eds.), *Nurse Anesthesia*. Philadelphia: W.B. Saunders.

138. ANSWER: **C**

Rationale: A blood sugar level of 500 mg/dL requires immediate attention. Regular insulin is the only formulation that should be given intravenously; therefore, it is the agent of choice for acute intervention.

Reference: Karlet, M.C. & Sebastian, L.A. (1997). Chapter 12: The Endocrine System. In J. Nagelhout & K. Zaglaniczny (Eds.), *Nurse Anesthesia*. Philadelphia: W.B. Saunders.

139. ANSWER: **C**

Rationale: Several potential complications are problematic, with vasospasm and rebleeding the most prominent. Rebleeding occurs in about 19% of the patients within 2 weeks of initial etiology. Vasospasms can occur in up to 70% of the patients.

Reference: DeVane, G.G. (1997). Chapter 37: Neurosurgical Anesthesia. In J. Nagelhout & K. Zaglaniczny (Eds.), *Nurse Anesthesia*. Philadelphia: W.B. Saunders.

140. ANSWER: **A**

Rationale: Cardiac arrhythmias occur at the usual rate regardless of whether the patient is in the sitting position. Hypotension, air embolism, and ischemia are much more problematic.

Reference: DeVane, G.G. (1997). Chapter 37: Neurosurgical Anesthesia. In J. Nagelhout & K. Zaglaniczny (Eds.), *Nurse Anesthesia*. Philadelphia: W.B. Saunders.

141. ANSWER: **A**

Rationale: Precordial Doppler is extremely sensitive for detecting air embolism. Incidence of embolism is 25% to 35% in the sitting position. Doppler evaluation can detect air in quantities as small as 0.25 mL.

Reference: DeVane, G.G. (1997). Chapter 37: Neurosurgical Anesthesia. In J. Nagelhout & K. Zaglaniczny (Eds.), *Nurse Anesthesia*. Philadelphia: W.B. Saunders.

142. ANSWER: **B**

Rationale: Elevating the head of the bed may allow air to enter the upper thorax and head, producing serious morbidity and mortality.

Reference: DeVane, G.G. (1997). Chapter 37: Neurosurgical Anesthesia. In J. Nagelhout & K. Zaglaniczny (Eds.), *Nurse Anesthesia*. Philadelphia: W.B. Saunders.

143. ANSWER: **D**

Rationale: Positive end-expiratory pressure or continuous positive airway pressure to the dependent lung helps increase oxygenation and prevent hypoxia by increasing Po_2.

Reference: Cafarelli, J.M. (1997). Chapter 39B: Thoracic Surgery. In J. Nagelhout & K. Zaglaniczny (Eds.), *Nurse Anesthesia*. Philadelphia: W.B. Saunders.

144. ANSWER: **D**

Rationale: It is not necessary to convert to a single-lumen tube because a double-lumen tube will ventilate both lungs if properly positioned.

Reference: Cafarelli, J.M. (1997). Chapter 39B: Thoracic Surgery. In J. Nagelhout & K. Zaglaniczny (Eds.), *Nurse Anesthesia*. Philadelphia: W.B. Saunders.

145. ANSWER: **D**

Rationale: Due to the coexistence of hypertension and tachycardia, labetolol will be the agent of choice because it will decrease both blood pressure and heart rate.

Reference: Alisoglu, R. (1997). Chapter 23: Cardiac Pharmacology. In J. Nagelhout & K. Zaglaniczny (Eds.), *Nurse Anesthesia*. Philadelphia: W.B. Saunders.

146. ANSWER: **C**

Rationale: Increasing fluids compensates for the rapid change in cardiac venous return after removal of the clamp. Adequate volume allows cardiac parameters to normalize.

Reference: McIntosh, L.S. (1997). Chapter 38C: Vascular Surgery. In J. Nagelhout & K. Zaglaniczny (Eds.), *Nurse Anesthesia*. Philadelphia: W.B. Saunders.

147. ANSWER: **B**

Rationale: Hypertension increases the load on the heart and would indicate possible problems with left ventricular function.

Reference: Aprile, A.E. & Aprile, F.D. (1997). Chapter 38B: Cardiac Anesthesia. In J. Nagelhout & K. Zaglaniczny (Eds.), *Nurse Anesthesia.* Philadelphia: W.B. Saunders.

148. ANSWER: **A**

Rationale: Strabismus repair is the most common pediatric eye operation. These patients have been observed to be susceptible to malignant hyperthermia, which reflects as local weakness in their eye musculature.

Reference: Harvey, R.R. (1997). Chapter 48: Anesthesia for Ophthalmic Procedures. In J. Nagelhout & K. Zaglaniczny (Eds.), *Nurse Anesthesia.* Philadelphia: W.B. Saunders.

149. ANSWER: **B**

Rationale: Goggles that absorb radiation should be worn because the eye is the most sensitive to damage from lasers. Moistened eyepads offer additional protection from both laser damage and fire.

Reference: DeVane, G.G. (1997). Chapter 51: Anesthesia and Laser Surgery. In J. Nagelhout & K. Zaglaniczny (Eds.), *Nurse Anesthesia.* Philadelphia: W.B. Saunders.

150. ANSWER: **C**

Rationale: Airway fire is the most common complication in this procedure. Endotracheal tubes with metal particles are more fire resistant, especially in the area of the cuff.

Reference: DeVane, G.G. (1997). Chapter 51: Anesthesia and Laser Surgery. In J. Nagelhout & K. Zaglaniczny (Eds.), *Nurse Anesthesia.* Philadelphia: W.B. Saunders.

151. ANSWER: **D**

Rationale: A double cuff provides adequate protection in case the laser accidentally deflates one of the cuffs.

Reference: DeVane, G.G. (1997). Chapter 51: Anesthesia and Laser Surgery. In J. Nagelhout & K. Zaglaniczny (Eds.), *Nurse Anesthesia.* Philadelphia: W.B. Saunders.

152. ANSWER: **A**

Rationale: CO_2 lasers have a helium-neon laser built into them to serve as a means of directing the CO_2 laser, which is normally invisible to the human eye.

Reference: DeVane, G.G. (1997). Chapter 51: Anesthesia and Laser Surgery. In J. Nagelhout & K. Zaglaniczny (Eds.), *Nurse Anesthesia.* Philadelphia: W.B. Saunders.

153. ANSWER: **B**

Rationale: Cisatracurium, atracurium, and mivacurium are examples of benzylisoquinoline chemical compounds. The other relaxants are steroidal except for succinylcholine.

Reference: Haas, R.E. & Erway, R.L. (1997). Chapter 22: Neuromuscular Blocking Agents, Reversal Agents, and Their Monitoring. In J. Nagelhout & K. Zaglaniczny (Eds.), *Nurse Anesthesia.* Philadelphia: W.B. Saunders.

154. ANSWER: **B**

Rationale: Hypertrophy represents a compensatory mechanism usually caused by an increase in pressure from mitral stenosis, aortic stenosis, and hypertension. Hypertrophied cardiac muscles function at lower inotropic states than normal.

Reference: Aprile, A.E., Serwin, J.P., & Boctor, B. (1997). Chapter 38A: Cardiac Pathophysiology. In J. Nagelhout & K. Zaglaniczny (Eds.), *Nurse Anesthesia.* Philadelphia: W.B. Saunders.

155. ANSWER: **A**

Rationale: Volume overload produces eccentric hypertrophy and is usually caused by mitral and aortic regurgitation. Dilation leads to an increased cardiac output by the Frank-Starling relationship; however, decreased cardiac efficiency is present.

Reference: Aprile, A.E., Serwin, J.P., & Boctor, B. (1997). Chapter 38A: Cardiac Pathophysiology. In J. Nagelhout & K. Zaglaniczny (Eds.), *Nurse Anesthesia.* Philadelphia: W.B. Saunders.

156. ANSWER: **D**

Rationale: SIADH is common with malignant tumors, pulmonary diseases, and central nervous system disorders. Plasma ADH concentration is generally not elevated but is inadequately suppressed relative to the decreased osmolarity in the plasma.

Reference: Karlet, M.C. & Sebastian, L.A. (1997). Chapter 12: The Endocrine System. In J. Nagelhout & K. Zaglaniczny (Eds.), *Nurse Anesthesia.* Philadelphia: W.B. Saunders.

157. ANSWER: **D**

Rationale: Antithrombin III is a circulating serine protease that irreversibly binds and inactivates thrombin.
Reference: Gerbasi, F.R. (1997). Chapter 41: Hematology and Anesthesia. In J. Nagelhout & K. Zaglaniczny (Eds.), *Nurse Anesthesia.* Philadelphia: W.B. Saunders.

158. ANSWER: **D**

Rationale: Coronary perfusion pressure is determined by the difference between aortic pressure and ventricular pressure, with the left ventricle being perfused almost entirely during diastole.
Reference: Morgan, R.O., Jr. (1997). Chapter 8: The Cardiovascular System. In J. Nagelhout & K. Zaglaniczny (Eds.), *Nurse Anesthesia.* Philadelphia: W.B. Saunders.

159. ANSWER: **D**

Rationale: This syndrome is a rare complication of antipsychotic therapy. It is related to dopamine blockade in the brain. Muscle rigidity, hyperthermia and rhabdomyolysis, autonomic instability, and altered consciousness occur.
Reference: Sherbinski, L. & Nagelhout, J.J. (1997). Chapter 24: Additional Drugs of Interest. In J. Nagelhout & K. Zaglaniczny (Eds.), *Nurse Anesthesia.* Philadelphia: W.B. Saunders.

160. ANSWER: **A**

Rationale: The normal dose of dantrolene is 2.5 mg/kg repeated up to a total dose of 10 mg/kg.
Reference: Karlet, M.C. (1997). Chapter 40: Musculoskeletal Pathophysiology and Anesthesia. In J. Nagelhout & K. Zaglaniczny (Eds.), *Nurse Anesthesia.* Philadelphia: W.B. Saunders.

161. ANSWER: **B**

Rationale: All local anesthetics have been shown to be safe in a patient who is susceptible to malignant hyperthermia.
Reference: Karlet, M.C. (1997). Chapter 40: Musculoskeletal Pathophysiology and Anesthesia. In J. Nagelhout & K. Zaglaniczny (Eds.), *Nurse Anesthesia.* Philadelphia: W.B. Saunders.

162. ANSWER: **C**

Rationale: Nitroprusside, a direct vasodilator, dilates both veins and arteries, thus reducing preload and afterload.
Reference: Alisoglu, R. (1997). Chapter 23: Cardiac Pharmacology. In J. Nagelhout & K. Zaglaniczny (Eds.), *Nurse Anesthesia.* Philadelphia: W.B. Saunders.

163. ANSWER: **A**

Rationale: Tyrosine hydroxylase is the rate-limiting enzyme that controls the quantity of catecholamines synthesized.
Reference: Alisoglu, R. (1997). Chapter 23: Cardiac Pharmacology. In J. Nagelhout & K. Zaglaniczny (Eds.), *Nurse Anesthesia.* Philadelphia: W.B. Saunders.

164. ANSWER: **C**

Rationale: Protamine interacts with platelets, fibrinogen, and other plasma proteins and may cause anticoagulation on its own.
Reference: Gerbasi, F.R. (1997). Chapter 41: Hematology and Anesthesia. In J. Nagelhout & K. Zaglaniczny (Eds.), *Nurse Anesthesia.* Philadelphia: W.B. Saunders.

165. ANSWER: **B**

Rationale: The drug acts by decreasing sarcoplasmic reticulum release of calcium or inhibiting excitation-contraction coupling at the transverse tubule level.
Reference: Karlet, M.C. (1997). Chapter 40: Musculoskeletal Pathophysiology and Anesthesia. In J. Nagelhout & K. Zaglaniczny (Eds.), *Nurse Anesthesia.* Philadelphia: W.B. Saunders.

166. ANSWER: **C**

Rationale: Acetylcholine is synthesized from acetylcoa plus choline, catalyzed by the enzyme choline acetyltransferase.
Reference: Karlet, M.C. (1997). Chapter 7: The Musculoskeletal System. In J. Nagelhout & K. Zaglaniczny (Eds.), *Nurse Anesthesia.* Philadelphia: W.B. Saunders.

167. ANSWER: **B**

Rationale: The most common tracheoesophageal fistula includes a combination of an upper esophagus that ends in a blind pouch and a lower esophagus that connects to the posterior trachea.
Reference: Dobbins, P. & Hall, S.M. (1997). Chapter 14: Pediatric Anesthesia. In J.

Nagelhout & K. Zaglaniczny (Eds.), *Nurse Anesthesia*. Philadelphia: W.B. Saunders.

168. ANSWER: **A**

Rationale: Increased urinary bladder tone is produced by the parasympathetic nervous system.

Reference: Alisoglu, R. (1997). Chapter 23: Cardiac Pharmacology. In J. Nagelhout & K. Zaglaniczny (Eds.), *Nurse Anesthesia*. Philadelphia: W.B. Saunders.

169. ANSWER: **B**

Rationale: Hypoxia or a decreased oxygen saturation usually precedes signs such as tachycardia and cyanosis. Bronchospasm can also occur as a later sign of aspiration.

Reference: Chipas, A. (1997). Chapter 33: Airway Management. In J. Nagelhout & K. Zaglaniczny (Eds.), *Nurse Anesthesia*. Philadelphia: W.B. Saunders.

170. ANSWER: **C**

Rationale: Parasympathetic side effects would be expected that include bradycardia, increased gastrointestinal function, and miosis.

Reference: Haas, R.E. & Erway, R.L. (1997). Chapter 22: Neuromuscular Blocking Agents, Reversal Agents, and Their Monitoring. In J. Nagelhout & K. Zaglaniczny (Eds.), *Nurse Anesthesia*. Philadelphia: W.B. Saunders.

171. ANSWER: **C**

Rationale: Laudanosine, acrylates, an alcohol, and an acid are the end products of atracurium metabolism. Laudanosine is not produced in sufficient numbers to elicit central nervous system effects.

Reference: Haas, R.E. & Erway, R.L. (1997). Chapter 22: Neuromuscular Blocking Agents, Reversal Agents, and Their Monitoring. In J. Nagelhout & K. Zaglaniczny (Eds.), *Nurse Anesthesia*. Philadelphia: W.B. Saunders.

172. ANSWER: **C**

Rationale: Nondepolarizers and phase II succinylcholine block, which resembles nondepolarizing block, both produce post-tetanic facilitation.

Reference: Haas, R.E. & Erway, R.L. (1997). Chapter 22: Neuromuscular Blocking Agents,

Reversal Agents, and Their Monitoring. In J. Nagelhout & K. Zaglaniczny (Eds.), *Nurse Anesthesia*. Philadelphia: W.B. Saunders.

173. ANSWER: **C**

Rationale: Meperidine causes the least amount of smooth muscle spasm; therefore, it is the drug of choice for the treatment of colic.

Reference: Fransden, J.L. (1997). Chapter 56: Pain Management. In J. Nagelhout & K. Zaglaniczny (Eds.), *Nurse Anesthesia*. Philadelphia: W.B. Saunders.

174. ANSWER: **B**

Rationale: Pharmacokinetics includes absorption, distribution, biotransformation, and elimination of drugs.

Reference: Troop, M. (1997). Chapter 16: Pharmacokinetics. In J. Nagelhout & K. Zaglaniczny (Eds.), *Nurse Anesthesia*. Philadelphia: W.B. Saunders.

175. ANSWER: **B**

Rationale: Morphine and the naturally occurring opiates are members of the phenanthrene chemical group.

Reference: Chick, M. (1997). Chapter 21: Opioid Agonists and Antagonists. In J. Nagelhout & K. Zaglaniczny (Eds.), *Nurse Anesthesia*. Philadelphia: W.B. Saunders.

176. ANSWER: **A**

Rationale: Blockade of dopamine in the brain depresses the vomiting center and produces a potent antiemetic effect.

Reference: Chick, M. (1997). Chapter 21: Agents and Antagonists. In J. Nagelhout & K. Zaglaniczny (Eds.), *Nurse Anesthesia*. Philadelphia: W.B. Saunders.

177. ANSWER: **D**

Rationale: Induction agents such as propofol wear off, owing to rapid redistribution from the brain to peripheral nonnervous sites.

Reference: Fallacaro, N.A. & Fallacaro, M.D. (1997). Chapter 19: Intravenous Induction Agents. In J. Nagelhout & K. Zaglaniczny (Eds.), *Nurse Anesthesia*. Philadelphia: W.B. Saunders.

178. ANSWER: **B**

Rationale: The combination of low blood gas coefficient and high lipid solubility would yield a rapid and very potent inhalation anesthetic.

Reference: Nagelhout, J.J. (1997). Chapter 17: Uptake and Distribution of Inhalation Anesthetics. In J. Nagelhout & K. Zaglaniczny (Eds.), *Nurse Anesthesia*. Philadelphia: W.B. Saunders.

179. ANSWER: **B**

Rationale: The blood/gas solubility coefficient is the main determinant of an anesthetic's speed of onset and offset.

Reference: Nagelhout, J.J. (1997). Chapter 17: Uptake and Distribution of Inhalation Anesthetics. In J. Nagelhout & K. Zaglaniczny (Eds.), *Nurse Anesthesia*. Philadelphia: W.B. Saunders.

180. ANSWER: **A**

Rationale: ALA synthetase is the rate-limiting enzyme for the synthesis of heme. It may be induced by barbiturates, leading to an excess production of porphyrins.

Reference: Fallacaro, N.A. & Fallacaro, M.D. (1997). Chapter 19: Intravenous Induction Agents. In J. Nagelhout & K. Zaglaniczny (Eds.), *Nurse Anesthesia*. Philadelphia: W.B. Saunders.

181. ANSWER: **D**

Rationale: 11-β-hydroxylase is a key enzyme for the conversion of cholesterol to cortisol and is inhibited by etomidate, resulting in steroid depression.

Reference: Fallacaro, N.A. & Fallacaro, M.D. (1997). Chapter 19: Intravenous Induction Agents. In J. Nagelhout & K. Zaglaniczny (Eds.), *Nurse Anesthesia*. Philadelphia: W.B. Saunders.

182. ANSWER: **D**

Rationale: Compound A is produced in the soda lime canister of the anesthesia machine; therefore, enzyme levels would not play a role.

Reference: Kossick, M.A. (1997). Chapter 18: Inhalation Anesthetics. In J. Nagelhout & K. Zaglaniczny (Eds.), *Nurse Anesthesia*. Philadelphia: W.B. Saunders.

183. ANSWER: **D**

Rationale: Fluoride ion is produced as a hepatic metabolite of sevoflurane. Car-

bon dioxide granules would play no role in this phenomenon.

Reference: Kossick, M.A. (1997). Chapter 18: Inhalation Anesthetics. In J. Nagelhout & K. Zaglaniczny (Eds.), *Nurse Anesthesia*. Philadelphia: W.B. Saunders.

184. ANSWER: **C**

Rationale: Production of acetylcholine both centrally and peripherally would be the treatment of choice for atropine poisoning. Physostigmine is the only anticholinesterase that has both central and peripheral effects.

Reference: Haas, R.E. & Erway, R.L. (1997). Chapter 22: Neuromuscular Blocking Agents, Reversal Agents, and Their Monitoring. In J. Nagelhout & K. Zaglaniczny (Eds.), *Nurse Anesthesia*. Philadelphia: W.B. Saunders.

185. ANSWER: **A**

Rationale: Increases in cardiac output would cause more anesthetic to soak into the blood. The more soluble an agent, the greater this phenomenon.

Reference: Kossick, M.A. (1997). Chapter 18: Inhalation Anesthetics. In J. Nagelhout & K. Zaglaniczny (Eds.), *Nurse Anesthesia*. Philadelphia: W.B. Saunders.

186. ANSWER: **B**

Rationale: Deficits will affect insoluble agents because they have the most rapid onset. They will be the most affected by lung disease.

Reference: Nagelhout, J.J. (1997). Chapter 17: Uptake and Distribution of Inhalation Anesthetics. In J. Nagelhout & K. Zaglaniczny (Eds.), *Nurse Anesthesia*. Philadelphia: W.B. Saunders.

187. ANSWER: **D**

Rationale: Nimodipine is a selective cerebral dilator and thus useful for the treatment of cerebrovascular disease.

Reference: DeVane, G.G. (1997). Chapter 37: Neurosurgical Anesthesia. In J. Nagelhout & K. Zaglaniczny (Eds.), *Nurse Anesthesia*. Philadelphia: W.B. Saunders.

188. ANSWER: **D**

Rationale: Verapamil affects primarily the atrioventricular node and thus is the most useful for the treatment of atrial tachyarrythmia.

Reference: Alisoglu, R. (1997). Chapter 23: Cardiac Pharmacology. In J. Nagelhout & K. Zaglaniczny (Eds.), *Nurse Anesthesia*. Philadelphia: W.B. Saunders.

189. ANSWER: **D**

Rationale: Variant angina is caused by spontaneous spasm of the coronary arteries, which occurs most often at rest.

Reference: Aprile, A.E., Serwin, J.P., Boctor, B. (1997). Chapter 38A: Cardiac Anesthesia. In J. Nagelhout & K. Zaglaniczny (Eds.), *Nurse Anesthesia*. Philadelphia: W.B. Saunders.

190. ANSWER: **C**

Rationale: Nitroglycerin produces a rapid tolerance that can occur during acute administration.

Reference: Alisoglu, R. (1997). Chapter 23: Cardiac Pharmacology. In J. Nagelhout & K. Zaglaniczny (Eds.), *Nurse Anesthesia*. Philadelphia: W.B. Saunders.

191. ANSWER: **C**

Rationale: Beta$_2$ stimulation produces vasodilation in skeletal muscle and splanchnic vascular beds and therefore decreases resistance.

Reference: Cafarelli, J.M. (1997). Chapter 39B: Thoracic Surgery. In J. Nagelhout & K. Zaglaniczny (Eds.), *Nurse Anesthesia*. Philadelphia: W.B. Saunders.

192. ANSWER: **C**

Rationale: Drugs that are eliminated through liver metabolism tend to have a low bioavailability because when taken orally they metabolize before reaching the systemic circulation.

Reference: Troop, M. (1997). Chapter 16: Pharmacokinetics. In J. Nagelhout & K. Zaglaniczny (Eds.), *Nurse Anesthesia*. Philadelphia: W.B. Saunders.

193. ANSWER: **D**

Rationale: Leukotrienes produce bronchoconstriction, and a new group of drugs called leukotriene antagonists are currently being prescribed for the chronic treatment of asthma.

Reference: Cafarelli, J.M. (1997). Chapter 39B: Thoracic Surgery. In J. Nagelhout & K. Zaglaniczny (Eds.), *Nurse Anesthesia*. Philadelphia: W.B. Saunders.

194. ANSWER: **B**

Rationale: Gastric toxicity and ulcers produced by the NSAIDs result from blockade of cyclooxygenase enzymes, which prevents the production of prostaglandin E$_2$.

Reference: Sherbinski, L. & Nagelhout, J.J. (1997). Chapter 24: Additional Drugs of Interest. In J. Nagelhout & K. Zaglaniczny (Eds.), *Nurse Anesthesia*. Philadelphia: W.B. Saunders.

195. ANSWER: **B**

Rationale: Mu receptors, the primary opiate site of action, are primarily supraspinal. Spinal analgesic actions result from interactions with kappa receptors.

Reference: Chick, M. (1997). Chapter 21: Opioid Agonists and Antagonists. In J. Nagelhout & K. Zaglaniczny (Eds.), *Nurse Anesthesia*. Philadelphia: W.B. Saunders.

196. ANSWER: **D**

Rationale: Endogenous analgesia at the spinal level is produced by the enkephalin-like substances. Endorphins and dynorphins work in the central nervous system and other peripheral nonspinal sites.

Reference: Harrigan, C. (1997). Chapter 6: The Central Nervous System. In J. Nagelhout & K. Zaglaniczny (Eds.), *Nurse Anesthesia*. Philadelphia: W.B. Saunders.

197. ANSWER: **C**

Rationale: Postural hypotension resulting from venous dilations is one of the most prominent actions of nitroglycerin.

Reference: Williams, J.R. (1997). Chapter 20: Local Anesthetics. In J. Nagelhout & K. Zaglaniczny (Eds.), *Nurse Anesthesia*. Philadelphia: W.B. Saunders.

198. ANSWER: **D**

Rationale: Improved urine output after digitalization results from the increased stroke volume, which produces increased renal blood flow and glomerular filtration rate.

Reference: Williams, J.R. (1997). Chapter 20: Local Anesthetics. In J. Nagelhout & K. Zaglaniczny (Eds.), *Nurse Anesthesia*. Philadelphia: W.B. Saunders.

199. ANSWER: C

Rationale: Furosemide and bumetanide are classified as loop diuretics. They block sodium and chloride reabsorption in the ascending limb of the loop.
Reference: Sherbinski, L. & Nagelhout, J.J. (1997). Chapter 24: Additional Drugs of Interest. In J. Nagelhout & K. Zaglaniczny (Eds.), *Nurse Anesthesia*. Philadelphia: W.B. Saunders.

200 ANSWER: A

Rationale: Quinidine is derived from a cinchona plant; thus, quinidine toxicity is often called cinchonism.
Reference: Williams, J.R. (1997). Chapter 20: Local Anesthetics. In J. Nagelhout & K. Zaglaniczny (Eds.), *Nurse Anesthesia*. Philadelphia: W.B. Saunders.

201. ANSWER: C

Rationale: Anticholinergic agents can block motion sickness through an action in the vestibular apparatus in the inner ear.
Reference: Sherbinski, L. & Nagelhout, J.J. (1997). Chapter 24: Additional Drugs of Interest. In J. Nagelhout & K. Zaglaniczny (Eds.), *Nurse Anesthesia*. Philadelphia: W.B. Saunders.

202. ANSWER: B

Rationale: The beta phase of drug elimination is referred to as the elimination phase because it results from the drug's metabolism and renal elimination.
Reference: Troop, M. (1997). Chapter 16: Pharmacokinetics. In J. Nagelhout & K. Zaglaniczny (Eds.), *Nurse Anesthesia*. Philadelphia: W.B. Saunders.

203. ANSWER: C

Rationale: Alpha phase of drug action refers to the distribution of the drug from the blood into the tissue sites of action.
Reference: Troop, M. (1997). Chapter 16: Pharmacokinetics. In J. Nagelhout & K. Zaglaniczny (Eds.), *Nurse Anesthesia*. Philadelphia: W.B. Saunders.

204. ANSWER: B

Rationale: The major difference between aspirin and acetaminophen is the inability of acetaminophen to produce an anti-inflammatory action.
Reference: Sherbinski, L. & Nagelhout, J.J. (1997). Chapter 24: Additional Drugs of Interest. In J. Nagelhout & K. Zaglaniczny (Eds.), *Nurse Anesthesia*. Philadelphia: W.B. Saunders.

205. ANSWER: D

Rationale: The greater the amount of protein binding of a local anesthetic agent, the longer it remains in the injected area and therefore the longer the duration of action.
Reference: Williams, J.R. (1997). Chapter 20: Local Anesthetics. In J. Nagelhout & K. Zaglaniczny (Eds.), *Nurse Anesthesia*. Philadelphia: W.B. Saunders.

206. ANSWER: C

Rationale: Ropivacaine, an analogue of bupivacaine, appears to have less binding to cardiac protein, rendering it safer as far as cardiac toxic effects.
Reference: Williams, J.R. (1997). Chapter 20: Local Anesthetics. In J. Nagelhout & K. Zaglaniczny (Eds.), *Nurse Anesthesia*. Philadelphia: W.B. Saunders.

207. ANSWER: A

Rationale: A phase 1 block is characterized by fasciculations, sustained tetanus, no train-of-four fade, and no post-tetanic facilitation.
Reference: Haas, R.E. & Erway, R.L. (1997). Chapter 22: Neuromuscular Blocking Agents, Reversal Agents, and Their Monitoring. In J. Nagelhout & K. Zaglaniczny (Eds.), *Nurse Anesthesia*. Philadelphia: W.B. Saunders.

208. ANSWER: B

Rationale: Remifentanil contains an ester link that allows for rapid hydrolysis in the plasma in a very short duration of action.
Reference: Chick, M. (1997). Chapter 21: Opioid Agonists and Antagonists. In J. Nagelhout & K. Zaglaniczny (Eds.), *Nurse Anesthesia*. Philadelphia: W.B. Saunders.

209. ANSWER: **A**

Rationale: Treatment of severe hyperna-tremia defined as a serum sodium level less than 120 mEq/L is 3% saline infused at a rate of less than 100 mL/hr.
Reference: Ouellette, S.M. (1997). Chapter 11: Renal Anatomy, Physiology, and Pathophysiology, and Anesthesia. In J. Nagelhout & K. Zaglaniczny (Eds.), *Nurse Anesthesia.* Philadelphia: W.B. Saunders.

210. ANSWER: **A**

Rationale: Distention of the abdomen with gas insufflation would produce de-creased respirations, leading to hypercap-nia and retention of CO_2.
Reference: Cafarelli, J.M. (1997). Chapter 39B: Thoracic Surgery. In J. Nagelhout & K. Zaglaniczny (Eds.), *Nurse Anesthesia.* Philadelphia: W.B. Saunders.

211. ANSWER: **C**

Rationale: H_2 receptors produce positive inotropic and chronotropic action and stimulate acid secretion in the stomach. H_1 receptors produce bronchoconstric-tion and gastrointestinal contractions.
Reference: Sherbinski, L. & Nagelhout, J.J. (1997). Chapter 24: Additional Drugs of Interest. In J. Nagelhout & K. Zaglaniczny (Eds.), *Nurse Anesthesia.* Philadelphia: W.B. Saunders.

212. ANSWER: **D**

Rationale: Alpha receptor stimulation causes intense vasoconstriction, raising blood pressure, which results in a reflex bradycardia as a compensatory mecha-nism.
Reference: Alisoglu, R. (1997). Chapter 23: Cardiac Pharmacology. In J. Nagelhout & K. Zaglaniczny (Eds.), *Nurse Anesthesia.* Philadelphia: W.B. Saunders.

213. ANSWER: **D**

Rationale: Ketamine raises both intra-cranial and intraocular pressures and must be avoided in patients with severe head injury or when increases in intra-cranial pressure are suspected.
Reference: Fallacaro, N.A. & Fallacaro, M.D. (1997). Chapter 19: Intravenous Induction Agents. In J. Nagelhout & K. Zaglaniczny (Eds.), *Nurse Anesthesia.* Philadelphia: W.B. Saunders.

214. ANSWER: **D**

Rationale: Cervical plexus block is usually for an operation on the lateral and ante-rior neck and is the preferred technique for carotid endarterectomy.
Reference: McIntosh, L.S. (1997). Chapter 38C: Vascular Surgey. In J. Nagelhout & K. Zaglaniczny (Eds.), *Nurse Anesthesia.* Philadelphia: W.B. Saunders.

215. ANSWER: **B**

Rationale: NSAIDs are well known for producing nephrotoxic side effects. These occur with chronic use of high doses.
Reference: Sherbinski, L. & Nagelhout, J.J. (1997). Chapter 24: Additional Drugs of Interest. In J. Nagelhout & K. Zaglaniczny (Eds.), *Nurse Anesthesia.* Philadelphia: W.B. Saunders.

216. ANSWER: **A**

Rationale: Stump pressures are measured to ensure adequate perfusion through the circle of Willis and must be maintained at a minimum of 60 mm Hg.
Reference: McIntosh, L.S. (1997). Chapter 38C: Vascular Surgery. In J. Nagelhout & K. Zaglaniczny (Eds.), *Nurse Anesthesia.* Philadelphia: W.B. Saunders.

217. ANSWER: **D**

Rationale: The circle of Willis receives its primary supply from the internal carotid and basilar arteries. The basilar artery receives its supply from the vertebral ar-teries.
Reference: Harrigan, C. (1997). Chapter 6: The Central Nervous System. In J. Nagelhout & K. Zaglaniczny (Eds.), *Nurse Anesthesia.* Philadelphia: W.B. Saunders.

218. ANSWER: **C**

Rationale: Decreases in pulse pressure in-dicate a decrease in stroke volume, an increase in systemic vascular resistance, or both. Hypovolemia would result in a decreased stroke volume.
Reference: Morgan, R.O., Jr. (1997). Chapter 8: The Cardiovascular System. In J. Nagelhout & K. Zaglaniczny (Eds.), *Nurse Anesthesia.* Philadelphia: W.B. Saunders.

219. ANSWER: **A**

Rationale: The second messenger cyclic adenosine monophosphate stimulates cardiac cells to release calcium, which is sometimes referred to as the third messenger.

Reference: Morgan, R.O., Jr. (1997). Chapter 8: The Cardiovascular System. In J. Nagelhout & K. Zaglaniczny (Eds.), *Nurse Anesthesia.* Philadelphia: W.B. Saunders.

220. ANSWER: **C**

Rationale: Spinal anesthesia has been reported to cause exacerbation of the disease; however, epidural and other regional techniques appear to be safe.

Reference: Karlet, M.C. (1997). Chapter 40: Musculoskeletal Pathophysiology and Anesthesia. In J. Nagelhout & K. Zaglaniczny (Eds.), *Nurse Anesthesia.* Philadelphia: W.B. Saunders.

221. ANSWER: **A**

Rationale: Fluoxetine is classified as a select serotonin reuptake inhibitor (SSRI). Reuptake inhibition results in an antidepressant effect.

Reference: Sherbinski, L. & Nagelhout, J.J. (1997). Chapter 24: Additional Drugs of Interest. In J. Nagelhout & K. Zaglaniczny (Eds.), *Nurse Anesthesia.* Philadelphia: W.B. Saunders.

222. ANSWER: **B**

Rationale: Hydralazine primarily dilates arterial circulation; therefore, its greatest influence is on afterload when producing its antihypertensive effect.

Reference: Alisoglu, R. (1997). Chapter 23: Cardiac Pharmacology. In J. Nagelhout & K. Zaglaniczny (Eds.), *Nurse Anesthesia.* Philadelphia: W.B. Saunders.

223. ANSWER: **C**

Rationale: Machine disconnect, hence airway disconnect with subsequent failure to ventilate, remains the most common critical adverse outcome associated with general anesthesia.

Reference: Dosch, M.P. (1997). Chapter 26: Anesthesia Equipment. In J. Nagelhout & K. Zaglaniczny (Eds.), *Nurse Anesthesia.* Philadelphia: W.B. Saunders.

224. ANSWER: **A**

Rationale: It is well established that the appearance of an S_3 gallop on auscultation of heart sounds is a sign of congestive heart failure.

Reference: Aprile, A.E. & Aprile, F.D. (1997). Chapter 38B: Cardiac Anesthesia. In J. Nagelhout & K. Zaglaniczny (Eds.), *Nurse Anesthesia.* Philadelphia: W.B. Saunders.

225. ANSWER: **A**

Rationale: A transtracheal block is performed by penetrating the cricothyroid membrane while the neck is extended. After air is aspirated the local anesthetic solution is injected into the trachea at the end of expiration.

Reference: Chipas, A. (1997). Chapter 33: Airway Management. In J. Nagelhout & K. Zaglaniczny (Eds.), *Nurse Anesthesia.* Philadelphia: W.B. Saunders.

226. ANSWER: **A**

Rationale: Most potent opioid drugs exert their main effect through mu receptors in the central nervous system. They are responsible for analgesia and respiratory depression as well as for other common actions of these drugs.

Reference: Chick, M. (1997). Chapter 21: Opioid Agonists and Antagonists. In J. Nagelhout & K. Zaglaniczny (Eds.), *Nurse Anesthesia.* Philadelphia: W.B. Saunders.

CHAPTER 5

Professional Issues

◆ ◆ ◆

1. What is the proper legal terminology used when an anesthetist's practice does not meet the level required by law?

   A. breach of duty
   B. breach of civil tort
   C. breach of statute
   D. breach of regulation

2. The person who earned international respect and the sobriquet "the mother of anesthesia" for her mastery of the open drop method of ether administration in the nineteenth century is:

   A. Florence Henderson
   B. Sister Secundina Mindrup
   C. Dinah Grahman
   D. Alice Magaw

3. The first president of the American Association of Nurse Anesthetists in 1931 was:

   A. Adeline Curtis
   B. Agatha Hodgins
   C. Alice Hunt
   D. Sophie Gran Winton

4. AANA educational standards were initially written at the behest of what person in 1934?

   A. Helen Lamb
   B. Major Julia O. Flikke
   C. Ann Penland
   D. Anna Marie S. Rose

5. The minimal degree required by the AANA for a student to graduate from a certified anesthesia program is:

   A. associate degree
   B. baccalaureate degree
   C. master's degree
   D. Ph.D. degree

6. CRNA practice scope is defined by all of the following except:

   A. parameters of state statute
   B. parameters of state regulation
   C. parameters of institutional policies
   D. parameters of the American Society of Anesthesiologists

7. For a CRNA to become recertified he or she is required by the AANA to have a total of how many continuing education units (CEUs) in a 2-year period?

   A. 20
   B. 30
   C. 40
   D. 50

8. Nurse anesthetists who knowingly sign forms indicating that procedures were performed when they actually were not are violating what type of law?

   A. criminal
   B. civil
   C. misdemeanor
   D. federal

9. The Latin statement *res ipsa loquitur* means:

   A. to prove a point beyond a doubt
   B. the thing speaks for itself
   C. the defendant is at fault
   D. the prosecutor is in error

10. A general rule is that expert testimony must be used for determining the standard of care in a case of professional malpractice. All of the following may be considered an expert except:

    A. nurse anesthetist
    B. medical physician
    C. layperson
    D. anesthesia textbook

11. What following points should be included when obtaining an informed consent for anesthesia?

    A. a signature with the patient's agreement to undergo a specified treatment by the CRNA
    B. the process in which the CRNA tells a patient not only about the proposed procedure but also about the probability of the procedure's success and its associated risks, as well as about reasonable alternatives to the procdure
    C. the process in which the CRNA makes recommendations on the basis of the surgeon's and the anesthetist's personal preferences and obtains the patient's signature of agreement.
    D. the process in which the CRNA guarantees the choice of the anesthesia plan to be safe and appropriate and avoids describing all details of the proposed procedure to decrease patient anxiety

12. Intentional touching of a patient without the patient's consent, even if it causes no harm, is considered:

    A. assault
    B. battery
    C. malpractice
    D. negligence

13. Examples of an emancipated minor, who is allowed to sign his or her own consent, include all of the following except:

    A. a minor who lives on his or her own
    B. a minor who is married
    C. a minor who is the parent of a child
    D. a minor who is older than 16 years of age

14. A patient is undergoing general anesthesia and a surgeon discovers a nonemergency problem that necessitates subsequent surgery. The most appropriate step to take is:

    A. have a member from the surgical team obtain consent from the spouse or closest relative and perform the procedure at that moment
    B. allow the surgeon, who is "captain of the ship," to legally decide and proceed in circumstances like this
    C. to delay the unanticipated procedure until consent by the patient can be obtained
    D. to wake the patient, obtain consent, and then proceed with the procedure

15. In a malpractice suit, who has the burden of proving that a deviation from the standard of care occurred?

    A. defendant
    B. plaintiff
    C. the state
    D. the hospital

16. The following points are true if a CRNA is involved in a deposition:

    A. Depositions are question and answer sessions during which only the lawyers for the plaintiff side question witnesses.
    B. Depositions are a forum for all sides to openly discuss errors and develop plans to prevent them.
    C. Depositions are informal and off-the-record with minimal notetaking.
    D. The deponents are under oath, and testimony given at the deposition can be presented during the trial.

17. Strikes and picketing by nurse anesthetists in a unionized labor organization can be legal if what requirements are met?

    A. The labor organization notifies the institution in writing, along with the Federal Mediation and Counciliation Service, that it intends to engage in any strike, picketing, or other concerted refusal to work not less than 10 days before the action.
    B. The labor organization notifies the workers in a verbal meeting that it intends to engage in any strike, picketing, or other concerted refusal to work 48 hours before the action.
    C. The labor organization has a 25% vote from the membership that the members desire to strike, picket, or refuse to work.
    D. It is illegal for CRNAs to strike and picket for any reason.

18. What organization makes regulations regarding universal precautions for health care professionals?

    A. Food and Drug Administration (FDA)
    B. Occupational Safety and Health Administration (OSHA)
    C. Patient Safety Commission
    D. United States Pharmacopoeia (USP)

19. According to claims made against St. Paul Insurance Company between 1992 and 1996, the most frequent claim submitted against CRNAs was:

    A. teeth damage
    B. adverse reaction
    C. baby-related incident
    D. equipment-related incident

20. One advantage of computer-generated anesthesia records is:

    A. statistical analysis
    B. medicolegal accuracy
    C. artifact deletion
    D. anesthetist removed from "information loop"

21. What is the correct order to follow in a research process:

    A. identify a problem, execute a plan, formulate a hypothesis, and review the literature
    B. identify a problem, review the literature, formulate a hypothesis, and execute a plan
    C. review the literature, analyze data, identify the problem, and execute a plan
    D. formulate a hypothesis, analyze data, develop a plan, and interpret the data

22. The AANA has established four separate autonomous councils that reside at the AANA's national office. Which one of the following is not a true council?

    A. Council on Accreditation of Educational Programs of Nurse Anesthesia
    B. Council on Certification
    C. Council on Misconduct of CRNAs
    D. Council for Public Interest in Nurse Anesthesia

23. Total quality management (TQM) was first introduced by:

    A. Dr. W. Edwards Deming
    B. Dr. John Coole
    C. Dr. Donna Ritz
    D. Dr. Mary Aspe

24. A case involving violation of state law or municipal ordinance that concerns the alleged violation of the rights of all the people will be based on the principle of:

    A. civil law
    B. common law
    C. corporate law
    D. criminal law

25. The four elements of a malpractice case include all of the following except:

    A. vigilance
    B. breach
    C. cause
    D. damage

26. In a study on preventable anesthesia mishaps in an urban teaching institution, it was determined that what percentage of the preventable accidents involved human error?

    A. 45%
    B. 65%
    C. 70%
    D. 80%

27. Which autonomous council of the AANA administers and oversees the certification exam?

    A. Council on Accreditation
    B. Council for Public Interest in Anesthesia
    C. Council on Certification
    D. Council on Recertification

28. The body that oversees anesthesia education with regard to clinical and academic requirements for certification is:

    A. Council on Accreditation
    B. Council for Public Interest in Anesthesia
    C. Council on Certification
    D. Council on Recertification

29. Currently, CRNAs administer approximately what fraction of the total anesthetics annually in this country?

    A. 45%
    B. 55%
    C. 65%
    D. 75%

30. Misconduct by CRNAs is which of the following:

    A. starting a case before a proper machine check
    B. error in judgment
    C. performing anesthesia without consent
    D. consuming alcohol when on "standby" call

ANSWERS
TO PRACTICE QUESTIONS
CHAPTER 5

1. ANSWER: **A**

   Rationale: A breach of duty may be an error in the performance of an act during the administration of anesthesia care. Such an error is known as an error of commission or omission.
   Reference: Kirsner, K. M. (1997). Chapter 57: Legal Aspects of Nurse Anesthesia Practice. In J. Nagelhout & K. Zaglaniczny (Eds.), *Nurse Anesthesia*. Philadelphia: W.B. Saunders.

2. ANSWER: **D**

   Rationale: Alice Magaw was a path-breaking scientist who published her findings in major international journals. In 1906, she reported the results of over 14,000 anesthetics, with her suggestions for further anesthesia practice.
   Reference: Gunn, I. P. (1997). Chapter 1: Nurse Anesthesia: A History of Challenge. In J. Nagelhout & K. Zaglaniczny (Eds.), *Nurse Anesthesia*. Philadelphia: W.B. Saunders.

3. ANSWER: **B**

   Rationale: Agatha Hodgins was a pioneer CRNA who helped develop the use of nitrous oxide and oxygen in early anesthesia machines. She was also involved in organizing the first anesthesia society.
   Reference: Gunn, I. P. (1997). Chapter 1: Nurse Anesthesia: A History of Challenge. In J. Nagelhout & K. Zaglaniczny (Eds.), *Nurse Anesthesia*. Philadelphia: W.B. Saunders.

4. ANSWER: **A**

   Rationale: Helen Lamb recognized the need for standardization and educational standards of excellence in order for nurse anesthetists to be recognized as professionals and advance in their careers. This led to certification of nurse anesthetists.
   Reference: Gunn, I. P. (1997). Chapter 1: Nurse Anesthesia: A History of Challenge. In J. Nagelhout & K. Zaglaniczny (Eds.), *Nurse Anesthesia*. Philadelphia: W.B. Saunders.

5. ANSWER: **C**

   Rationale: As of 1998, graduation from an accredited program requires a master's degree as entry into practice.
   Reference: Garde, J. F. (1997). Chapter 2: Specialty Practice of Nurse Anesthesia. In J. Nagelhout & K. Zaglaniczny (Eds.), *Nurse Anesthesia*. Philadelphia: W.B. Saunders.

6. ANSWER: **D**

   Rationale: Nurse anesthetists practice under nurse practice acts and therefore are subject to state nursing regulations. Institutional practice privileges also play a major role in clinical situations. The American Society of Anesthesiologists has nothing to do with the practice scope of nurse anesthetists.
   Reference: Garde, J. F. (1997). Chapter 2: Specialty Practice of Nurse Anesthesia. In J. Nagelhout & K. Zaglaniczny (Eds.), *Nurse Anesthesia*. Philadelphia: W.B. Saunders.

7. ANSWER: **C**

   Rationale: The Council on Recertification requires proof of continued education of nurse anesthetists. This includes a requirement for 40 continuing education credits to be obtained every 2 years, along with practice requirements in order to become recertified.
   Reference: LaPointe, G. (1997). Chapter 3: Management of an Anesthesia Department. In J. Nagelhout & K. Zaglaniczny (Eds.), *Nurse Anesthesia*. Philadelphia: W.B. Saunders.

8. ANSWER: **A**

   Rationale: Falsifying documents regarding anesthesia care is a violation of criminal law. This includes the patient's medical chart and, of course, the anesthesia record itself.
   Reference: Kirsner, K. M. (1997). Chapter 57: Legal Aspects of Nurse Anesthesia Practice. In J.

Nagelhout & K. Zaglaniczny (Eds.), *Nurse Anesthesia*. Philadelphia: W.B. Saunders.

9. ANSWER: **B**

Rationale: *Res ipsa loquitur* is a doctrine that allows circumstantial evidence to prove negligence. For example, if a person is walking by a window and something falls out of it and hits him or her in the head and causes injury, it is obvious things shouldn't be thrown out of windows; and even though it was not witnessed, the act speaks for itself.

Reference: Kirsner, K. M. (1997). Chapter 57: Legal Aspects of Nurse Anesthesia Practice. In J. Nagelhout & K. Zaglaniczny (Eds.), *Nurse Anesthesia*. Philadelphia: W.B. Saunders.

10. ANSWER: **C**

Rationale: An expert is a person who has special skill and knowledge about a subject related to the case. Textbooks can be used to determine the standard of care.

Reference: Kirsner, K. M. (1997). Chapter 57: Legal Aspects of Nurse Anesthesia Practice. In J. Nagelhout & K. Zaglaniczny (Eds.), *Nurse Anesthesia*. Philadelphia: W.B. Saunders.

11. ANSWER: **B**

Rationale: Consent is the patient's agreement to undergo a specific treatment. A patient must be given all reasonable choices and complications so that he or she may make an informed decision. Not every possible risk must be disclosed but enough should be understood by the patient to make a reasonable judgment.

Reference: Kirsner, K. M. (1997). Chapter 57: Legal Aspects of Nurse Anesthesia Practice. In J. Nagelhout & K. Zaglaniczny (Eds.), *Nurse Anesthesia*. Philadelphia: W.B. Saunders.

12. ANSWER: **B**

Rationale: Battery is the unwanted touching of an individual, and assault is placing someone in fear of an unwanted touching. They can describe both a civil and a criminal offense.

Reference: Kirsner, K. M. (1997). Chapter 57: Legal Aspects of Nurse Anesthesia Practice. In J. Nagelhout & K. Zaglaniczny (Eds.), *Nurse Anesthesia*. Philadelphia: W.B. Saunders.

13. ANSWER: **D**

Rationale: An emancipated minor is one who, for the purposes of the law, is not a minor despite his or her being younger than the usual age of majority. This may include a minor who lives on his or her own, is married, or who has a child.

Reference: Kirsner, K. M. (1997). Chapter 57: Legal Aspects of Nurse Anesthesia Practice. In J. Nagelhout & K. Zaglaniczny (Eds.), *Nurse Anesthesia*. Philadelphia: W.B. Saunders.

14. ANSWER: **C**

Rationale: Because it is a nonemergency procedure the patient should be allowed to decide on the appropriateness of treatment after he or she has awakened from anesthesia.

Reference: Kirsner, K. M. (1997). Chapter 57: Legal Aspects of Nurse Anesthesia Practice. In J. Nagelhout & K. Zaglaniczny (Eds.), *Nurse Anesthesia*. Philadelphia: W.B. Saunders.

15. ANSWER: **B**

Rationale: The injured party, the patient, who filed the suit has the burden to prove that malpractice occurred.

Reference: Kirsner, K. M. (1997). Chapter 57: Legal Aspects of Nurse Anesthesia Practice. In J. Nagelhout & K. Zaglaniczny (Eds.), *Nurse Anesthesia*. Philadelphia: W.B. Saunders.

16. ANSWER: **D**

Rationale: Attorneys for both sides are present and may ask questions when a person is deposed. The deposition is used as evidence in a subsequent trial if it occurs.

Reference: Kirsner, K. M. (1997). Chapter 57: Legal Aspects of Nurse Anesthesia Practice. In J. Nagelhout & K. Zaglaniczny (Eds.), *Nurse Anesthesia*. Philadelphia: W.B. Saunders.

17. ANSWER: **A**

Rationale: The National Labor Relations Board under section 8(g) requires what is called the 10-day rule before any strikes, picketing, or refusal to work is undertaken.

Reference: Kirsner, K. M. (1997). Chapter 57: Legal Aspects of Nurse Anesthesia Practice. In J. Nagelhout & K. Zaglaniczny (Eds.), *Nurse Anesthesia*. Philadelphia: W.B. Saunders.

18. ANSWER: **B**

Rationale: The Occupational Safety and Health Administration is a federal agency that promulgates and enforces regulations designed to promote worker safety.
Reference: Kirsner, K. M. (1997). Chapter 57: Legal Aspects of Nurse Anesthesia Practice. In J. Nagelhout & K. Zaglaniczny (Eds.), *Nurse Anesthesia*. Philadelphia: W.B. Saunders.

19. ANSWER: **A**

Rationale: Inadvertent damage to teeth during airway management and intubation is the most common adverse claim against nurse anesthetists.
Reference: Kirsner, K. M. (1997). Chapter 57: Legal Aspects of Nurse Anesthesia Practice. In J. Nagelhout & K. Zaglaniczny (Eds.), *Nurse Anesthesia*. Philadelphia: W.B. Saunders.

20. ANSWER: **A**

Rationale: Automated record keeping allows for statistical analysis across cases when a particular incident is being studied. For example, all cases of hypotension can be generated and statistically analyzed.
Reference: Dosch, M. P. (1997). Chapter 58: Statistics and Computers. In J. Nagelhout & K. Zaglaniczny (Eds.), *Nurse Anesthesia*. Philadelphia: W.B. Saunders.

21. ANSWER: **B**

Rationale: The research process is an orderly process guided by scientific thinking. You first must identify the problem, study it, formulate a hypothesis, and execute a research study.
Reference: Biddle, C. (1997). Chapter 59: Nurse Anesthesia Research: Science of an Orderly, Purposeful, and Systematic Nature. In J. Nagelhout & K. Zaglaniczny (Eds.), *Nurse Anesthesia*. Philadelphia: W.B. Saunders.

22. ANSWER: **C**

Rationale: The fourth council is the Council on Recertification. These councils have been established to govern and oversee the practice of nurse anesthesia.
Reference: Garde, J. F. (1997). Chapter 2: Specialty Practice of Nurse Anesthesia. In J. Nagelhout & K. Zaglaniczny (Eds.), Nurse Anesthesia. Philadelphia: W.B. Saunders.

23. ANSWER: **A**

Rationale: Dr. Deming became fascinated with process and quality control while working in the Department of Agriculture. He defined *quality* as meeting or exceeding the customer's expectations in every function that the organization performed.
Reference: LaPointe, G. (1997). Chapter 3: Management of an Anesthesia Department. In J. Nagelhout & K. Zaglaniczny (Eds.), *Nurse Anesthesia*. Philadelphia: W.B. Saunders.

24. ANSWER: **A**

Rationale: Civil law is a body of legality that functions to protect society as a whole.
Reference: Kirsner, K. M. (1997). Chapter 57: Legal Aspects of Nurse Anesthesia Practice. In J. Nagelhout & K. Zaglaniczny (Eds.), *Nurse Anesthesia*. Philadelphia: W.B. Saunders.

25. ANSWER: **A**

Rationale: Vigilance is not required; however, the other three answers are. The fourth requirement is that there is a legal *duty* that the practitioner owes the patient.
Reference: Kirsner, K. M. (1997). Chapter 57: Legal Aspects of Nurse Anesthesia Practice. In J. Nagelhout & K. Zaglaniczny (Eds.), *Nurse Anesthesia*. Philadelphia: W.B. Saunders.

26. ANSWER: **D**

Rationale: Obviously, most preventable accidents are due to human error. Occasionally, it may involve equipment failure or some nonhuman event.
Reference: Kirsner, K. M. (1997). Chapter 57: Legal Aspects of Nurse Anesthesia Practice. In J. Nagelhout & K. Zaglaniczny (Eds.), *Nurse Anesthesia*. Philadelphia: W.B. Saunders.

27. ANSWER: **C**

Rationale: Initial certification of a registered nurse anesthetist when he or she graduates from school as well as disciplinary functions throughout his or her career is administered by the Council on Certification.
Reference: Garde, J.F. (1997). Chapter 2: Specialty Practice of Nurse Anesthesia. In J. Nagelhout & K. Zaglaniczny (Eds.), *Nurse Anesthesia*. Philadelphia: W.B. Saunders.

28. ANSWER: **A**

> **Rationale:** The Council on Accreditation of Nurse Anesthesia Programs oversees clinical requirements, academic and classroom requirements, and program accreditation to ensure high-quality nurse anesthesia providers.
>
> *Reference:* Garde, J. F. (1997). Chapter 2: Specialty Practice of Nurse Anesthesia. In J. Nagelhout & K. Zaglaniczny (Eds.), *Nurse Anesthesia.* Philadelphia: W.B. Saunders.

29. ANSWER: **C**

> **Rationale:** CRNAs, practicing alone or in the anesthetic care team, are involved in approximately 65% of all anesthetic procedures in the United States.
>
> *Reference:* Garde, J. F. (1997). Chapter 2: Specialty Practice of Nurse Anesthesia. In J. Nagelhout & K. Zaglaniczny (Eds.), *Nurse Anesthesia.* Philadelphia: W.B. Saunders.

30. ANSWER: **B**

> **Rationale:** Although each of the listed examples would represent improper conduct, true professional misconduct is defined as an error in judgment.
>
> *Reference:* Kirsner, K. M. (1997). Chapter 57: Legal Aspects of Nurse Anesthesia Practice. In J. Nagelhout & K. Zaglaniczny (Eds.), *Nurse Anesthesia.* Philadelphia: W.B. Saunders.

CHAPTER 6

Comprehensive Examination

• • •

1. The rationale for adding epinephrine to local anesthetics is:

   A. decreased metabolism of local anesthetic
   B. increased rate of metabolism of local anesthetic after absorption
   C. decrease toxicity by decreasing rate of absorption
   D. increased rate of absorption therefore faster onset

2. Blood levels of local anesthetic drugs are the highest after which regional technique?

   A. intercostal
   B. spinal
   C. epidural
   D. brachial plexus

3. Mendelson's syndrome is most likely after aspiration of gastric contents with one of the following characteristics:

   A. volume less than 40 mL and a pH greater than 2.5
   B. volume greater than 25 mL and a pH less than 2.5
   C. volume greater than 40 mL and a pH greater than 2.5
   D. volume less than 25 mL and a pH less than 2.5

4. Management of patients undergoing diagnostic laparoscopies includes:

   A. kidney rest to facilitate abdominal exposure
   B. maintenance of anesthesia by mask due to shortness of procedure
   C. positioning in reverse Trendelenburg to aid surgeon's visualization
   D. intubation and controlled ventilation to prevent aspiration and because of high intraperitoneal pressure

5. Air blowing over an exposed portion of a patient's body results in what type of heat loss?

   A. evaporation
   B. convection
   C. conduction
   D. radiation

6. According to ASA classification, type 2 diabetes should result in:

   A. class 1
   B. class 2
   C. class 3
   D. class 4

7. Occlusion of the innominate artery during mediastinoscopy can be detected by:

   A. monitoring the left pulse
   B. monitoring the right pulse
   C. Doppler
   D. ECG changes

8. Expansion of gases from an O_2 cylinder when it is opened is an example of:

   A. Reynold's law
   B. Dalton's law
   C. Boyle's law
   D. Henry's law

9. In the laminar flow of gases through a horizontal tube, the rate of flow is:

   A. most dependent on the viscosity of the gas
   B. most dependent on the amount of the gas
   C. most dependent on the molecular weight of the gas
   D. most dependent on the temperature of the gas

10. The total amount of epinephrine in 10 mL of a 1:200,000 solution is:

    A. 50 μg
    B. 50 mg
    C. 5 mg
    D. 500 μg

11. The flow of fluids through tubes of varying diameters indicates that the pressure of a fluid is least where its speed is greatest. These laws were formulated by:

    A. Charles
    B. Bernoulli
    C. Gay-Lussac
    D. Poiseuille

12. Which factor relates to Graham's law?

    A. density of a liquid
    B. molecular weight of a gas
    C. blood solubility of a gas
    D. oil solubility of a gas

13. Which gas law states that the pressure of a gas in a liquid is proportional to the pressure of a gas above the liquid?

    A. Dalton's
    B. Boyle's
    C. Henry's
    D. Charles'

14. An indicator in soda lime changes color in response to the production of:

    A. NaCl
    B. $Ca(OH)_2$
    C. NAOH
    D. Na_2CO_3

15. Doubling the radius of a tube will increase flow by how many times?

    A. 4
    B. 6
    C. 16
    D. 32

16. What volume in liters will 1 mole of a gas occupy at standard temperature and pressure?

    A. 22.4
    B. 11.2
    C. 44.8
    D. 6.023×10^{23}

17. Which gas law justifies the use of Wood's metal?

    A. Dalton's
    B. Charles'
    C. Gay-Lussac
    D. Boyle's

18. During spinal anesthesia, which function would you expect to lose last?

    A. motor
    B. sensory
    C. propioception
    D. sympathetic

19. The frequency of pneumothorax is the highest when performing which of the following blocks?

    A. intercostal
    B. thoracic epidural
    C. supraclavicular
    D. intrascalene

20. Which of the following signs would you expect to see first in the patient with malignant hyperthermia?

    A. increased $PaCO_2$
    B. increased temperature
    C. tachypnea
    D. hypotension

21. The most common cause of coagulopathies in a patient receiving massive blood transfusion is:

    A. low platelets
    B. deceased factor VIII
    C. decreased factor V
    D. dilutional thrombocytopenia

22. When profound hypotension develops suddenly during placement of the prosthesis in a patient having total hip replacement, it is most likely due to:

    A. blood loss
    B. fat embolism
    C. air embolism
    D. the cement used to secure the hip

23. The most common complication associated with mediastinoscopy is:

    A. brachial plexus injury
    B. innominate artery occlusion
    C. recurrent laryngeal nerve injury
    D. blood loss

24. The proper diluent for mixing dantrolene sodium is:

A. distilled sterile water
B. sterile sodium chloride
C. mannitol
D. dextrose

25. Which of the following is a sign of a phase II block?

A. sustained tetanus
B. post-tetanic count of 11
C. no post-tetanic facilitation
D. train of four fade

26. Which of the following therapies are indicated for a patient with von Willebrand's disease?

A. cryoprecipitate and desmopressin
B. cryoprecipitate and fresh-frozen plasma
C. desmopressin and fresh-frozen plasma
D. factor VIII and platelets

27. All of the following regarding citrate phosphate dextrose adenine (CPDA-1)–stored blood are true except:

A. reduces risk of hepatitis
B. citrate affects calcium binding
C. phosphate acts as a buffer
D. type and crossmatching are unaffected

28. The most common blood transfusion reaction is:

A. acute hemolytic reaction
B. delayed hemolytic reaction
C. febrile reaction
D. Rh antibody reaction

29. A common clinical finding in a patient with a fat embolus is:

A. S_3 murmur
B. increased PaO_2
C. bradycardia
D. petechiae on the chest wall

30. What is the most common cause of mortality with respiratory failure from burn injury?

A. respiratory failure
B. hypoxia
C. hyperkalemia
D. sepsis

31. What virus is transmitted most often after blood transfusions?

A. hepatitis A virus
B. human immunodeficiency virus
C. hepatitis B virus
D. cytomegalovirus

32. The major reason for the drop in blood pressure with sympathetic blockade after a spinal administration is:

A. reflex vasoconstriction
B. bradycardia
C. decreased preload
D. myocardial depression

33. Which is the most important determinant of the level of a spinal anesthetic?

A. speed of injection
B. addition of epinephrine
C. baricity and position
D. dose

34. Discontinuing total parenteral nutrition before surgery can lead to:

A. delayed hypotension
B. hypoglycemia
C. hyperglycemia
D. metabolic acidosis

35. Which type of laser is most frequently associated with eye damage?

A. infrared
B. argon
C. Nd:YAG
D. CO_2

36. Spinal headache is characterized by:

A. exacerbation in the supine position
B. frontal and temporal pain
C. onset immediately postoperatively
D. a definite dependence on posture

37. Cardiovascular effects of spinal anesthesia include:

    A. decreased myocardial oxygen consumption
    B. increased pulmonary vascular resistance
    C. increased total peripheral vascular resistance
    D. an absolute increase in preload

38. Which of the following would be an indication of a venous air embolism?

    A. decreased end-tidal carbon dioxide
    B. increased end-tidal carbon dioxide
    C. decreased pulmonary artery pressure
    D. increased arterial blood pressure

39. In a patient with a spinal cord lesion at T5 or above, distention of a hollow viscus such as the bladder or rectum will frequently produce:

    A. hypotension with tachycardia
    B. hypertension with tachycardia
    C. hypertension with bradycardia
    D. hypotension with bradycardia

40. One of the fastest ways to decrease intracranial pressure in the acute situation is:

    A. osmotic dehydration
    B. corticosteroid administration
    C. cerebrospinal fluid drainage/diversion
    D. hyperventilation

41. For most neurosurgical cases where a reduction in brain bulk is desired, optimal ventilation should be aimed at:

    A. P_{CO_2} of 25 to 30 mm Hg
    B. P_{CO_2} of 30 to 35 mm Hg
    C. P_{CO_2} of 28 to 32 mm Hg
    D. P_{CO_2} of 32 to 38 mm Hg

42. The major cause of postoperative complications associated with deliberate hypertension is:

    A. ischemia to organs
    B. hypovolemia
    C. cerebral edema
    D. vasospasm

43. Which of the following statements is not true of hypoxic pulmonary vasoconstriction (HPV)?

    A. HPV results in an increase in pulmonary vascular resistance in the atelectatic lung.
    B. HPV is an autoregulatory mechanism that protects the P_{CO_2} from rising to levels associated with arrhythmias.
    C. HPV decreases the amount of shunt flow through the hypoxic lung.
    D. Vasodilating drugs are associated with an inhibition of the HPV response.

44. Which of the following is not an advantage of double-lumen tubes?

    A. Placement is relatively easy.
    B. They allow repeated conversion from one- to two-lung ventilation and vice versa.
    C. They allow constant positive pressure to be applied to the nonventilated lung.
    D. The oval-shaped lumina decrease airway resistance, facilitating ventilation and suction.

45. Transesophageal echocardiography:

    A. cannot be used in a continuous mode
    B. can only be used in the closed chest and therefore is not useful in the cardiac patient
    C. gives poor delineation of the right ventricle
    D. gives good delineation of the left ventricle

46. Goals for anesthetic management of a patient with severe coronary artery disease include all except:

    A. maintain low to normal afterload
    B. maintain contractility
    C. maintain sinus rhythm
    D. maintain high heart reate

47. Which of the following factors is not associated with "good" left ventricular function?

A. ejection fraction > 50%
B. left ventricular end-diastolic pressure < 12 mm Hg
C. ejection fraction < 40%
D. normal cardiac output
E. hypertension and obesity

48. Which of the following is not associated with an aortic dissection?

    A. Marfan's syndrome
    B. hypertension and left ventricular hypertrophy
    C. trauma
    D. diabetes mellitus

49. Of the following conditions, which is associated with the poorest perioperative prognosis?

    A. evidence of congestive heart failure
    B. heart rate of 100 to 110 beats per minute with induction of anesthesia
    C. preoperative serum glucose level of 300 mg/dL
    D. evidence of chronic obstructive pulmonary disease

50. A woman presents for an emergent cesarean section for fetal distress. The number one cause of maternal mortality in the perioperative period is:

    A. aspiration
    B. failed intubation
    C. hypovolemic shock
    D. amniotic fluid embolism

51. Cardiac output in the parturient is greatest at what point in her pregnancy?

    A. immediately post partum
    B. at 10 to 12 weeks' gestation
    C. immediately after conception
    D. at 20 weeks' gestation

52. An absolute contraindication to the administration of heparin for cardiopulmonary bypass is:

    A. increased antithrombin III activity
    B. carotid disease
    C. recent cerebrovascular accident
    D. previous streptokinase therapy

53. "Second dose" administration of a nondepolarizing muscle relaxant during cardiopulmonary bypass is used mainly to:

    A. assist in the prevention of recall
    B. prevent microshivering
    C. prevent movement
    D. reverse the effect of hemodilution on the induction dose of nondepolarizing muscle relaxant

54. How would you ventilate a newborn undergoing an emergency repair of congenital diaphragmatic hernia?

    A. use normal mechanical ventilation parameters for neonates
    B. hand ventilate using small tidal volume, rate of approximately 60 breaths per minute, and positive inspiratory pressure < 20 cm H_2O
    C. mechanical ventilation with small tidal volume, rate of 20 breaths per minute, and positive inspiratory pressure of 20 cm H_2O
    D. hand ventilate, applying positive pressure approximately 20 cm H_2O to expand lungs

55. When using a Jackson-Rees system, how can you prevent rebreathing and accomplish CO_2 washout?

    A. by assisting ventilation on every single breath
    B. by using fresh gas flows equal to the minute volume of the patient
    C. by using fresh gas flows two to three times the patient's minute volume
    D. by incorporating a CO_2 absorption system into the circuit

56. During an unsuccessful laryngoscopy attempt after an inhalation induction on a 6-month-old infant, the patient's heart rate dropped to 56 beats per minute. How would you handle this situation?

    A. continue with laryngoscopy attempt
    B. hand ventilate with mask and 100% O_2, and start an intravenous line
    C. give atropine immediately by intramuscular route
    D. give succinylcholine, 15 mg, intramuscularly to facilitate intubation

57. Which of the following statements is most correct when considering the ventilatory response to spinal anesthesia?

    A. diaphragmatic activity is usually impaired

    B. the phrenic nerve will be affected by mid-thoracic levels of anesthesia

    C. exhalation may become impaired by high thoracic levels of anesthesia

    D. inspiratory volumes are affected as a result of intercostal paralysis

58. The correct sequence of anatomic demarcation for the formation of the brachial plexus is:

    A. roots, trunks, cords, divisions, branches

    B. roots, cords, trunks, divisions, branches

    C. roots, branches, trunks, cords, divisions

    D. roots, trunks, divisions, cords, branches

59. All of the following terminal nerve branches are found "outside" the brachial plexus at the level of the axilla except:

    A. musculocutaneous

    B. intercostobrachial

    C. medial brachial cutaneous

    D. medial antebrachial cutaneous

60. Which of the following nerves is anesthetized by producing a superficial skin wheal over the pulsation of artery in the axilla (when performing an axillary block)?

    A. medial antebrachial cutaneous

    B. axillary

    C. intercostobrachial

    D. musculocutaneous

61. The main site of action of local anesthetics in producing a nerve block is likely the:

    A. nerve sheath

    B. phospholipid of axonal membrane

    C. intracellular end of the Na^+ channel

    D. extracellular end of the Na^+ channel

62. Which of the following statements regarding the recovery phase of local anesthetics from nerve blockade is most correct?

    A. Regression of analgesia takes place initially in the core fibers and lastly in the muscle fibers.

    B. Mantle fibers retain a higher anesthetic concentration than core fibers.

    C. Diffusion and absorption of local anesthetic account for termination of blockade.

    D. Lipophilic solubility of the local anesthetic is not important to duration.

63. The five major laser hazards are:

    A. eye injuries, fire, skin and tissue burns, radiation exposure, and electrical hazards

    B. argon gas poisoning, carbon dioxide toxicity, eye injuries, skin and tissue burns, and electrical hazards

    C. toxic fumes and smoke inhalation, radiation exposure, eye injuries, electrical hazards, and skin and tissue burns

    D. eye injuries, skin and tissue burns, fire, toxic fume and smoke inhalation, and electrical injuries

64. The cuff of a laser endotracheal tube should:

    A. be made of laser reflective silicone

    B. be wrapped with laser reflective tape by the surgeon

    C. be a double cuff and be filled with sterile normal saline and methylene blue

    D. be a double cuff and be filled with sterile water and indigo carmine

65. The CO_2 laser beam is:

    A. white

    B. red

    C. blue-green

    D. invisible

66. Lubricants used on endotracheal tubes and in patients' eyes during laser surgery should be:

    A. petroleum-based non–water-soluble

    B. non–petroleum-based water-soluble

    C. petroleum-based water-soluble

    D. non–petroleum-based non–water-soluble

67. The intravenous infusion therapy for a 20-year-old trauma patient with positive urine findings of myoglobin should be:

    A. kept at keep-vein-open rate
    B. titrated to replace prior hour's urine output
    C. kept at a rate to a ensure the patient is kept well hydrated
    D. Myoglobinuria should not influence intravenous therapy.

68. Disruption of the blood-brain barrier:

    A. is caused by constriction of the cerebral capillary bed and lysis of the tight junctions
    B. can be due to hypertension and hypocarbia
    C. can be therapeutically induced by the use of corticosteroids
    D. leads to the development of vasogenic cerebral edema and increased intracranial pressure

69. Cerebral blood flow:

    A. is determined by cerebral perfusion pressure and cerebrovascular resistance
    B. is primarily dependent on changes in intracranial pressure and cerebral venous pressure
    C. is controlled by an intrinsic autoregulatory mechanism that in theory is under neurogenic control
    D. is directly related to cerebrovascular resistance

70. Inverse steal:

    A. results in an increase in flow to the normal brain when $PaCO_2$ is reduced
    B. occurs in response to hypercarbia and is also known as luxury perfusion
    C. happens when the $PaCO_2$ is elevated and blood supply is increased to normal areas of the brain
    D. may occur when the $PaCO_2$ is reduced and vasoconstriction of the normal vessels results, shunting blood to the ischemic areas

71. Which statement is true regarding the action of mannitol?

    A. The rebound phenomenon will occur when mannitol is infused over 2 to 5 minutes.
    B. A transient hypervolemia can occur as water is drawn into the intravascular space.
    C. It works more efficiently and decreases intracranial pressure more when given in larger doses
    D. mannitol crosses the blood-brain barrier by carrier-mediated transport

72. Fluid management in the neurosurgical patient dictates that:

    A. fluid administration should be done slowly and the patient should be given minimal amounts to prevent edema
    B. optimal hematocrit for cerebral perfusion in the presence of ischemia is 35% to 38%
    C. neurosurgical patients should be given glucose-free solutions to avoid increasing free water formation in the brain
    D. rapid fluid infusions will cause disruption of the blood-brain barrier and cytotoxic cerebral edema

73. Epidural hematoma:

    A. is a collection of blood between the dura and arachnoid membrane
    B. develops slowly, often occurring in elderly or alcoholic patients without history of traumatic injury
    C. is a fairly common traumatic injury with a mortality of 40% to 60%
    D. classically presents as clinical signs of a transient loss of consciousness followed by a lucid interval

74. According to the Monro-Kellie doctrine, if intracranial pressure increases during hypotension:

    A. cerebral perfusion pressure will decrease
    B. cerebral perfusion pressure will increase
    C. mean arterial pressure will decrease
    D. mean arterial pressure will increase

75. One of the important signals for antidiuretic hormone release is:

A. decreased serum sodium concentration
B. increased extracellular fluid osmolarity
C. increased plasma volume
D. none of the above

76. The glomerular filtration rate of a normal kidney is:

A. 75 mL/mm Hg/min
B. 125 mL/min
C. 650 mL/mm Hg/min
D. 650 mL/min

77. The osmolarity of a solution depends on the:

A. size of the solute molecules
B. number of solute particles
C. degree of ionization
D. weight of solute molecules

78. Which of the following would be most useful in determining a defect in platelet function?

A. thrombin time
B. prothrombin time
C. partial thromboplastin time
D. bleeding time

79. At a pH of 7.4, a drug with a pK_a of 7.4 would be ionized approximately:

A. 20%
B. 30%
C. 50%
D. 70%

80. To make a 10-mL epinephrine solution 1:100,000 from ampules containing 1 mL of 1:1,000 epinephrine, how many milliliters of epinephrine 1:1,000 must be added to the saline diluent?

A. 0.10 mL
B. 0.15 mL
C. 0.20 mL
D. 0.25 mL

81. Anesthetic partial pressure in the brain depends on:

A. solubility of the agent
B. anesthetic partial pressure in the alveoli
C. minimal alveolar concentration of the agent
D. second gas effect

82. How many milligrams per milliliter will result if 1% tetracaine hydrochloride is added to 1 mL of 10% dextrose for use in a spinal anesthetic?

A. 20
B. 15
C. 10
D. 5

83. The antimuscarinic drug with the most limited ability to cross the blood-brain barrier is:

A. atropine
B. scopolamine
C. glycopyrrolate
D. hyoscine

84. The most prevalent serious incident associated with anesthesia is?

A. sore throat
B. awareness
C. airway disconnect
D. esophageal intubation

85. Unauthorized videotaping of a patient's operation would be?

A. assault
B. battery
C. negligence
D. vicarious liability

86. A patient suffers nerve injury due to negligence by a certified registered nurse anesthetist. The hospital and the surgeon are sued for damages under the doctrine of:

A. *res ipsa loquiter*
B. *respondent superior*
C. vicarious liability
D. assault and battery

87. The purpose of an electrocautery grounding plate is to:

A. divert the electric current to a larger area
B. act as a ground
C. form a complete circuit
D. act as a conductor

88. The pulse pressure is the greatest at which of the following sites?

A. carotid artery
B. radial artery
C. dorsalis pedis artery
D. brachial artery

89. Which of the following symptoms would one expect to see in a patient with cyanide poisoning?

A. low arterial PO_2 and metabolic acidosis
B. high venous PO_2 and metabolic acidosis
C. low venous PO_2 and metabolic alkalosis
D. high arterial PO_2 and metabolic acidosis

90. Arterial waveform damping is most commonly caused by:

A. kinking of the catheter
B. air bubbles
C. vasopressors
D. hypotension

91. With the lateral approach to a spinal anesthetic, which structure other than skin and subcutaneous tissue is punctured first?

A. supraspinous ligament
B. interspinous ligament
C. ligamentum flavum
D. dura

92. Monoamine oxidase is found in what part of the cell?

A. nucleus
B. endoplasmic reticulum
C. Golgi apparatus
D. mitochondria

93. The second messenger in parasympathetic innervated cells is:

A. cyclic adenosine monophosphate
B. cyclic guanosine monophosphate
C. calcium
D. magnesium

94. The primary effect of antidiuretic hormone is exerted on the:

A. distal convoluted tubule
B. ascending collecting duct
C. loop of Henle
D. proximal convoluted tubule

95. The primary function of thyroid gland is to control:

A. enzyme activity
B. hormone release
C. cardiovascular tone
D. metabolic rate

96. Sumatriptan, which is used to treat migraine headaches, works primarily on what receptors?

A. norepinephrine
B. epinephrine
C. dopamine
D. serotonin

97. Which of the following agents exhibits a modest antiemetic effect?

A. thiopental
B. ketamine
C. propofol
D. etomidate

98. Beta-receptor antagonists are contraindicated in a patient with:

A. glaucoma
B. hyperthyroidism
C. asthma
D. migraine

99. The kidney reabsorbs approximately what percent of the filtrate product?

A. 99%
B. 75%
C. 25%
D. 50%

100. What spinal anesthetic level is required for cesarean section?

    A. T2
    B. T4
    C. T6
    D. T8

101. Which of the following inhalation anesthetics is metabolized to the greatest extent?

    A. isoflurane
    B. sevoflurane
    C. desflurane
    D. nitrous oxide

102. Hepatic enzyme induction may be responsible for:

    A. increased oral bioavailability
    B. increased hepatic extraction ration
    C. increased plasma half-life (elimination phase)
    D. increased drug efficacy

103. Which of the following agents exhibits the fastest induction and emergence?

    A. halothane
    B. desflurane
    C. isoflurane
    D. sevoflurane

104. Tissue uptake of an anesthetic agent will be greater when:

    A. blood flow to the tissue is high
    B. tissue capacity is low
    C. solubility coefficient is low
    D. minimal alveolar concentration of the agent is high

105. All of the following are common side effects of beta blocker therapy except?

    A. reflex tachycardia
    B. bronchoconstriction
    C. peripheral vasoconstriction
    D. hypoglycemia

106. Exocytotic release of neuronal norepinephrine is inhibited physiologically by which of the following presynaptic actions of norepinephrine?

    A. activation of $alpha_2$ adrenoceptors
    B. inhibition of $alpha_2$ adrenoceptors
    C. activation of $alpha_1$ adrenoceptors
    D. blockage of Ca^{2+} channels

107. Patients with congestive heart failure may show reduced rates of narcotic elimination because such patients may exhibit:

    A. digitalis-induced hepatic enzyme inhibition
    B. reduced hepatic blood flow
    C. reduced plasma albumin levels
    D. increased liver function

108. Nitroglycerin is effective in treating the anginal symptoms of ischemic heart disease primarily because the drug causes a reduced:

    A. coronary arterial resistance
    B. systemic venous tone
    C. sinoatrial heart rate
    D. cardiac sympathetic tone

109. The most serious complication involved in the use of thiazides as diuretics in patients being treated for heart failure is:

    A. acidosis
    B. hypocalcemia
    C. hypokalemia
    D. peripheral vasoconstriction

110. The prostaglandins are derived from which of the following substances?

    A. arachidonic acid
    B. glutathione
    C. cholesterol
    D. glucuronic acid

111. During cardiopulmonary bypass, the activated clotting time should be maintained:

    A. above 200 seconds
    B. above 300 seconds
    C. above 400 seconds
    D. above 500 seconds

112. All are characteristics of Cushing's triad except:

    A. intracranial hypertension
    B. hyperventilation
    C. arterial hypertension
    D. reflex bradycardia

113. Which of these changes do not occur during the storage of banked blood?

    A. increased potassium
    B. increased pH
    C. deceased platelets
    D. increased 2,3-diphosphoglycerate

114. Metoclopramide does not:

    A. increase lower esophageal sphincter tone
    B. inhibit gastric acid secretion
    C. speed gastric emptying time
    D. have antiemetic properties

115. Von Willebrand's disease has a deficiency of:

    A. Factor VII
    B. Factor VIII
    C. Factor IX
    D. Factor X

116. Which of the following does not cause error in pulse oximetry readings?

    A. carboxyhemoglobin
    B. methemoglobin
    C. methylene blue
    D. fetal hemoglobin

117. Where is the pressure regulator located in the anesthesia machine?

    A. high pressure system
    B. intermediate pressure system
    C. low pressure system
    D. flowmeter assembly system

118. Why is the oxygen flowmeter downstream for all other gases?

    A. to allow proper vapor pressure
    B. because it is part of the low pressure system
    C. so that oxygen is farthest from the common gas outlet
    D. so a leak will result in a loss of anesthetic gas rather than oxygen

119. Induced hypotension is least likely to be used for which of the following?

    A. vagotomy and antrectomy
    B. Harrington rodding
    C. cerebral aneurysm clipping
    D. maxillofacial surgery

120. "Quantitatively" the most important buffer in the body is:

    A. erythrocytes
    B. proteins
    C. phosphates
    D. bicarbonate

121. The duration of spinal anesthesia is primarily dependent on:

    A. fatigue of the nerve fiber causing a regeneration of nerve impulses
    B. breakdown of the agent in the cerebrospinal fluid and removal through venous sinuses
    C. removal of the agent via the vascular and lymphatic supply of the spinal cord
    D. facilitated removal of the local anesthetic agent from the nerve trunks by an increase in acetylcholine

122. The temperature at which the vapor pressure exceeds atmospheric pressure is the:

    A. boiling point
    B. critical temperature
    C. latent heat of vaporization
    D. absolute temperature

123. According to national standards, the anesthesia machine should be checked for internal leaks:

    A. before every case
    B. daily
    C. weekly
    D. monthly

124. In the midline approach to a subarachnoid block, the following sequence of ligaments are pierced:

    A. interspinous, supraspinous, ligamenta flava, dura
    B. supraspinous, anterior longitudinal, interspinous, dura
    C. posterior longitudinal, supraspinous, ligamenta flava, dura
    D. supraspinous, interspinous, ligamenta flava, dura

125. Using first-order kinetics, the percent of drug eliminated after two elimination half-lives is:

    A. 25
    B. 50
    C. 75
    D. 100

126. The method of regulating the output concentration with agent-specific vaporizers is:

    A. bubble-through
    B. flow-over
    C. measured flow
    D. variable bypass

127. Using the peripheral nerve stimulator, a stimulus at 50 or 100 Hz for 5 seconds would result in:

    A. twitch
    B. train-of-four
    C. tetanus
    D. post-tetanic stimulation

128. Cerebral vessels contract and expand to maintain a constant blood supply over a wide range of mean arterial pressure. This process is called:

    A. autoregulation
    B. cerebral perfusion
    C. cerebral blood flow
    D. a cerebral spasm

129. Central venous pressure measurements best determine the status of:

    A. afterload
    B. preload
    C. contractility
    D. stroke volume

130. The nerve responsible for sensory innervation of the larynx down to the vocal cord is:

    A. recurrent laryngeal nerve
    B. internal branch of the superior laryngeal nerve
    C. glossopharyngeal nerve
    D. external branch of the superior laryngeal nerve

131. The nerve responsible for sensory innervation of the larynx below the vocal cord is:

    A. recurrent laryngeal nerve
    B. internal branch of the superior laryngeal nerve
    C. glossopharyngeal nerve
    D. external branch of the superior laryngeal nerve

132. In order to decrease conduction of static electricity the operating room floor resistance should be between:

    A. 10,000 and 20,000 ohms
    B. 2000 and 10,000 ohms
    C. 25,000 and 1 million ohms
    D. 1 million and 10 million

133. Total air exchange in the operating room should occur:

    A. 10 times per hour
    B. 15 times per hour
    C. 20 times per hour
    D. 5 times per hour

134. The agent of choice for use against human immunodeficiency virus is:

    A. 70% alcohol
    B. alkaline glutaraldehyde
    C. sodium hypochlorite
    D. 100% alcohol

135. The volume of dissolved gas is independent of pressure if the temperature is constant. This is:

A. Boyle's law
B. Henry's law
C. Laplace's law
D. Bohr effect

136. The maximum PaO_2 that may be achieved in a patient ventilated by a mask is:

A. 115
B. 93
C. 105
D. 75

137. The usual dose of local anesthetic for an epidural block is:

A. 1.5 mL per dermatone
B. 0.75 mL per dermatone
C. 0.5 mL per dermatone
D. 0.25 mL per dermatone

138. The CO_2 beam is:

A. red
B. blue-green
C. invisible
D. white

139. The part of the body most susceptible to damage from the CO_2 laser is the:

A. cornea
B. lungs
C. retina
D. mucous membrane

140. A patient is undergoing CO_2 laser micro-laryngoscopic vocal cord surgery under general anesthesia. The endoscopic tube of choice would be:

A. silicone
B. red rubber
C. metal
D. polyvinyl chloride

141. One of the most feared hazards during laser surgery of the airway is:

A. damage to adjacent tissues
B. an airway and endotracheal tube fire
C. vocal cord damage
D. patient movement

142. If the endotracheal tube is ignited during laser surgery, the most appropriate immediate action is to:

A. flood the area with irrigation solution
B. hyperventilate the patient with oxygen
C. decrease the rate of laser bursts
D. remove the oxygen source

143. When a vaginal hysterectomy is performed on a patient using regional anesthesia, the suggested dermatone level to obtain motor/sensory paralysis would be:

A. C4–C5
B. T3–T4
C. T6–T8
D. L1–L2

144. Anesthetic implications of bleomycin in patients undergoing gynecologic procedures include which of the following?

A. The patient should not receive greater than 30% oxygen.
B. The patient must be kept on 100% O_2 during the case.
C. The end-tidal CO_2 levels must be maintained at greater than 46 mm Hg.
D. The end-tidal CO_2 levels must be maintained at less than 34 mm Hg.

145. Which of the following would be instituted for treatment of a gas embolism during an abdominal laparoscopic procedure?

A. placement of the patient in the left lateral, head-down position
B. placement of a central venous pressure line to remove the gas
C. insufflation of carbon dioxide
D. administration of intravenous fluids

146. The oculocardiac reflex may cause all of the following except:

A. decreased intensity with subsequent stimulation
B. nodal rhythm
C. ventricular fibrillation
D. cardiac arrest

147. The oculocardiac reflex is triggered by what nerve pathway?

A. efferent, trigeminal nerve and afferent, vagus nerve

B. afferent, optic nerve and efferent, trochlear nerve

C. afferent, trigeminal nerve and efferent, vagus nerve

D. efferent, optic nerve and afferent, trochler nerve

148. The surgeon is about to instill the sulfur hexafluoride bubble before the completion of a scleral buckling. Appropriate actions include:

A. deepening the anesthetic

B. turning off the N_2O for the remainder of the case

C. administering atropine 0.2 mg IV

D. checking the patient's peak airway pressures

149. Characteristics of an ideal continuous irrigation fluid administered to patients undergoing transurethral prostatic resection would include all of the following except:

A. It is inexpensive.

B. It is iso-osmolar.

C. It is highly ionized.

D. It is nonhemolytic.

150. The most common continuous irrigation solution currently used for transurethral prostatic resection is:

A. Cytosol

B. glycine 1.5% in water

C. distilled water

D. lactated Ringer's solution

151. The gastroesophageal sphincter remains competent up to _____ cm H_2O.

A. 10

B. 20

C. 30

D. 40

152. A 78-year-old patient presents to the operating room for the insertion of a feeding jejunostomy. On physical examination you discover findings consistent with a moder-

ate degree of dehydration. These would include all of the following except:

A. narrow pulse pressure

B. decreased urine output

C. poor skin turgor

D. orthostatic hypotension

153. What is the ASA physical status classification of a moribund patient not expected to survive 24 hours because of a severe condition such as a ruptured aneurysm or head trauma with increasing intracranial pressure?

A. ASA 2

B. ASA 3

C. ASA 4

D. ASA 5

154. The presence of a bubble in an arterial line:

A. is not significant if it is small

B. leads to an artificially high reading

C. leads to damping of the tracing

D. affects only the diastolic pressure

155. The largest amount of heat loss occurs in the surgical patient due to:

A. radiation

B. evaporation

C. convection

D. conduction

156. The least reliable site for central temperature monitoring is the:

A. rectum

B. nasopharynx

C. tympanic membrane

D. skin on forehead

157. Of the following choices, the best way to maintain body temperature and possibly raise the core temperature is by using what device?

A. radiant heat unit

B. heat and moisture exchanger

C. forced air warmer

D. water circulating mattress

158. What color of nail polish would have the greatest effect on the accuracy of dual-wavelength pulse oximeters?

A. red
B. blue
C. green
D. white

159. Purposes of capnography include all of the following except:

A. confirm endotracheal intubation
B. detect exhaustion of CO_2 absorber
C. aid in the diagnosis of severe atelectasis
D. aid in the diagnosis of pulmonary embolism

160. Hypoxemia in the recovery room may be due to all of the following except:

A. increased vital capacity
B. pulmonary edema
C. shivering
D. atelectasis

161. The most common reason for admitting outpatients to the hospital after general anesthesia is:

A. hypotension
B. nausea and vomiting
C. respiratory complications
D. inability to ambulate

162. The _____ nerve is the best indicator of adequacy of intubation conditions while the _____ nerve is the best indicator of adequacy for extubation.

A. adductor pollicis, orbicularis oculi
B. peroneal, posterior tibial
C. posterior tibial, peroneal
D. orbicularis oculi, adductor pollicis

163. Conventional peripheral nerve stimulators deliver four twitches of the train-of-four at how many hertz and how many seconds apart?

A. 2 Hz, 0.5 second
B. 4 Hz, 1 second
C. 2 Hz, 5 seconds
D. 4 Hz, 0.1 second

164. Which change does not occur in the gastrointestinal system of the near-term woman in labor?

A. decreased lower esophageal sphincter tone
B. slower emptying of stomach contents
C. increased intragastric pressure
D. increased incidence of heartburn

165. Factors that influence a drug's ability to cross the placental barrier include:

A. rate of injection, pH, tissue affinity
B. alkalinity, volume of distribution, timing of injection
C. molecular weight, lipid solubility, ionization
D. beta half-life, rate of injection, solubility

166. During delivery, a lower dose of local anesthetic is required for regional anesthesia because:

A. pregnant women have greater pain tolerance
B. the pain fibers are more superficial in the spinal canal
C. the epidural and subarachnoid spaces are distended
D. maternal hyperventilation decreases pain

167. Which is not a contraindication for regional anesthesia?

A. seizure disorder
B. acute fetal distress
C. maternal hemorrhage
D. abscess at insertion site

168. Pain in the first stage of labor is innervated through:

A. the pudendal nerve
B. the sacral plexus
C. S2–S4
D. T10–L1

169. The antihypertensive agent used most often to treat blood pressure is:

A. nitroprusside
B. hydrazine
C. nitroglycerin
D. methyldopa

170. You are performing postoperative rounds and find a patient who had regional anesthesia performed and is now complaining of a postpuncture headache. Which statement is false regarding postpuncture headaches?

A. They are better in the supine position.
B. They are of lower incidence after puncture with a 25-gauge needle.
C. They are less prevalent in the obstetric female.
D. They are lessened if the patient is hydrated.

171. A patient presents in preterm labor who was on ritodrine to stop labor. Treatment was unsuccessful, and the patient is to be given a spinal block for cesarean section. What might you expect to see in this patient?

A. hypoglycemia
B. hyperkalemia
C. tachycardia
D. bradycardia

172. Pharmacokinetic qualities of the elderly include:

A. decreased plasma protein binding
B. decreased percentage of total body water
C. decreased receptor activity
D. decreased hepatic function

173. Initial airway management for the head-injured patient includes all of the following except:

A. to provide supplemental oxygen to the patient while the airway and ventilation are evaluated
B. to evaluate the patient's airway including full range of motion, atlanto-occipital joint function, temporomandibular joint function, and thyromental distance.
C. to provide "in-line" stabilization during the use of a fiberoptic intubation
D. to remember that all patients must be considered to have a full stomach after the trauma incident

174. An 81-year-old woman is undergoing a craniotomy in the sitting position. Suddenly the patient becomes hypotensive and air is heard on the precordial Doppler. All are appropriate actions except:

A. discontinue the N_2O
B. aspirate fluid from the central venous catheter
C. place the patient in the right lateral decubitus position with a slight head-up position
D. apply 8 cm PEEP

175. The neuromuscular disorder involving lower motor neurons and muscle fibers that is characterized by abnormal fatigability and fluctuating motor weakness of voluntary skeletal muscles that worsens with repetitive use and improves with rest is:

A. Eaton-Lambert syndrome
B. muscular dystrophy
C. multiple sclerosis
D. myasthenia gravis

176. Anesthetic implications for the patient with muscular dystrophy include:

A. performing a rapid sequence induction with increased dosage of succinylcholine
B. preparing for potential malignant hyperthermia
C. performing a "heavy" inhalational technique
D. performing a deep extubation

177. Early signs and symptoms of malignant hyperthermia include all of the following except:

A. tachycardia
B. skeletal muscle rigidity
C. fever
D. hypercarbia

178. The first step in the treatment of malignant hyperthermia involves:

A. internal and external cooling of the patient
B. hyperventilation with 100% oxygen
C. discontinuation of all triggering agents
D. administration of dantrolene, 1.0 to 2.5 mg/kg

179. What monitoring device would provide the most sensitive information regarding myocardial ischemia/myocardial infarction during the intraoperative period?

    A. wall-motion abnormalities on the transesophageal echocardiogram
    B. ST-segment changes in lead V_5 of the electrocardiogram
    C. appearance of V waves on the pulmonary capillary wedge pressure tracing
    D. elevation of the pulmonary capillary wedge pressure tracing

180. You visit a patient preoperatively and note that she is on propranolol 40 mg daily. This drug:

    A. should be stropped immediately and the procedure performed the next day
    B. should be stopped and surgery postponed for 2 weeks
    C. should be continued as per schedule
    D. must always be discontinued, but gradually over 4 weeks

181. A mechanical obstruction to ventricular ejection resulting in a chronic pressure load on the left ventricle is characteristic of:

    A. mitral regurgitation
    B. aortic stenosis
    C. mitral stenosis
    D. aortic insufficiency

182. A 38-year-old female was delivered of her second child 4 months ago. She has recently been diagnosed with mitral stenosis. Which of the following drugs would you not expect this patient to be taking?

    A. a beta blocker
    B. digoxin
    C. an anticoagulant
    D. a corticosteroid

183. The plasma protein with the greatest effect on colloid osmotic pressure is:

    A. hemoglobin
    B. albumin
    C. fibrinogen
    D. globulin

184. Which of the following substances diffuses readily across the capillary membrane?

    A. hemoglobin
    B. glucose
    C. albumin
    D. fibrinogen

185. The percentage of the cardiac output that perfuses the coronary arteries is:

    A. 0.5%
    B. 15%
    C. 5%
    D. 20%

186. The venous drainage system that collects 75% of the coronary blood flow and empties into the right atrium is the:

    A. great coronary vein
    B. posterior cardiac vein
    C. anterior descending vein
    D. coronary sinus

187. Despite having an extensive arterial blood vessel network, this layer of the heart is most vulnerable to decreases in coronary blood flow:

    A. visceral pericardium
    B. epicardium
    C. subendocardium
    D. parietal pericardium

188. A prime candidate for local vasodilator of the coronary arteries is:

    A. endothelin
    B. atrial natriuretic peptide
    C. angiotensin
    D. adenosine

189. Which of the following factors will increase myocardial O_2 supply:

    A. increased left ventricular end-diastolic pressure
    B. increased aortic diastolic pressure
    C. coronary artery vasoconstriction
    D. increased myocardial wall tension

190. In patients homozygous for hemoglobin S, a situation that can initiate or exacerbate red blood cells "sickling" includes:

    A. high oxygen tension in the blood
    B. alkalosis
    C. hyponatremia
    D. hypothermia

191. Which of the following white blood cells behave as mast cells, releasing histamine, bradykinin, and serotonin when stimulated?

    A. eosinophils
    B. lymphocytes
    C. basophils
    D. none of the above

192. Identify the class of antibody (immunoglobin) often elevated in patients with a history of asthma or allergies:

    A. IgG
    B. IgE
    C. IgA
    D. IgM

193. Which of the following is the major spinal cord tract for voluntary, purposeful movement:

    A. reticulospinal
    B. spinocerebellar
    C. corticospinal
    D. spinothalamic

194. Preganglionic sympathetic fibers:

    A. are mostly unmyelinated
    B. enter the sympathetic chains via gray rami communicantes
    C. on the average diverge to several postganglionic sympathetic fibers
    D. all of the above

195. Which of the following is an effect of parasympathetic stimulation?

    A. vasodilation of most systemic arterioles
    B. increased basal metabolic rate
    C. glycogenolysis and increased blood glucose
    D. copious secretion from nasal, lacrimal, gastric, and pancreatic glands

196. Which of the following is not a beta-adrenergic response?

    A. cardioacceleration
    B. glycogenolysis
    C. vasoconstriction
    D. uterine relaxation

197. A drug that stimulates the parasympathetic nervous system may produce:

    A. bradycardia
    B. pupillary dilation
    C. bronchodilation
    D. copious sweating

198. The average blood flow through the brain is:

    A. 3.5 mL/100 g/min
    B. 20 to 25 mL/100 g/min
    C. 50 to 55 mL/100 g/min
    D. 750 mL/100 g/min

199. Marked hyperventilation can produce cerebral ischemia when the $PaCO_2$ is less than:

    A. 20 mm Hg
    B. 35 mm Hg
    C. 45 mm Hg
    D. 50 mm Hg

200. Cerebrospinal fluid is secreted into the cerebral ventricles by the:

    A. arachnoid villi
    B. pia mater
    C. arachnoid trabecula
    D. choroid plexuses

201. A posterior convexity of the spine is termed:

    A. scoliosis
    B. kyphosis
    C. pectus excavatum
    D. lordosis

202. The trachea extends from:

    A. C6 to T5
    B. C1 to C4
    C. C2 to C3
    D. T1 to T7

203. Bronchodilation is commonly induced by:

A. histamine
B. leukotrienes
C. mast cell activation
D. sympathetic nervous system activation

204. Which of the following muscles moves the sternum forward and increases the antero-posterior diameter of the chest cavity during inspiration?

A. sternocleidomastoid
B. external intercostal
C. abdominal
D. internal intercostal

205. Surfactant is produced by:

A. the alveolar macrophages
B. mast cells
C. type II alveolar epithelial cells
D. alveolar lymphocytes

206. Alveoli that are ventilated but not perfused by the adjacent pulmonary capillaries contribute to the:

A. physiologic shunt
B. anatomic deadspace
C. absolute shunt
D. alveolar deadspace

207. The smallest diameter in a child's airway is the:

A. tracheal ring
B. vocal cord aperture
C. hyoid bone
D. cricoid ring

208. When a Macintosh laryngoscope is used, the:

A. epiglottis is lifted directly
B. laryngoscope is held in the right hand
C. blade enters the mouth on the right side
D. instrument is manufactured in various sizes

209. A nasopharyngeal airway is contraindicated in all of the following patients except:

A. patients with nasal polyps
B. patients with a very low platelet count
C. patients with the jaw wired shut
D. patients with a basilar skull fracture

210. Cool air flowing over an exposed patient in the operating room results in what type of heat loss?

A. evaporation
B. conduction
C. radiation
D. convection

211. Which of the following statements are true regarding the electrical outlets in the operating room?

A. The electrical outlet in the operating room is grounded.
B. The operating room power supply is always grounded.
C. In the operating room there is not direct connection from the power to the ground.
D. The voltage of the operating room is always 240 volts.

212. Wood's metal is:

A. an alloy used in fusible plugs of cylinders
B. used in flowmeters
C. used in vaporizers
D. used in circle systems to conduct heat

213. In classification of risks for transmitting infections in anesthesia, critical risk items should all be:

A. sterile
B. intermediate-level disinfected
C. low-level disinfected
D. clean

214. The purpose of cracking an oxygen cylinder is to:

A. remove gaseous impurities
B. establish that there is gas in the tank
C. establish that the gas in the tank is oxygen
D. remove dust or other flammable substances from the yoke

215. Which of the following occur when laminar flow changes to turbulent flow?

    A. viscosity increases
    B. flow increases
    C. temperature increases
    D. resistance increases

216. The reaction of CO_2 with soda lime is:

    A. oxidation
    B. reduction
    C. neutralization
    D. acidification

217. If the partial pressure of a gas over a liquid doubles, the amount of gas dissolved in the liquid will:

    A. halve
    B. double
    C. remain the same
    D. increase 16 times

218. The amount of energy it takes to convert a liquid to a gas is referred to as:

    A. latent heat of vaporization
    B. specific heat
    C. evaporation
    D. vapor pressure

219. The rate of diffusion of a gas across the alveolar capillary membrane is inversely proportional to the:

    A. partial pressure of the gas
    B. thickness of the membrane
    C. surface area of the membrane
    D. solubility of the gas

220. Which of the following monitors measures the most accurate core body temperature?

    A. rectal
    B. esophageal
    C. skin
    D. tympanic

221. A major disadvantage of laryngeal mask airway is:

    A. more postoperative coughing
    B. tracheal trauma
    C. does not prevent aspiration of gastric contents
    D. requires postoperative mechanical ventilation

222. The glomerular filtration rate becomes fully mature at what age?

    A. 5 days
    B. 3 months
    C. 6 months
    D. 1 to 2 years

223. Which of the following statements are true regarding uncuffed endotracheal tubes?

    A. used on children younger than age 2 only
    B. provides less risk of postextubation edema
    C. an air leak at 5 cm H_2O is indicative of an adequate fit
    D. fits snugly on the vocal cords

224. All of the following are true regarding NPO status in children except:

    A. clear liquids 2 to 3 hours before surgery
    B. breast feeding 6 hours before surgery
    C. solid/semisolid foods 6 to 8 hours before surgery
    D. NPO 8 hours before surgery for both solids and clear liquids

225. ECG criteria for diagnosing ischemia in the anesthetized patient include all of the following except:

    A. ST-segment elevation
    B. T-wave inversion
    C. isoelectric ST segment
    D. downsloping ST segment greater than 1 mV from the isoelectric line

226. A shift of the oxyhemoglobin dissociation curve to the right is produced by:

    A. alkalosis
    B. acidosis
    C. hypothermia
    D. carbon monoxide

1. ANSWER: C

2. ANSWER: A

3. ANSWER: B

4. ANSWER: D

5. ANSWER: B

6. ANSWER: B

7. ANSWER: B

8. ANSWER: C

9. ANSWER: A

10. ANSWER: A

11. ANSWER: B

12. ANSWER: B

13. ANSWER: C

14. ANSWER: D

15. ANSWER: D

16. ANSWER: A

17. ANSWER: C

18. ANSWER: C

19. ANSWER: C

20. ANSWER: A

21. ANSWER: D

22. ANSWER: B

23. ANSWER: D

24. ANSWER: A

25. ANSWER: D

26. ANSWER: A

27. ANSWER: A

28. ANSWER: C

29. ANSWER: D

30. ANSWER: D

31. ANSWER: D

32. ANSWER: C

33. ANSWER: C

34. ANSWER: B

35. ANSWER: B

36. ANSWER: D

37. ANSWER: **A**

38. ANSWER: **A**

39. ANSWER: **C**

40. ANSWER: **D**

41. ANSWER: **A**

42. ANSWER: **A**

43. ANSWER: **C**

44. ANSWER: **A**

45. ANSWER: **D**

46. ANSWER: **D**

47. ANSWER: **C**

48. ANSWER: **D**

49. ANSWER: **A**

50. ANSWER: **B**

51. ANSWER: **A**

52. ANSWER: **A**

53. ANSWER: **B**

54. ANSWER: **B**

55. ANSWER: **C**

56. ANSWER: **B**

57. ANSWER: **D**

58. ANSWER: **D**

59. ANSWER: **A**

60. ANSWER: **C**

61. ANSWER: **C**

62. ANSWER: **C**

63. ANSWER: **D**

64. ANSWER: **C**

65. ANSWER: **A**

66. ANSWER: **B**

67. ANSWER: **C**

68. ANSWER: **D**

69. ANSWER: **A**

70. ANSWER: **C**

71. ANSWER: **B**

72. ANSWER: **C**

73. ANSWER: **D**

74. ANSWER: **A**

75. ANSWER: **B**

76. ANSWER: **B**

77. ANSWER: **B**

78. ANSWER: **D**

79. ANSWER: C

80. ANSWER: A

81. ANSWER: B

82. ANSWER: C

83. ANSWER: C

84. ANSWER: C

85. ANSWER: B

86. ANSWER: B

87. ANSWER: A

88. ANSWER: C

89. ANSWER: B

90. ANSWER: B

91. ANSWER: C

92. ANSWER: D

93. ANSWER: B

94. ANSWER: A

95. ANSWER: D

96. ANSWER: D

97. ANSWER: C

98. ANSWER: C

99. ANSWER: A

100. ANSWER: B

101. ANSWER: B

102. ANSWER: B

103. ANSWER: B

104. ANSWER: A

105. ANSWER: A

106. ANSWER: A

107. ANSWER: B

108. ANSWER: B

109. ANSWER: C

110. ANSWER: A

111. ANSWER: C

112. ANSWER: B

113. ANSWER: D

114. ANSWER: B

115. ANSWER: B

116. ANSWER: D

117. ANSWER: A

118. ANSWER: D

119. ANSWER: A

120. ANSWER: B

121. ANSWER: C

122. ANSWER: A

123. ANSWER: A

124. ANSWER: D

125. ANSWER: C

126. ANSWER: D

127. ANSWER: C

128. ANSWER: A

129. ANSWER: B

130. ANSWER: B

131. ANSWER: A

132. ANSWER: C

133. ANSWER: B

134. ANSWER: B

135. ANSWER: A

136. ANSWER: C

137. ANSWER: A

138. ANSWER: C

139. ANSWER: A

140. ANSWER: C

141. ANSWER: B

142. ANSWER: D

143. ANSWER: C

144. ANSWER: A

145. ANSWER: B

146. ANSWER: A

147. ANSWER: C

148. ANSWER: B

149. ANSWER: C

150. ANSWER: B

151. ANSWER: B

152. ANSWER: A

153. ANSWER: D

154. ANSWER: C

155. ANSWER: A

156. ANSWER: D

157. ANSWER: C

158. ANSWER: B

159. ANSWER: C

160. ANSWER: A

161. ANSWER: B

162. ANSWER: D

163. ANSWER: A

164. ANSWER: B

165. ANSWER: C

166. ANSWER: C

167. ANSWER: A

168. ANSWER: D

169. ANSWER: B

170. ANSWER: C

171. ANSWER: C

172. ANSWER: D

173. ANSWER: B

174. ANSWER: C

175. ANSWER: D

176. ANSWER: B

177. ANSWER: C

178. ANSWER: C

179. ANSWER: A

180. ANSWER: C

181. ANSWER: B

182. ANSWER: D

183. ANSWER: B

184. ANSWER: B

185. ANSWER: A

186. ANSWER: D

187. ANSWER: C

188. ANSWER: D

189. ANSWER: B

190. ANSWER: D

191. ANSWER: C

192. ANSWER: B

193. ANSWER: C

194. ANSWER: C

195. ANSWER: D

196. ANSWER: C

197. ANSWER: A

198. ANSWER: C

199. ANSWER: A

200. ANSWER: D

201. ANSWER: B

202. ANSWER: A

203. ANSWER: D

204. ANSWER: B

205. ANSWER: C

206. ANSWER: D

207. ANSWER: C

208. ANSWER: D

209. ANSWER: C

210. ANSWER: D

211. ANSWER: C

212. ANSWER: A

213. ANSWER: A

214. ANSWER: D

215. ANSWER: D

216. ANSWER: C

217. ANSWER: B

218. ANSWER: A

219. ANSWER: B

220. ANSWER: D

221. ANSWER: C

222. ANSWER: D

223. ANSWER: B

224. ANSWER: D

225. ANSWER: C

226. ANSWER: B